GENETIC DISEASE

Diagnosis and Treatment

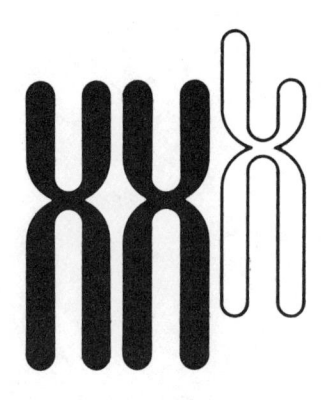

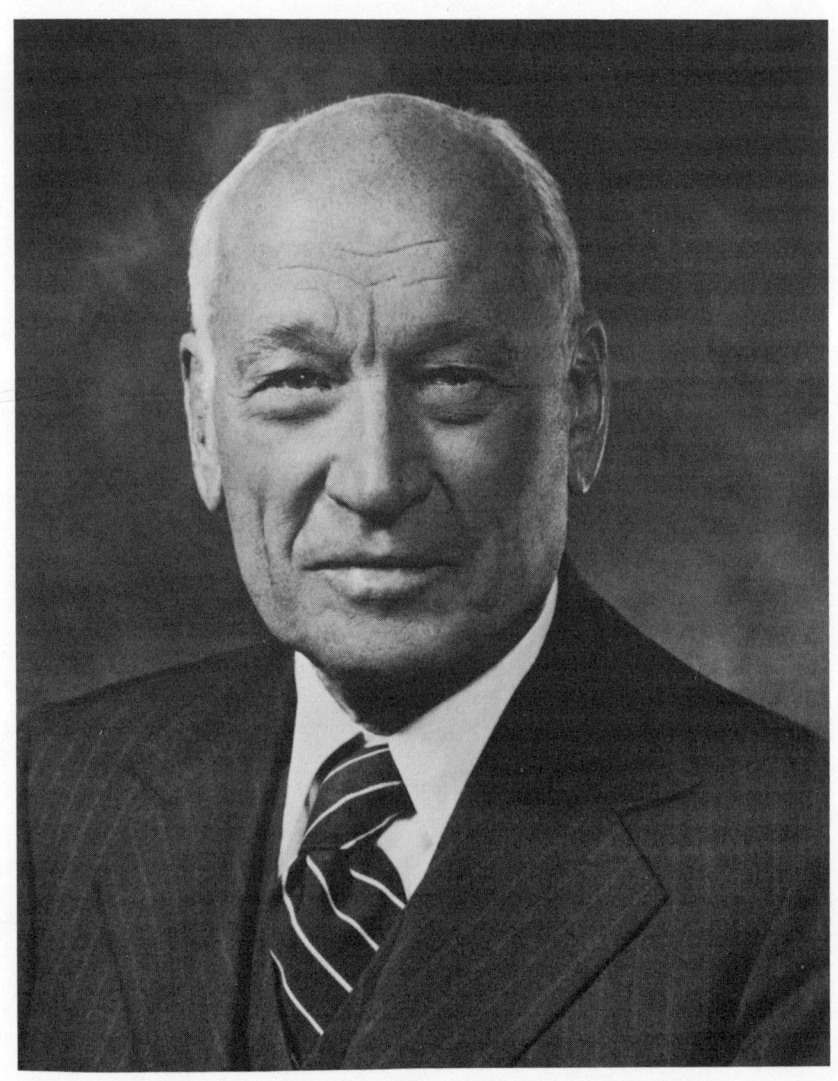

Arnold O. Beckman, Founder and Chairman of the Board, Beckman Instruments, Inc.

GENETIC DISEASE
Diagnosis and Treatment

Proceedings of the Fifth Arnold O. Beckman
Conference in Clinical Chemistry

Edited by
Albert A. Dietz

Executive Editor
Virginia S. Marcum

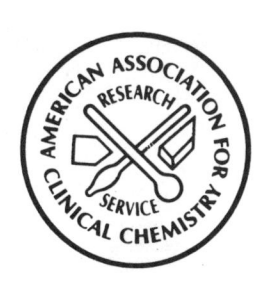

The American Association for Clinical Chemistry

1725 K Street, N.W.
Washington, DC 20006

Previous Proceedings of Arnold O. Beckman Conferences in Clinical Chemistry, published by the American Association for Clinical Chemistry:

1, Clinician and Chemist: The Relation of the Laboratory to the Physician
2, The Clinical Biochemistry of Cancer
3, Aging—Its Chemistry
4, Human Nutrition: Clinical and Biochemical Aspects

Library of Congress Cataloguing in Publication Data

Arnold O. Beckman Conference in Clinical Chemistry
(5th: 1981: Monterey, Calif.)
Genetic disease: diagnosis and treatment:
proceedings of the Fifth Arnold O. Beckman Conference
in Clinical Chemistry.

Includes index.
1. Medical genetics—Congresses. I. Dietz,
Albert Arnold Clarence, 1910–1982. II. Marcum,
Virginia S. III. American Association for Clinical
Chemistry. IV. Title. [DNLM: 1. Hereditary
diseases—Diagnosis—Congresses. 2. Hereditary
diseases—Therapy—Congresses. W3 AR719 5th 1981g
QZ 50 A761 1981g]

RB155.A73 1981   616'.042   82-20576
ISBN 0-915274-20-5

Printed in the United States of America.
© 1983, by the American Association for Clinical Chemistry, Inc.
All rights reserved. No part of this book may be reproduced by any means, nor transmitted, nor translated into a machine language without the written permission of the publisher.

Contents

Preface   vii
Conference Participants and Attendees   ix

I. Perspective

An Overview of Human Genetics
    Robert S. Sparkes   3

Legal Liability in Genetic Screening, Genetic Counseling, and Prenatal Diagnosis
    Ellen E. Wright and Margery W. Shaw   17

Cytogenetic Abnormalities Related to Mental Retardation
    Park S. Gerald   43

II. Clinical Diagnosis

Tay–Sachs Disease: A Model for Genetic Disease Control
    Michael M. Kaback   59

Cancer Susceptibility as a Birth Defect
    Richard A. Gatti   72

Genetic Disorders of the Endocrine Glands
    David L. Rimoin   88

III. New Diagnostic Procedures

Most Cancers May Have a Chromosomal Defect
    Jorge J. Yunis   105

A Role for DNA Repair Mechanisms in the Genetics of Aging
    Kathleen Y. Hall   120

Molecular Approaches to Human Immune Functions and Disorders
    Randolph Wall and Andrew Saxon   131

IV. Therapeutic Aspects

Diagnosis and Treatment of Inborn Errors of Organic Acid Metabolism
    Stephen D. Cederbaum   147

Liver Transplantation and Portacaval Shunt in Genetic Diseases
    Thomas E. Starzl   167

Treatment of Inherited Metabolic Diseases: Current Status and Prospects
    Robert J. Desnick   183

V. Prospects

Progress in Bone Marrow Transplantation
    Robert A. Good   263

Ethical Aspects of Therapy for Genetic Diseases
    Marc Lappé   282

Gene Therapy—Is It Inevitable or Necessary?
    Theodore Friedmann   302

Index   311

Preface

Until recently, a diagnosis of genetic disease commonly meant that the affected individual was condemned to a premature, often painful, death. Most such persons could not expect to survive past childhood, and only a few ameliorative measures could be taken to alleviate some of the symptoms in the meantime.

Today, however, some genetic diseases can be treated, and we are on the threshold of developing effective treatment for others. Diseases involving the metabolism of dietary components are being treated by altering the diet (e.g., for phenylketonuria), by altering how the deficient nutrients are supplied (e.g., parenteral nutrition or intragastric infusion to bypass the liver), and by gross surgical intervention (e.g., liver transplantation).

More exciting still is the prospect of correcting genetic defects at the cellular, or even the molecular, level. Preliminary work is underway on such approaches, but conclusive success has not yet been reported. Further progress probably must await the development and refinement of new techniques of gene and chromosomal study; however, this is a field in which new findings are being announced rapidly. In fact, between the date of this Conference and the publication of these Proceedings, Dr. Friedmann has announced the isolation and copying of the gene that apparently is involved in the Lesch–Nyhan syndrome, a debilitating disorder involving mental retardation, spastic cerebral palsy, and self-mutilating biting. The only gene deciphered so far in which malfunctions affect behavior and produce retardation, this breakthrough offers the first possibility for learning how genes work on the brain to affect intelligence and behavior. A comparison of the structure of functioning genes and defective ones is already in progress, with the long-term goal of being able to use recombinant DNA techniques for effective treatment of a currently incurable disease.

As the ability to detect, diagnose, and treat genetic diseases increases, so also will the complexity of the nonscientific issues related to these diseases: the moral, legal, and even species survival ramifications. Morality is involved because human life is involved, both its quality and the possibility of its negation. Close behind morality, but not necessarily in parallel with it, are the legal questions regarding the responsibilities of the family physician, the diagnostic center, and the genetic counselor in cases of genetic diseases. And finally, what are the effects on *Homo sapiens* as a species if its gene pool is altered, either by improving the treatment of persons with heritable disorders so that they live long enough to reproduce, or by trying to eliminate all bearers of "defective" genes? If one also considers the possibility that life span is genetically determined, it is clear that problems involving genetic disorders are not confinable to the laboratory.

Once again, we at the American Association for Clinical Chemistry are grateful to Arnold O. Beckman for supporting an exciting conference of broad interest. The topics touched on above, and others relating the role of the clinical laboratory to the diagnosis of genetic disease, were presented by well-known investigators who are also stimulating speakers. A sense of the interest sparked by these presentations is reflected in the question-and-answer discussions that followed the speeches (and included in these proceedings). As those attending can testify, the fruitful interaction between speakers and members of the audience fulfilled a principal aim of these Conferences in Clinical Chemistry. For the success of the conference and of its arrangements, credit must be given to the organizing committee: Frank A. Ibbott (*Chairman*), James A. Demetriou, and Denis O. Rodgerson.

In closing, I note with sorrow the death of Albert A. Dietz, whose tireless work was instrumental in getting these proceedings assembled and published, and whose numerous contributions to the AACC and other scholarly and professional organizations have been substantial. A hard worker, a dedicated leader, and a good man, he will be sadly missed.

V. S. Marcum

Conference Participants
(1, speaker; 2, co-author; 3, session moderator)

Stephen D. Cederbaum, M.D.[1]
Departments of Psychiatry and Pediatrics
Mental Retardation Research Center
University of California
Los Angeles CA 90024

James A. Demetriou, Ph.D.[3]
Bio-Science Laboratories
Van Nuys CA 91405

Robert J. Desnick, M.D., Ph.D.[1]
Professor of Pediatrics and Genetics
Chief, Division of Medical Genetics
Mt. Sinai School of Medicine
New York NY 10029

Martin Fleisher, Ph.D.[3]
Memorial Sloan-Kettering Cancer Center
New York NY 10021

Theodore Friedmann, M.D.[1]
Department of Pediatrics
University of California, San Diego
La Jolla CA 92093

Richard A. Gatti, M.D.[1]
Department of Pathology
University of California
Los Angeles CA 90024

Park S. Gerald, M.D.[1]
Chief, Clinical Genetics Division
Children's Hospital Medical Center
Harvard Medical School
Boston MA 02115

Robert A. Good, M.D., Ph.D.[1]
Oklahoma Medical Research Foundation
Oklahoma City OK 73104

Kathleen Y. Hall, Ph.D.[1]
Department of Pathology
University of California
Los Angeles CA 90024

Frank A. Ibbott, Ph.D.[3]
Bio-Science Laboratories
Van Nuys CA 91405

Michael Kaback, M.D.[1]
Departments of Pediatrics and Medicine
University of California School of Medicine
Division of Medical Genetics
Harbor-UCLA Medical Center
Los Angeles CA 90024

Marc Lappé, Ph.D.[1]
School of Public Health
Department of Social & Administrative Health Sciences
University of California
Berkeley CA 94720

David L. Rimoin, Ph.D.[1]
Departments of Pediatrics and Medicine
Chief, Division of Medical Genetics
Harbor-UCLA Medical Center
Torrance CA 90509

Denis O. Rodgerson, Ph.D.[3]
Department of Pathology
Center for Health Sciences
University of California
Los Angeles CA 90024

Andrew Saxon[2]
Department of Medicine
University of California School of Medicine
Los Angeles CA 90024

Margery W. Shaw, M.D., J.D.[1]
Institute for the Study of International Health Law
University of Texas Medical Genetics Center
Houston TX 77030

Robert S. Sparkes, M.D.[1]
Department of Medicine
Center for Health Sciences
University of California
Los Angeles CA 90024

Thomas E. Starzl, M.D., Ph.D.[1]
Department of Surgery
University of Pittsburgh
Pittsburgh PA 15261

Randolph Wall, Ph.D.[1]
Departments of Microbiology and Immunology
Molecular Biology Institute
University of California School of Medicine
Los Angeles CA 90024

Ellen E. Wright, J.D.[2]
Brookline MA 02146

Jorge J. Yunis, M.D.[1]
Department of Laboratory Medicine and Pathology
University of Minnesota Medical School
Minneapolis MN 55455

Attendees

Thomas H. Adams
Hybritech Inc.
La Jolla CA

Ada May Ames
San Jose CA

F. Philip Anderson
Ruston LA

Arnold O. Beckman
Beckman Instruments, Inc.
Fullerton CA

Laszlo Beres
New England Nuclear
Boston MA

James Berkman
New York NY

Edward W. Bermes, Jr.
Loyola University Hosp.
Maywood IL

George E. Bernett
Buena Park CA

Paige K. Besch
Baylor College of Med.
Houston TX

William N. Bigler
San Francisco State University
San Francisco CA

Roger L. Boeckx
Childrens Hosp. Natl. Med.
  Center
Washington DC

Lemuel Bowie
Evanston Hosp.
Evanston IL

Ira A. Budwig, Jr.
El Paso Rehabilitation Center
El Paso TX

George F. Bulbenko
Princeton Biomedix
Princeton NJ

Thorne J. Butler
Southern Nevada Memorial Hosp.
Las Vegas NV

Robert J. Carrico
Miles Laboratories, Ames Div.
Elkhart IN

Willard R. Centerwall
University of California
Sacramento CA

Wai-Yee Chan
University of Oklahoma
Oklahoma City OK

Larry W. Clark
Norton-Children's Hosp.
Louisville KY

Teresita B. Coligado
Roosevelt Hosp.
New York NY

Ann Copeland
Northwest Hosp.
Seattle WA

Diana Copsey
International Med. News Group
Rockville MD

Lin Cowan
University of California
Sacramento CA

Robert V. Coyne
Citrus Heights CA

Stephan Crothers
SmithKline Instruments
Sunnyvale CA

Sr. Jo Clare Daloisio
St. Mary's Health Center
St. Louis MO

Rogelio Decanio
Charleston Area Med. Center
Charleston WV

Albert A. Dietz
VA Hospital
Hines IL

Myra Di Salvo
Valley Children's Hosp.
Fresno CA

Patricia K. Dowling
MetPath Laboratories
Hackensack NJ

Louis Dunka, Jr.
Syva Co.
Cupertino CA

John W. Eastman
Berkeley CA

Klara Efron
Stanford University Med. Center
Stanford CA

Russell J. Eilers
Bio-Science Laboratories
Van Nuys CA

Joseph R. Elliott
St. Lukes Hosp.
Kansas City MO

Earl Ettiene
Fairfax CA

Michael Everitt
University of Washington
Seattle WA

Lilian M. Ewen
Royal Columbian Hosp.
New Westminster BC
Canada

Agnes Fakete
Chicago IL

Frances Finkelstein
Westbury NY

Nancy E. Fitzmaurice
Orinda CA

Alfred Free
Miles Laboratories, Ames Div.
Elkhart IN

Herbert Fritsche
MD Anderson Hosp.
Houston TX

Gerry Gallwas
Beckman Instruments
Brea CA

Philip Garry
University of New Mexico
Albuquerque NM

Spencer B. Gilbert
Placentia-Linda Community
   Hosp.
Placentia CA

Linda Glanville
SmithKline Instruments, Inc.
Sunnyvale CA

Candy Goday
Salinas CA

Barbara Goldsmith
Richmond VA

Manuel J. Gordon
Beckman Instruments, Inc.
Palo Alto CA

Harold J. Grady
Baptist Memorial Hosp.
Kansas City MO

I. J. Greenblatt
Woodmere NY

Bill Gregory
Beckman Instruments, Inc.
Fullerton CA

Linda Greve
University of California
Sacramento CA

Hanns-Dieter Gruemer
Med. College of Virginia
Richmond VA

Aida Gutierrez
Alexandria VA

Robert L. Habig
Duke Med. Center
Durham NC

Bill H. Haden
Beckman Instruments, Inc.
Brea CA

Keith B. Hammond
University of Colorado Health Sci.
  Center
Denver CO

Scinichi Hamushige
Irvine CA

Albert Hanok
Hawthorne NY

Jocelyn M. Hicks
Children's Hosp. Natl. Med.
  Center
Washington DC

J. Gilbert Hill
Hosp. for Sick Children
Toronto Ontario
Canada

Earle W. Holmes, Jr.
Loyola University Hosp.
Maywood IL

Vernon N. Houk
Centers for Disease Control
Atlanta GA

Harvey J. Hoyt
Miami FL

Ray Inman
American Scientific Products
McGaw Park IL

Steven Kaye
Los Angeles CA

W. J. Keenan
Roseville CA

Terry Kenny
Oregon Health Sci. University
Portland OR

Julius Kerkay
Cleveland State University
Cleveland OH

Mary Ellen King
Med. College of Virginia
Richmond VA

J. Y. Kiyasu
Roosevelt Hosp.
New York NY

Edward C. Knoblock
Mt. Airy MD

Anthony Koller
Michael Reese Hosp. & Med.
  Center
Chicago IL

Kenneth G. Krul
Technicon Instruments Co.
Tarrytown NY

Frank Kung
Cetus Corp.
Berkeley CA

Dennis E. Leavelle
Mayo Clinic
Rochester MN

Chung-Mei Ling
Abbott Laboratories
North Chicago IL

Joseph L. Longtin
St. Mary's General Hosp.
Lewiston ME

Penn Lupovich
Washington DC

Herbert Malkus
Providence Med. Center
Seattle WA

Gilbert B. Manning
Instrumentation Laboratory, Inc.
Spokane WA

Virginia S. Marcum
Clinical Chemistry
Winston-Salem NC

James H. McBride
Newhall CA

Michael McNeely
Victoria BC
Canada

Samuel Meites
Children's Hospital
Columbus OH

Anna Meriwether
Clinical Chemistry News
Washington DC

Janina W. Michalowska
Aurora CO

Curtis E. Miller
Beckman Instruments, Inc.
Fullerton CA

Greg Miller
Med. College of Virginia
Richmond VA

Linda S. Miller
Valley Children's Hosp.
Fresno CA

Razia S. Muneer
University of Oklahoma Health
  Sci. Center
Oklahoma City OK

Ted Namm
W. Chelumsford MA

Richard A. Nesbit
Beckman Instruments, Inc.
Fullerton CA

Karen L. Nickel
Bio-Science Laboratories
Van Nuys CA

John T. Ning
Arlington MA

Ron Obernolte
Valley Children's Hosp.
Fresno CA

Emelie H. Ongcapin
St. Barnabas Med. Center
Livingston NJ

José Planas
Puerto Rico

Popkin
Royal Jubilee Hosp.
Victoria BC
Canada

George Reed
Monterey CA

Mohamed A. Remtulla
Toronto Ontario
Canada

Jose P. Resendes
Cincinnati OH

Lawrence A. Reynolds
Syva Co.
Cupertino CA

Jo Rickard
Lopez WA

J. Richard Riese
SmithKline Instruments, Inc.
Sunnyvale CA

Morris Rockenmacher
Downey CA

Guilford G. Rudolph
Louisiana State University Med.
    Center
Shreveport LA

Lawrence Samec
Woodland Hills CA

Ilene Schneider
Beckman Instruments, Inc.
Fullerton CA

Roberta L. Schoderbeck
SmithKline Instruments, Inc.
Sunnyvale CA

Carol J. Schwarzott
Sunnyvale CA

Lorne E. Seargeant
Health Sci. Centre
Winnipeg Manitoba
Canada

Barbara E. Shearer
Toronto Ontario
Canada

Charlotte E. Shideler
Wesley Med. Center
Wichita KS

Elizabeth K. Smith
Children's Orthopedic Hosp.
    Med. Center
Seattle WA

Melvin Soule
Terumo Medical Corp.
Elkton MD

Salma Styles
Royal Jubilee Hosp.
Victoria BC
Canada

Jane V. Sun
SmithKline Instruments, Inc.
Sunnyvale CA

J. Robert Swanson
Oregon Health Sci. University
Portland OR

Doug Sweet
Syva Co.
Palo Alto CA

Ramesh C. Trivedi
Syva Co.
Palo Alto CA

Charles P. Turley
Little Rock AR

Nicholas VanBrunt
Reid Memorial Hosp.
Richmond IN

Z. H. Verjee
Hosp. for Sick Children
Toronto Ontario
Canada

Sr. Leo Rita Volk
St. Mary's Health Center
St. Louis MO

Anna N. Vorkoeper
Carmel CA

W. H. C. Walker
McMaster University
Hamilton Ontario
Canada

Robert J. Walton
Oakwood Hosp.
Dearborn MI

Judy M. Walton
Oakwood Hosp.
Dearborn MI

Graham M. Widdowson
Institutes of Med. Sci.
San Francisco CA

Rodney E. Willard
Loma Linda University Med.
    Center
Loma Linda CA

Will Wright
University of California
San Diego CA

Alan Wu
Hartford Hosp.
Hartford CT

Donald S. Young
Mayo Clinic
Rochester MN

Ben Zinser
Beckman Instruments, Inc.
Fullerton CA

I
PERSPECTIVE

An Overview of Human Genetics

Robert S. Sparkes

In this paper I present background information that will be important for a full understanding of the other, more detailed presentations to follow, and cover some areas not otherwise discussed in this conference.

Genetic disease is often assumed to result only from aberrant genetic processes. However, all phenotypes result from the interaction of genetic and environmental factors. Conditions in which the genetic component appears to be the major determining factor are often called genetic disorders, but even in many of these conditions environmental factors play a role. For example, although our understanding of the genetic and biochemical basis of sickle cell disease is extensive, there is no effective form of therapy that modifies the expression of the abnormal gene; this is one of the few conditions in which the mutant gene appears to be predominant without recognizable environmental factors modifying its expression. At the other end of the spectrum are certain types of trauma, such as bone fractures, that result from environmental stress; some people, however, have mutant genes that lead to brittle bones, which fracture with very little stress from the environment. Aside from these extreme examples, most normal and abnormal (disease) phenotypes result from the interaction of genetic and environmental factors. Good examples of these are the inborn errors of metabolism, such as phenylketonuria and galactosemia, in which the affected person must have the appropriate genetic makeup for the disease to manifest, but in which also the full expression of the abnormal gene can be prevented by appropriate dietary management. Thus, it is important to remember that most diseases result from the interaction of genetic and environmental factors and that the relative contribution of each varies from disease to disease.

Biochemical and Molecular Genetics

To understand genetic mechanisms, one must consider basic biology and biochemistry. With few exceptions, e.g., erythrocytes, each cell in the body contains in the cell nucleus a full complement of genes to control the metabolic processes of the cytoplasm. The genes contain information encoded in the DNA. From the DNA, messages (messenger RNA) are transcribed and delivered to the cytoplasm of the cell, where they interact with ribosomes and transfer RNAs to synthesize proteins. The primary structure of the gene determines the primary structure (amino acid sequence) of the protein, which in turn determines the function of the protein.

This constitutes one of the two important functions of the DNA. Its second important function is to replicate itself in a true fashion; otherwise, mutations occur. The information in the DNA is encoded in the purine and pyrimidine bases in the DNA molecule. The linear sequence of each three bases forms a code word, the triplet code, for a given amino acid. The messenger RNA transcribed from the DNA contains the same information as found in the DNA code words. These code words in the messenger RNA attract specific transfer RNAs based on a complementary structure in the transfer RNA, the anticodon. The anticodon of the transfer RNA is closely correlated with a specific amino acid, which attaches to another part of the transfer RNA molecule. Thus, specific transfer RNAs line up in a linear sequence, determined by their anticodons, to pair with the codons found in the messenger RNA. This determines the sequence of the amino acids, hence forming the primary structure of the protein.

This relatively simple model of how the gene controls cell metabolism has recently become more complicated as we have gained new insights into the structure of genes and the processing of messenger RNA. Within most genes, the regions that code for specific parts of a protein (exons) are separated by other sequences of DNA (introns). When the messenger RNA is first transcribed from the DNA, both exons and introns are transcribed. However, mature messenger RNA contains only the information found in the exons. Therefore, there has to be a processing of the primary messenger RNA to remove the introns. Although this processing mechanism is not fully understood, it probably involves several different steps, and an alteration in one could lead to an aberrant expression of the structural gene. Thus, not only can a change in the structure of the gene itself lead to an abnormal function, but also an abnormality in the processing of the messenger RNA may lead to an abnormal expression of an otherwise apparently normal gene. There is also still the possibility of some type of regulatory function, to determine whether a specific gene will be transcribed at all. The reasons for all this complexity are not clear, but it is evident that the abnormal expression of the gene depends on several factors and not simply a change in its structure.

Inborn Errors of Metabolism

Our understanding of the biochemistry of inborn errors of metabolism is one of the most complete for any of the genetic problems. The majority of these disorders involve the so-called metabolic blocks. A given substance in the body is processed through a metabolic pathway of many steps, each of which is under the control of an enzyme, which in turn is under the control of one or more genes. Hence, the biochemical basis of most of these metabolic blocks is a defective or absent enzyme, the result of a mutation affecting the structural gene or perhaps some processing step of its messenger. When a metabolic block occurs, disease can result from accumulation of the substrate before the blocked step, from lack of the normally formed product, or perhaps from increased functioning of an alternative metabolic pathway for the substrate (which in turn may lead to an increased concentration of a disease-causing substance).

The metabolic pathway for the metabolism of phenylalanine provides examples of each of these possibilities. Normally, phenylalanine is metabolized to tyrosine. In phenylketonuria the enzyme phenylalanine hydroxylase (EC 1.14.16.1), which converts phenylalanine to tyrosine, is absent; with this metabolic block, phenylketones accumulate and are excreted in urine, producing a positive result for the ferric chloride test. Also, phenylalanine accumulates in the blood, which is the basis for the screening test for phenylketonuria in the newborn. Currently, it is not clear whether the increased phenylalanine itself leads to the mental retardation characteristic of this disease or whether the increased production of products from the alternative pathway may lead to the disease. In the next step of the metabolic pathway, tyrosine can be transformed to melanin, which produces the coloring of the skin. In albinism there is a metabolic block in the transformation of tyrosine to melanin; in this instance, the absence of the product beyond the metabolic block results in disease. Alternatively, tyrosine can be metabolized to homogentisic acid through another pathway; the accumulation of the homogentisic acid in tissue such as the joints leads to the disease alkaptonuria.

Inheritance Patterns

Autosomal recessive. Most metabolic blocks are transmitted as recessive disorders. In most of the recessive disorders for which the biochemical basis is understood, there is an absence of enzyme activity. These recessive disorders can be either X-linked or autosomal. A characteristic of autosomal recessive inheritance is that the responsible gene is located on one of the autosomal chromosomes; increasingly, we are able to locate these genes on specific chromosomes.

For these disorders to manifest, the affected individual must have a double dose of the mutant gene; i.e., both members of the gene pair must be of the abnormal type (homozygosity). In general, the affected persons in a family are limited to a single generation because both of the parents must be heterozygous carriers. Usually carriers do not manifest disease, although the abnormality may be detectable by appropriate biochemical studies, such as studies of enzyme activity. In some of the rare genetic traits, the parents of an affected child are related, i.e., consanguineous. This is not unexpected because, if the disease is rare, the gene also is uncommon, and the likelihood that two people will carry the same uncommon gene is increased if the individuals are biologically related. As is well known, on the average a mating between two carrier (heterozygous) parents carries the risk of 25% that a child will be homozygous for the mutant gene and have the disease, 25% that he or she will neither have the disease nor be a carrier for the mutant gene, and 50% that a child will be a carrier like the parents. Homozygosity in one parent will lead to a greater proportion of abnormalities in the offspring.

The hemoglobin problems illustrate some difficulties in classifying the inheritance of a genetic disorder on the basis of the criteria used to define the presence or absence of a gene. For example, the sickle cell trait rarely produces clinical disease, and only a person with the sickle cell disease has the clinical manifestations of the abnormal gene. Thus, clinically the disease behaves like a recessive trait. However, the heterozygote carrier (sickle cell trait) can readily be detected by electrophoresis of hemoglobin, which implies that sickle cell trait behaves like a dominant disorder. This apparent confusion results from the use of the terms *dominant* and *recessive* to describe clinical manifestations, whereas with newer biochemical techniques these conditions might now be reclassified. This represents only a semantic problem, however, not a biological problem. If the sickle cell disease does represent an autosomal recessive problem, it is one of the few recessive problems that is not due to the alteration of an enzyme protein, but rather to the alteration of the nonenzyme protein, hemoglobin.

Autosomal dominant. The characteristics of autosomal dominant inheritance are as follows. As with the autosomal recessive problems, the genes involved are located on one of the autosomes. In contrast to the recessive problems, however, the gene is generally present in the heterozygous state; i.e., only one member of the allelic gene pair is of the mutant type. Because only one member of the gene pair need be abnormal, the disorder is found in successive generations. On the average, 50% of the children of an affected parent will get the abnormal gene; if the gene is fully penetrant, then all of those 50% will be affected. Moreover, on the average, both males and females are equally affected.

In contrast to the recessive problems, where most recognized defects involve enzymes, the basic biochemical alteration in dominant traits is largely unknown. Theoretically, alterations affecting genetic regulatory processes, cell structures, or increased enzyme activities could all be expressed in a dominant fashion.

X-linked. The third type of single-gene inheritance pattern is the sex-linked pattern, perhaps better called X-linked, because in these problems the affected gene is located on the X chromosome. Most of the disorders that have been recognized are recessive traits; therefore, generally the male is affected and the female, with two X chromosomes, is a carrier. Such traits thus tend to skip generations: affected males have asymptomatic carrier daughters, who in turn transmit the gene to half of their sons. Also, for a given patient, one often finds affected males on the mother's side of the family. The most definitive characteristic for X-linked inheritance is the complete lack of transmission from father to son, because if the offspring is going to be male, the father supplies the Y chromosome but not his X chromosome, whether it contains an abnormal gene or not.

Polygenic inheritance. Some traits occur or recur in certain families more often than in the general population. Unless due to chance, this is often attributed to polygenic inheritance plus interaction with environmental factors, leading to multifactorial etiology of the trait. In these instances, several genes contribute to the presence or absence of a given trait. Secondly, there is assumed to be a threshold beyond which a trait is manifest, such that several mutant genes are needed to push past this threshold. Closely related individuals, having more genes in common, are more likely to be affected than individuals more distantly related.

Chromosomes

Human chromosomes can be readily viewed under the light microscope, but the genes are too small to be seen with this technique. Thus, a chromosome analysis can detect a gross abnormality of a chromosome but tells nothing about the alteration in a single gene.

Human chromosomes are usually studied in somatic cells, such as from the peripheral blood. A few drops of blood are put into tissue culture medium and phytohemagglutinin is added to stimulate the T lymphocytes to divide. After three days of culture, dividing cells are accumulated by exposing the cells to a mitosis-inhibiting agent, e.g., Colcemid (demecolcine), for the last hour of culture. The cells are then processed through a hypotonic solution, which causes the cells to expand and the chromosomes to separate from each other. After exposure to a fixative, the cells are placed on a microscope slide for staining.

Several staining techniques with specific objectives and uses are currently available. First, the homogeneous staining technique with Giemsa stain provides a uniform staining of the chromosomes. This stain does not permit identification of each individual chromosome nor does it permit recognition of small chromosome changes. For those objectives, differential staining techniques are used, most commonly quinacrine (Q) or Giemsa (G) banding techniques, which give similar results. There is also a reverse-banding technique in which the banding pattern is similar to those obtained with the two stains but with the brightness or darkness of the stain reversed. This stain is particularly useful in looking for changes at the ends of the chromosomes, which tend to stain lightly with the G stain. The centromeric heterochromatin region stains with the C band technique. There is also a silver stain, which primarily stains the nucleolus organizer regions, where the ribosomal genes are. With high-resolution banding techniques the chromosomes can be studied in their more extended state before they enter metaphase. This technique, which is very effective for recognizing very small chromosome changes, is discussed in a later chapter by Dr. Yunis.

For most chromosomal analyses, chromosomes are examined and photographed under the light microscope. For the full karyotype analysis, the chromosomes in the photographs are cut out and studied.

Chromosome abnormalities. Numerous human chromosome abnormalities have been found, including abnormalities in both the number and the structure of chromosomes. When all cells in the body contain abnormal numbers of chromosomes, the conception has probably resulted from one gamete, an egg or a sperm, that had an abnormal number of chromosomes. In turn, the abnormal gamete was produced by a nondisjunction during meiosis, in which the usual segregation of members of an homologous pair of chromosomes did not occur. One of the few clues we have for understanding nondisjunction is the incidence of advanced maternal age in Down's syndrome, but even here we do not understand how this leads to the presumed nondisjunction.

In general we do not know how chromosome imbalance leads to the phenotypic abnormality. However, there is a good correlation between a chromosome imbalance and certain clinical problems. For example, although all persons with Down's syndrome are not identical, they appear sufficiently alike that a clinical diagnosis usually is possible without resorting to chromosomal analysis. This clinical picture is different from that associated with other autosomal trisomies (tripled chromosomes instead of paired), such as trisomy 13 or trisomy 18, which are also readily distinguished from each other.

Most of the abnormalities of the autosomal chromosomes are associated with mental retardation, as discussed extensively in the chapter by Dr. Gerald.

Abnormalities of the sex chromosomes show a less clear relationship to mental retardation. Most patients with Turner's syndrome have only 45 chromosomes (only one X chromosome) and usually are not retarded; however, on IQ tests many of them show a wide disparity between the verbal component, which tends to be good, and the performance part, which tends to be relatively poor. Hence, most of these individuals do satisfactorily in society or in a job if they select activities with a strong verbal component. They are females, short, and have primary amenorrhea. Females with extra X chromosomes have few physical stigmata, but with an increasing number of X chromosomes, mental retardation is increased. In addition, these women have a greater problem with infertility than normal women. An extra X chromosome in the male produces the Klinefelter syndrome, characterized by small testes and infertility. As with the females, an extra X chromosome produces a tendency toward mental retardation. Finally, there is the XYY syndrome, which is probably a chromosomal syndrome not associated with a specific phenotype. Early studies suggested that this chromosome change was associated with an increased tendency toward criminal behavior; subsequent studies, however, have not clearly demonstrated such a relationship, and the present feeling is that some such persons may have a slightly increased risk for criminal behavior but most do not demonstrate this problem. These persons may also be taller than their siblings, but very tall persons are not more significantly involved with this chromosome change.

The sex chromatin bodies reflect the sex chromosome makeup. The Barr body or the X chromatin body is thought to represent an inactivated X chromosome. The Lyon hypothesis indicates that under normal circumstances only one X chromosome remains genetically active and any additional X chromosomes are genetically inactivated. Thus, the male, with only one X chromosome, does not have an X chromatin body, whereas the female, with two X chromosomes, has a single X chromatin body. More recently, a Y chromatin body, a brightly fluorescent region on the distal end of the Y chromosome, has been described in the cells of a normal male at interphase. Tests for both the X and Y chromatin bodies are relatively simple, but both have technical and biological limitations and probably should not be used as the sole basis for establishing the sex chromosome makeup of an individual.

Gene mapping. Recent developments have greatly expanded our knowledge of the human gene map, which can be used to help diagnose chromosome problems. Our experience with a recent example illustrates this point (*1*). In a patient with sporadic retinoblastoma, mental retardation, and short stature, but without other physical abnormalities, chromosome studies revealed a chromosome deletion affecting the middle part of the long arm of a chromosome 13 (*1*). Earlier studies by others (*2, 3*) had indicated that the genetic locus for the enzyme esterase D was on chromosome 13. Because the quantitative expression of a number of genes is related to the number of genes for that trait, we evaluated the expression of the esterase D activity in this patient. She had approximately one-half the normal enzyme activity, which, on the basis of a gene-dose relationship, suggested that the gene for this enzyme would have been located in the deleted part of the chromosome. Studies of additional patients with retinoblastoma, who had similar but not exactly the same chromosome deletion, suggested that the genetic factor involved with the retinoblastoma is in band 13q14; enzyme studies also indicated that the gene for the esterase D is in this same band. In our subsequent studies of additional patients, there is so far a close correlation with the deletion of this chromosome band and the presence of only 50% enzyme activity, indicating that the determination of enzyme activity could be useful in interpreting a chromosome deletion in the long arm of chromosome 13.

The esterase D enzyme also shows genetic polymorphism on electrophoresis (*2, 3*). We have used this information to try to determine whether the gene for the inherited form of retinoblastoma is also closely linked to the esterase D. Our studies to date suggest this may be the case, but we still do not have enough information to state with statistical assurance that there is genetic linkage of the esterase D with the inherited form of retinoblastoma.

A second instance in which gene mapping information helped in cytogenetic interpretation is as follows (4). We studied chromosomes in a patient who had an extra chromosome that appeared to comprise duplicated short arms of a chromosome 9. Earlier studies (5, 6) had suggested that the locus for galactose-1-phosphate uridylyltransferase (EC 2.7.7.10) is on the short arm of chromosome 9. Our patient had twice the normal activity of this enzyme, which is what one would expect if there were four representations of the gene, as would be found in the presence of four short arms of chromosome 9. Here, the enzyme study confirmed the interpretation of the cytogenetics.

There has been considerable interest in the association of chromosome abnormalities with leukemia and other neoplastic processes. The classic example of this is the Philadelphia chromosome in chronic myelogenous leukemia. Initially, part of the long arm of one of the G group chromosomes (21 or 22) was thought to be deleted. Banding chromosome studies showed that the affected chromosome was indeed chromosome 22. Subsequent studies demonstrated that there is not a simple deletion in the long arm of chromosome 22 but rather a translocation of part of the long arm of one chromosome 22 to the distal end of a chromosome 9, although other chromosomes may be involved as well. More extensive studies suggest that chromosome abnormalities are common in various tumors; further, these changes tend to be relatively nonrandom, suggesting that there could be an important intimate relationship between the chromosome change and the neoplastic process. However, it is not clear as to how this relationship operates—whether it is a cause-and-effect relationship or just a marker for the tumor. Chromosome changes in cancer are discussed extensively by Dr. Yunis.

Prevention of Genetic Problems

Because there are no effective forms of therapy for many genetic disorders, there has been an interest in preventing them. Some approaches involve prenatal diagnosis and selective abortion of affected fetuses. The two most commonly used techniques for prenatal diagnosis are ultrasound and amniocentesis. With amniocentesis, amniotic fluid is obtained at about the 16th week of pregnancy. The amniotic cells, which are primarily from the fetus, are grown in tissue culture and analyzed for chromosomes or for specific inborn errors of metabolism. Most such studies are directed toward detecting chromosome abnormalities. Unfortunately, some inborn errors are not expressed in the amniotic cells; moreover, each metabolic defect requires its own specific test to determine whether the fetus is affected.

Because some of the inherited disorders are not expressed in the amniotic cells, recombinant DNA techniques have been applied to determine the presence or absence of a specific gene. One such approach focuses on the prenatal diagnosis of sickle cell disease (7). A radioactive probe, complementary DNA (cDNA), is used to detect the presence of a β-globin gene (the sickle cell gene is a mutation of the β-globin gene) by extracting the DNA from cells, treating the DNA with restriction endonuclease, and electrophoresing the DNA fragments. A relatively high proportion of persons with the sickle cell mutation have a DNA fragment larger than that for the normal β-globin gene. Because electrophoresis separates the DNA fragments primarily on the basis of their size, one can determine whether a normal β-globin gene or a sickle cell globin gene is present. By applying this technique to the study of amniotic cells, one can tell in some families whether the fetus has the normal or the sickle cell gene and whether the gene is present in the homozygous or the heterozygous state. Thus, we can now detect the presence of genes directly and not have to depend on their expression in the amniotic cells.

Treatment of Genetic Diseases

Some areas of current treatment will be discussed in detail in some of the other presentations. Therefore, I will only briefly review some of the general approaches to treatment of genetic problems. First, there is the dietary form of therapy, which includes restriction of substances in the diet to manage a genetic problem; examples are restriction of phenylalanine in phenylketonuria and galactose in galactosemia. In other conditions, a product that is absent because of a genetic defect can be replaced; for example, the adrenogenital syndrome can be managed by giving steroid replacement. Some genetic conditions are due to increased accumulation or deposits of substances in the tissues, e.g., the deposition of copper in Wilson's disease; through the use of penicillamine, copper can be removed from at least some of the tissues.

Sometimes a genetic problem is related to drug exposure, as in glucose-6-phosphate dehydrogenase deficiency (EC 1.1.1.49); prevention of exposure to the responsible drug can prevent the problem from manifesting. Surgery, such as splenectomy in hereditary spherocytosis, can prevent many of the manifestations of an abnormal gene. Prophylactic removal of the colon from patients with polyposis coli can prevent the development of life-threatening tumors of the colon. Tissue transplantation, such as renal transplantation to treat cystic disease of the kidney, can prove effective.

Thus, for a limited number of genetic disorders specific forms of therapy are available. The form of therapy has to be specific to make the therapy effective, and this is a major limitation in the treatment of genetic diseases. Even in conditions in which the basic molecular defect is known, such as the sickle cell disease, we have still not developed a rational form of therapy based on this knowledge. With increased knowledge of genetic problems, we can anticipate that improved therapies will become available for an increasing number of genetic disorders.

References

1. Sparkes, R. S., Sparkes, M. C., Wilson, M. G., Towner, J. W., Benedict, W., Murphree, A. L., and Yunis, J. J., Regional assignment of genes for human esterase D and retinoblastoma to chromosome band 13q14. *Science* **208**, 1042–1044 (1982).
2. van Heyningen, V., Bobrow, M., Bodner, W. F., Gardiner, S. E., Povey, S., and Hopkinson, D. A., Chromosome assignment of some human enzyme loci: Mitochondrial malate dehydrogenase to 7, manosephosphate isomerase and pyruvate kinase to 15, and probably esterase D to 13. *Ann. Human Genet.* **38**, 295–303 (1975).
3. Chen, S., Creagan, R. P., Nichols, F. A., and Ruddle, F. H., Assignment of esterase-D gene to chromosome 13. *Birth Defects* **11**, 99–102 (1975).
4. Moedjono, S. J., Crandall, B. F., and Sparkes, R. S., Tetrasomy 9p: Confirmation by enzyme analysis. *J. Med. Genet.* **17**, 227–229 (1980).
5. Ghymers, D., Hermann, B., Disteche, C., and Frederic, J., Tetrasomie partielle du chromosome 9, à l'ètat de mosaique, chez un enfant porteur de malformations multiples. *Human Genet.* **20**, 273–282 (1973).
6. Abe, T., Morita, M., Kawai, K., Misawa, S., Takino, T., Mashimota, H., and Nakagome, Y., Partial tetrasomy 9(9pter9q2101) due to an

extra iso-dicentric chromosome. *Ann. Genet. (Paris)* **20,** 273–282 (1977).
7. Kan, Y. W., and Dozy, A. M., Antenatal diagnosis of sickle-cell anemia by DNA analysis of amniotic-fluid cells. *Lancet* **ii,** 910–912 (1978).

General References

Vogel, F., and Motulsky, A. G., *Human Genetics: Problems and Approaches,* Springer Verlag, New York, NY, 1979.

Thompson, J. S., and Thompson, M. W., *Genetics and Medicine,* W. B. Saunders Co., Philadelphia, PA, 1980.

Discussion

Q: What is the status of in utero blood sampling?

DR. SPARKES: Much of the early impetus for in utero blood sampling came from the desire to make a prenatal diagnosis of hemoglobin problems. Because the hemoglobin gene is not expressed in amniotic cells, it is necessary to sample the blood of the fetus. Unfortunately, fetal blood sampling still carries a 5–10% risk of associated miscarriages. Because of this and the skills required, the test is available in only a few centers. Alternative approaches such as the use of cDNA probes for hemoglobin will probably replace fetal blood sampling.

Q: Can esterase D activity be evaluated in amniotic cells?

DR. SPARKES: We know that esterase D is present in amniotic cells, but most of our studies have been done on erythrocytes. Studies on fibroblasts with which we have some experience show a considerably broader range of enzyme activity than found for erythrocytes. As a result, the assay of esterase D activity will probably have limited application in retinoblastoma, although with increased experience we may develop better techniques. Qualitative electrophoresis of esterase D will probably become more useful in familial studies.

DR. IBBOTT: In those conditions where the number of chromosomes is altered, as in trisomies, is it true that certain chromosomes, e.g., 21, seem to be more subject to alterations?

DR. SPARKES: This is a somewhat complicated question because it involves both the frequency of conception of individuals with chromosome abnormalities as well as their ability to survive to the point of detection. Most chromosome trisomies can be found in early spontaneous abortuses, while only a few of these survive to be detected in the postnatal period. For example, trisomy 16 is found quite commonly in spontaneous abortuses but seldom postnatally. The XO karyotype of Turner's syndrome appears also to occur very commonly in spontaneous abortuses, but statistical studies suggest to only 1 in 100 individuals conceived with XO abnormalities survives. Why this should be, we do not know because the phenotype with Turner's syndrome is relatively mild in terms of life-threatening problems in the postnatal period. Thus, it seems we cannot tell whether certain chromosomes are more prone than others to abnormalities, but clearly only a small portion of fetuses with chromosome abnormalities survive.

Q: Is retinoblastoma associated with mental retardation?

DR. SPARKES: In those few instances of retinoblastoma associated with partial deletion of the long arm of chromosome 13, mental retardation is common. In most other instances of sporadic cases of retinoblastoma, as well as the inherited variety, mental retardation is not increased.

Legal Liability in Genetic Screening, Genetic Counseling, and Prenatal Diagnosis

Ellen E. Wright and Margery W. Shaw

Recent scientific and medical developments have caused the obstetrician to become increasingly concerned about the legal implications of genetic counseling and screening. Liability in this area exists only when one can predict the possibility of defective children. Thus physicians' potential legal exposure grew dramatically as pedigree analysis and empiric risk figures were supplemented by techniques for detecting mutant gene carrier states in the parents and genetic disorders in the fetus. The legalization of abortion further increased the options available to prospective parents. At the same time, malpractice litigation virtually exploded, reflecting patients' increasing expectations of high-quality, disappointment-free medical care. The scarcity of settled legal precedent in this field makes it especially difficult in genetic counseling cases to establish guidelines for future practice. As if this were not enough, it is likely that scientific advances will continue at a rapid pace, posing legal quandaries not yet addressed or even imagined.

Yet despite all the pressures that favor legal liability, doctors are *not* required to compensate all patients' dissatisfactions with the counseling or screening process. This article seeks to acquaint the obstetrician with the legal rules that determine when a physician's actions or nonactions may give rise to liability. This analysis will focus on the elements of a cause of action—that is, which events as alleged by aggrieved patients are ones for which the law provides a remedy. Specific legal issues arising both in current genetic counseling and screening practices as well as from some foreseeable scientific developments and new reproductive options will be explored. Finally, the authors' views on relevant judicial trends anticipated in the future will be presented.

The following comments represent only the authors' opinions based on the legal principles followed by most jurisdictions. The law on any given issue may vary among the states and is not finally settled in any state until it is decided by that state's highest court.

The Cause of Action for Undisclosed Genetic Risks

The elements of a cause of action can be best described in the context of the prototypical genetic counseling case, one in which the parents say that had their obstetrician told them about their genetic risk, they would have prevented the birth of their defective child. This encompasses negligence in both prenatal diagnosis and genetic screening. The latter is here defined as any efforts, whether made in widespread programs or individual physicians' offices, to detect parents at an increased risk for having defective children.

The Requirement of Contract

While most genetic counseling cases are won or lost in the area of medical negligence law, the law of contracts provides both a first step in the legal analysis and, on occasion, an independent basis for liability. The threshold question is whether the physician entered into a contract to treat one or both parents as patients. The answer is usually yes. Generally, a contract exists between two people only when one person makes an offer that the other accepts and both people understand the terms of the agreement. In addition, each person must promise to exchange something of value with the other. From this description, it would seem relatively difficult to prove the existence of a physician–patient contract. Yet in areas such as medicine, wherein one relatively uninformed person is likely to rely on the actions and statements of another more knowledgeable person, the law is quick to find that a contract was made. Thus, a prospective patient's request for aid may be construed as an implied offer to pay for necessary medical care that is implicitly accepted as soon as the physician begins discussions toward providing either advice or actual treatment (79).

The physician's duties based solely on contract are relatively few. If the physician promises, as part of the contract, to provide specified services or, more significantly, to obtain certain results, he/she must live up to the promise (28). Indeed, patients frequently sue in contract, alleging that their physicians "guaranteed," for example, that a vasectomy or tubal ligation would prevent any chance of pregnancy or that there was no chance that subsequent children would be born defective (65). Although the courts do occasionally find that a physician promised to achieve a specific result, they generally view such "breach of warranty" actions with disfavor, either finding that the physician intended merely to reassure the patient or recasting the complaint as one in medical malpractice.

The Role of Torts

The relevance of the physician–patient contract is to show the existence of a legal relationship between the parties. So long as the contract is in effect, the physician's duties are determined not only by specific contractual promises, but more significantly also by the law of medicine malpractice, a branch of tort law. A tort is a legal harm or injury caused by the actions of another person. Tort law encompasses *intentional wrongdoing* such [as] battery, if consent was not obtained for performing an operation or treatment; *nonintentional wrongdoing*, which includes negligence (e.g., medical malpractice); and *strict liability*, such as liability without fault of drug companies for adverse side effects of their products. To oversimplify greatly, a physician will be liable in tort when he/she breaches a duty to the patient, thereby proximately causing the patient to suffer an injury for which the law provides a remedy.

The Physician's Duty

Who are the recipients of a physician's tortious acts? In the typical genetic counseling case, the obstetrician's clearest duty is to the prospective mother since she usually is the actual patient. The physician may also owe a duty to the prospective father because the father may be injured by the additional support responsibilities for a defective child and by his own and the mother's emotional suffering (*4*). This obligation will be especially clear in those instances in which it is necessary to examine or take a genealogic history from the prospective father in order to make an assessment of the couple's genetic risks. By contrast, the courts have almost uniformly rejected claims by siblings that they were deprived of parental care by the birth of a defective child (*1, 17*).

The court may also be asked to determine whether the physician owed a duty to the defective child in a case in which the parents or the child say that the child should never have been born. The few courts and judges that have addressed this issue found that the child came within the physician's duty of care (*18*). Most courts, however, do not reach the question of duty to the unborn child, but rather rely on other grounds for denying the child's cause of action (*4, 19*).

The Standard of Care

The next inquiry concerns the standard of care required of a physician's performance. One of the obstetrician's obligations is to detect an increased risk of having defective children. In this, as in much of medical practice, a physician is required to use only that degree of skill and care that would have been exercised by other physicians in the same or similar circumstances (*80*). So long as one meets the appropriate degree of care, there can be no legal liability. Yet any failure to comply with this standard, even an honest mistake, can constitute negligence. There is no requirement of "neglect" or moral culpability. In addition, findings of negligence can be based not only on inappropriately performed actions but also on unreasonable failures to act. Indeed, errors of omission, such as failures to take a family history or to offer diagnostic tests (*4, 6, 32, 39*), are far more prevalent than errors of commission (*18*).

There are some important corollaries and limitations to this standard. The first is that the skill and knowledge required varies with the extent of the physician's training. Thus a specialist practicing within his/her area of expertise must provide a higher level of medical care than a general practitioner (*48, 60*). At the same time, however, a physician with less particularized expertise has a duty to refer patients to a specialist or to a genetic counseling clinic if, in the exercise of due care, problems arise that he/she cannot handle (*43*). For example, any physician who works with women of childbearing age should be aware that older women have a higher incidence of children with chromosome anomalies and that such defects can be diagnosed prenatally. As a result, the physician should be able either to perform amniocentesis or to explain this procedure and know where to refer the patients who wish to use it.

In addition, while there is an overwhelming trend to hold specialists to a nationally uniform standard of care (*60*), many courts still require nonspecialists to exercise only the degree of skill common to general practitioners in their own communities (*69*). This "locality rule," however, is eroding, due in part to both the emerging speciality of family practice and rapid developments in communication (*68*).

Even the national standard is not entirely uniform. For example, the law recognizes different approaches to practice so long as each particular view is espoused by at least a "respectable minority" of the medical profession (*2, 31*). Thus, physicians will probably be considered to have exercised the necessary degree of care whether they disclose the risks reported in the Canadian and American studies as to the safety and reliability of amniocentesis (*45, 49*) or the higher risk figures of the United Kingdom study (*59*). The uniform rule may also be modified in instances in which the incidence of specific genetic disorders varies throughout the country. For example, an obstetrician practicing in Manhattan, where there are many Ashkenazi Jews and people of Mediterrenean descent, has a higher duty to know about the risks of Tay–Sachs disease and α-thalassemia than does a physician working in rural Texas (*52*).

The required standard of care may be modified in two other ways. The first is by statute. Although none currently does, a state could require, for example, that serum α-fetoprotein be assayed in all pregnant women. Such a statutory requirement would then represent the minimum acceptable standard of care. Thus, if a person who was the object of the law's protection were injured by its violation—in this case, if parents bore a child with a neural tube defect due to a failure to test—negligence could be shown simply by showing violation of the statute. Unlike most malpractice cases, the care exercised by other physicians would be irrelevant. In other words, violation of the statutory standards would be negligence per se, and the injured patient would be required to prove only the extent of damages (*58*).

Second, even exercising the same degree of skill as other similar doctors does not always immunize the physician from a risk of malpractice. On rare occasions, the courts find that some procedure normally omitted by the "reasonable practitioner" nonetheless should have been offered and that failure to do so was negligent. Generally, such omissions are found to be substandard only when the costs and risks of providing the service are very low and the harm to be avoided is very great. For instance, the Supreme Court of the State of Washington held that ophthalmologists reasonably should test for glaucoma in all patients, not just those over 40 (*30*). By analogy, a physician in the District of Columbia would be well advised to test newborns for phenylketonuria even though that procedure is no longer required by statute.

Two aspects of the duty to detect genetic risks deserve special emphasis. First, the physician who has access to the patient before conception should take a careful family history and offer heterozygote detection tests when available (*32*). The second is the duty to keep up with developments in the field (*48*). For example, physicians should know that there have been large published surveys in the United Kingdom recommending α-fetoprotein (AFP) and acetylcholine esterase (AChE) screening of maternal serum in all pregnancies (*8, 12, 72*). AFP and AChE levels in the amniotic fluid should be determined any time a woman has amniocentesis for any reason or when there is a family history of neural tube defect. Further, the standard of care may soon include the use of recombinant DNA probes to detect various hemoglobinopathies (*38*) and it has been predicted that in the not too distant future diagnosis of *all* mendelian diseases will be possible in the fetus by family studies of restriction endonuclease polymorphisms (*7*).

The Standard of Disclosure

Once a physician discerns that specific prospective parents are at an increased genetic risk, what is the scope of his/her duty to convey that information? Under the law of informed consent, as it is currently developing in many jurisdictions, a prospective parent must be given, or at least offered, all the information that a reasonable person would want to know before making a decision (*9, 14, 77*). The physician's duty extends beyond merely answering patients' direct questions (*9*). Information sufficient to afford the basis for a logical decision must be given even though the patient's ultimate choice may not be entirely rational. In addition, whatever justifications may be offered for the "therapeutic privilege" exception to the general law of informed consent (*77*), the courts should reject any physician's argument that he/she did not provide genetic risk information because he/she thought that the prospective parents would somehow have been "better off" without it.

The "reasonable patient" standard, on its face, is more advantageous to the counselee than is a "reasonable practitioner" rule. For instance, it could well require counselors to convey more information than they think is appropriate (*52*). Perhaps more significantly, it permits the jury to decide solely on the basis of its own experience which information should have been disclosed (*77*). This is in distinct contrast to most issues in medical malpractice, in which the jury must rely on experts' testimony about what should or should not have been done.

This approach to informed consent, however, provides the patient with only limited protection since the law at present focuses only on what information must be disclosed. It ignores important issues of whether the patients actually understand the information given and whether, in light of the complex psychologic interactions at work in the physician–patient relationship, the patients are truly free to make their own choices or whether the physicians' attitudes play a significant role in these decisions (*40*). These overlooked questions may be especially important in genetic counseling, both because of the difficulties that many prospective parents have in assimilating the reality of their genetic risk and because of the directive approach taken by some counselors (*66*).

In summary, physicians have duties at least to detect and to inform their patients about increased genetic risks. These obligations are governed by either the performance of other physicians or the needs of the patients. If a physician's actions meet the standards of care, there can be no legal liability (*36*). Even if aggrieved parents can show that their physicians negligently failed to detect a genetic risk or to disclose some relevant information, there are still other hurdles to surmount before liability can be imposed. The parent must show that an injury occurred that is compensable at law. The parent must also prove that the physician's breach of duty proximately caused the injury and that the injury was a reasonably foreseeable risk of the act or omission.

Foreseeability

To demonstrate the role of foreseeability, a physician who prescribed diethylstilbestrol (DES) to pregnant women 25 years ago should not be liable to their daughters who develop clear cell carcinoma because there was no reasonable way one could have foreseen that sort of risk. By contrast, the manufacturers of DES may be held strictly liable under legal theories that do not apply to physicians (71). In the area of genetic counseling, if the physician fails either to detect or to disclose risks that are reasonably foreseeable, then he/she could be held liable in negligence. Parents of infants with genetic tragedies that are not foreseeable have no valid claim for damages.

Proximate Cause

The proof of proximate cause in malpractice actions is more problematic. This requires that the negligence was sufficiently related to the injury that the law [w]ill impose liability. As a result, a negligent act can be a proximate cause even though it is not the *sole* cause of the events that follow (58). This distinction is well illustrated in cases concerning the birth of genetically defective children. Obviously, physicians do not "cause" the disorders in the usual sense because the underlying cause is either a new mutation, a chromosomal error, or a defective gene in one or both of the parents' germ cells. Yet a physician's failure to detect or to disclose genetic information can proximately cause such births if the mother can show that had she been correctly informed, she would have avoided conception or aborted the fetus.

Legal Remedies

Even if the people who bring genetic counseling suits can prove negligence and proximate causation, they still face one final obstacle to recovery—the problem of injury and damages. The courts frequently rule that, as a matter of law, no compensation may be provided for some or all of the injuries suffered in these cases. The reasons given for these rulings are of three general types.

The courts often believe that the injuries themselves are too speculative, too difficult to measure, or too atypical to be compensable (*35*). In some cases, they think that awarding damages would be contrary to public policy (*25*). And occasionally they hold that there was no injury because the claimant was not deprived of anything to which he/she had a legally protectable right (*1*). In addition, for those injuries deemed to be legally cognizable, plaintiffs still bear the burden of showing the extent of their damages.

The possible injuries suffered in genetic counseling fall into three broad categories: economic injuries sustained by the parents, emotional pain and suffering by the parents, and physical pain and suffering by the defective child. In recent decisions, the courts have consistently held that the parents of genetically defective children may state a claim for some damages, although they differ widely as to whether the parents may recover the entire cost of supporting the child, or only the extraordinary medical expenses, or compensation for their own emotional pain and suffering.

The courts have been mixed in their responses to claims by defective children. The highest state courts, however, have uniformly rejected such claims, saying either that it is impossible to determine whether life with defects is worse than no life at all or that recognition of such claims is simply contrary to public policy. Notably, however, many judges and legal commentators favor the recognition of such claims (*6, 10, 15*). Indeed, one appellate court not only upheld the child's claims but also allowed punitive damages if fraud, oppression, or malice could be shown (*18*).

The legal decisions in several recently reported cases involving genetic conditions are summarized in Table 1. This is not a complete listing because most trial court cases and all out-of-court settlements are not published.

Other Legal Problems in Genetic and Reproductive Contexts

Injuries from Techniques in Prenatal Diagnosis

Using the framework set forth in the analysis above, we can now turn to the legal implications of other specific situations that

Table 1. Malpractice Suits Involving Genetic Conditions

Name of case (reference) state/date/court[a]	Defect; indications of risk	Birth date; alleged malpractice	Parents' claims — Economic loss	Parents' claims — Emotional pain and suffering	Child's claims — Physical pain and suffering from defects
Karlsons v. Guerinot (39) NY 4/15/77 (I)	Down's syndrome; mother's age—37, thyroid condition, previous deformed child	b. 1/9/74; failure to warn	Unanimously upheld claim for expenses of care and support	3 upheld claim; 2 would deny claim	Claim denied—relying on precedental issue that nonexistence cannot be compared with existence with defects
Howard v. Lecher (32) NY 6/16/77 (H)	Tay-Sachs; Ashkenazi Jewish parents	b. 8/21/72; failure to warn	Medical and funeral expenses allowed but not raised on appeal	4 denied claim on grounds that parents were bystanders; 3 would award damages to mother	Child did not bring suit
Gildiner v. Thomas Jefferson Hosp. (24) PA 5/25/78 (T)	Tay-Sachs; Ashkenazi Jewish parents	b. 8/14/74; false-negative amniocentesis	Upheld claim citing policy in favor of accurate testing	Issue not raised by parents	Claim denied—damages not cognizable at law
Elliot v. Brown (19) AL 8/18/78 (H)	"Serious deformities"	Birth date unknown; failed vasectomy	Issue not raised by parents	Issue not raised by parents	Unanimously denied—impossible to measure damages, would lead to duty to abort, no proximate cause between negligence and deformity
Becker v. Schwartz (4) NY 12/27/78 (H)	Down's syndrome; mother's age—38	b. 11/3/74; failure to warn	5 upheld claim; 2 would deny claim	Unanimously denied claim for pain of rearing defective child; 2 would permit claim for stress relating to pregnancy	Unanimously denied claim—3 cited public policy, need for legislation, injury not cognizable at law, inability to measure damages; 2 claimed courts not capable to decide; 2 held they were bound by precedent

Park v. Chessin (53) NY 12/27/78 (H)	Polycystic kidney disease (autosomal recessive); previous affected child	b. 7/70; parents told no risk of recurrence	Same result as Becker v. Schwartz	Same result as Becker v. Schwartz	Same result as Becker v. Schwartz
Berman v. Allen (6) NJ 6/26/79 (H)	Down's syndrome; mother's age—38	b. 11/3/74; failure to warn	Unanimously denied; disproportionate to doctor's culpability; parents reap benefits	Unanimously upheld; 1 judge expressed broader view of damages available	6 denied claim—not cognizable at law, cannot measure damages, child's ability to love and be loved; 1 would uphold claim for impaired childhood
Speck v. Finegold (74) PA 7/25/79 (I)	Neurofibromatosis in father and 2 sibs (autosomal dominant)	b. 4/29/75; failed vasectomy and failed abortion	Unanimously allowed expense of abortion and sterilization; 5 upheld claim for care and treatment of child; 1 would offset expenses by benefit of child; 1 would deny expenses for care and treatment of child	6 denied claim; 1 would allow claim	Unanimously denied claim—injury not cognizable at law, unable to measure damages, no fundamental right to be born as a "whole, functional human being"
Curlender v. Bio-Science Laboratories (18) CA 6/11/80 (I)	Tay-Sachs; Ashkenazi Jewish parents	Birthdate unknown; false-negative Tay-Sachs carrier test on both parents 1/21/77; child diagnosed 5/10/78; Lab on notice that test [was] inaccurate	Suit pending by parents	Suit pending by parents	Unanimously upheld claim for child's physical pain and suffering during life and special pecuniary loss; would uphold punitive damages if fraud, oppression, or malice is shown

^a T = trial court, I = intermediate appellate court, H = highest state court

may arise in genetic counseling or screening. For instance, either the mother or the fetus may be injured during the process of amniocentesis, fetoscopy, or placentesis. If the physician negligently used substandard techniques, the mother's injuries, if they were at all foreseeable, are surely cognizable. Injuries to fetuses who would otherwise have been born healthy, however, are more problematic. The overwhelming trend in this country is to treat such cases as traditional personal injury actions and to compensate such mishaps only if the child is subsequently born alive (*61*).

By contrast, most jurisdictions provide no remedy if the fetus is injured so severely that it dies before birth. This seemingly inequitable distinction reflects the fact that actions for wrongful death, which are brought on behalf of the survivors, are based solely on statutes written by legislatures, while the law of personal injuries has evolved by judicial decision. The vast majority of states hold that their wrongful death statutes require either that the child be born alive (*20, 37*) or at least have become viable at the time of the negligent act (*11, 47*). Indeed, only two states suggest that negligence before fetal viability can give rise to a cause of action if the fetus dies before birth (*56, 57*). Yet when substandard prenatal diagnostic techniques clearly cause fetal loss without any significant physical injury to the mother, some courts may well read wrongful death statutes broadly in order to provide a meaningful recovery to the parents (*61*).

The Problem of False-Positive Tests

Although most genetic counseling cases involve assertions that physicians or laboratories negligently failed to detect some risk, problems also arise when counselees, in reliance on false-positives, either become sterilized or abort unaffected fetuses. In order to prevail, the patients need to show only that the incorrect results were due to negligence and that they would not have undergone the sterilization or abortion had they been correctly informed. If they can provide such proof, there are no public policy reasons why damages should not be awarded for the deprivation of their opportunity to procreate.

Plaintiffs in cases involving false-positives do face one peculiar procedural problem that may, in some instances, bar their claims. Every state has defined certain periods of time, which usually begin immediately after the alleged wrongful act, during which claimants must file suit. Failure to file within this period means that the claim is lost. The major purpose of these statutes of limitation is to enable defendants to put together their defenses while evidence is still relatively available. The limitation periods, however, cause problems in medical malpractice because many tortious acts—here, the negligent diagnoses—may not be discovered until some time after they occur.

In response, many state legislatures (*51*) and courts (*26, 29*) have said that these periods will not begin to run until the claimants know or should have known of the wrongful acts. These "discovery rules," of course, give greater protection to patients. However, courts may differ in deciding when patients should have known about mistaken diagnoses of genetic risks (*54*).

Conscientious Objections to Provide Reproductive Alternatives

Some physicians refuse to provide prenatal diagnosis or even genetic screening. The legal implications of these refusals turn largely on the physicians' reasons. For instance, in suits involving the birth of a defective child, a physician might argue in defense that because genetic counseling may result in preventing the birth of some children, requiring him/her to give information about genetic risks would contravene his/her religious objections to the use of contraception or abortion (*39*). Federal law protects the conscientiously objecting physician's right to refuse to provide either contraception or abortion (*13*). This right, however, should not be expanded to protect physicians's refusals to alert patients about possible genetic risks. First, prospective parents have few other ways to learn about their risks. By contrast, people who desire contraception or abortion for purposes of family planning need not be educated by all physicians because they know of their need to seek those who will provide the desired services. In addition, the burden placed on the physician's religious beliefs is relatively slight. They need not provide the genetic counseling themselves. Rather, a physician must simply exercise reasonable care in detecting indications of genetic risk, such as a positive family history, advanced maternal age, or various ethnic backgrounds, among his/her patients and, when indicated, refer them elsewhere for further diagnosis and counseling (*46, 52*).

Failure to Provide Services in Low-Risk Pregnancies

When a defective child is born after an objectively low-risk pregnancy, such as the birth of a child with Down's syndrome to a woman in her twenties, the physician may argue that prenatal diagnosis was not offered because the dangers of the procedures were higher than the risk of defect. Although the birth of a defective child is compensable in other circumstances, the physician would probably prevail on such a defense, largely because it currently is not standard practice to offer prenatal diagnosis in low-risk pregnancies. This is particularly true when the diagnostic techniques entail substantial danger to the mother or fetus, such as fetoscopy. In order to avoid liability in the future, however, genetic clinics should develop guidelines for deciding who will receive services and apply them uniformly. In addition, individual practitioners should keep records of their reasons for deciding not to offer genetic tests or refusing to perform prenatal diagnosis (*79*).

Refusal to Provide Sex Selection

Many physicians refuse to perform amniocenteses solely for the purpose of sex selection because they believe that such a goal is inappropriate. Although parents may sue when such refusals lead to the birth of children of the unwanted sex, their claims should fail for several reasons. First, prenatal diagnosis for sex selection is not required by the standard of care of reasonable practitioners. Second, if objective proximate causation is required, the judge or jury might find that "reasonable" prospective parents would not abort a fetus simply because it is the "wrong" sex. Third, the parents would find it virtually impossible to prove that they had suffered an injury by having a child of the undesired sex. Finally, even if these were overcome, awarding damages in such a case would contravene the overriding national policy of eliminating sex discrimination. Even though there is, therefore, little chance that liability will be imposed for refusing to provide prenatal diagnosis in this situation, the prospective parents should at least be given counseling or referred to another facility that will provide the testing (*79*).

Whether or not sex selection is an undesirable societal goal, at least one author has argued that since the US Supreme Court has ruled the pregnant women have the freedom of choice to abort for any reason during the first trimester, sex choice is the prerogative of the parents (22, 62). In addition, when fetal sex can be determined by analysis of fetal cells in the mother's bloodstream or when separation of X and Y sperm becomes a feasible mechanism for determining sex at conception, other ethical and legal arguments will apply, which might ultimately invalidate many attempts to prevent sex selection.

Breach of Confidentiality in Family Studies

Issues of confidentiality may also arise in genetic counseling. For instance, a physician may wish to contact a patient's relatives either to obtain further information regarding the patient's genetic risk or to warn the relatives that they may be carriers of some deleterious genetic trait. Although counselees usually agree to such communication, some people for any number of reasons will not want their family members to know about the possible risks. If a physician talks with the relatives of an unconsenting patient anyway, the patient may bring suit for invasion of privacy, alleging that he/she reasonably believed that the private information disclosed or lab tests revealed in the counseling process would be held confidential. Particularly since physicians are generally bound by the AMA code of medical ethics and statutes to keep patients' confidences (76), such claims in many instances may be upheld.

Yet in the name of moral obligation and the public interest, the courts have excused breaches of confidentiality when such actions avert the risk of serious harm to third persons. For example, some states hold that psychotherapists must use reasonable care in determining which of their patients are likely to be violent to third parties and either warn the potential victims, if known, or take steps to detain the patient (41, 44, 75). Other courts encourage or even require the revelation of confidences when that is the only way to prevent the spread of highly infectious diseases (70). Similar analyses classically are used to uphold statutes requiring physicians to report the names and addresses of persons with certain contagious diseases (50).

In light of such precedents, a physician may have a right to make unconsented disclosures when the relatives do not otherwise know that they have a substantial risk of bearing a child with a major genetic defect. For instance, contact may be justifiable when a patient has a chromosome translocation or when there are sisters or other female relatives who may carry an X-linked gene for a very burdensome disease, such as Lesch–Nyhan syndrome, Duchenne's muscular dystrophy, or hemophilia A. It could even be argued from the psychiatric and infectious disease case that a physician has a duty to breach patient confidence if a third party is endangered by not being warned and the psychiatric and infectious disease cases that a physician has a duty to breach court's view on whether, in any given situation, the relatives' genetic risks are substantial enough to warrant disclosure against the counselee's wishes. As a result, the safer course of action is to establish criteria for deciding when relatives should be sought out and to tell all patients about these guidelines at the beginning of the counseling process. So long as any subsequent disclosures and inquiries are narrow and made with due care, there can be no liability because the initial warning will dispel any expectation of privacy that the counselee might have had (*10, 79*).

Artificial Insemination by Donor (AID) and in Vitro Fertilization (IVF)

Artificial insemination by donor, although predominantly used in cases of male infertility, is an important option for avoiding genetic risks. Some indications for its use include 1) the actual or suspected presence of a deleterious autosomal dominant gene, 2) a chrom[o]somal rearrangement in the prospective father, or 3) the existence of the same recessive gene in both prospective parents. This alternative is especially valuable when either the feared defect is not detectable in utero or the counselees are opposed to selective abortion.

Since the techniques involved in AID are relatively risk-free, the risk of liability realistically arises only when the physician does not adequately screen semen donors. The standard of care generally exercised in selecting sperm donors has been notoriously lax. Although this situation is improving slowly even for use of AID for infertility, "nonselection" of donors should be inexcusable in the context of genetic counseling no matter what other physicians normally do. Thus there may well be a duty to take genealogic histories of donors. Indeed, special attention is warranted when the risk to be avoided is a recessive trait carried by the prospective mother. If a heterozygote test is available, it should be done on the male donor. Moreover, in case the child who is born should need genetic counseling in the future, a physician should keep the donor's genealogic history and perhaps even provide the prospective parents with a copy from which the donor's name has been deleted.

In vitro fertilization may also be used to avoid genetic risks (67). Implanting into the wife an ovum from a donor that has been fertilized by the husband's sperm may become a reproductive option when the wife has a chromosome rearrangement, autosomal or X-linked dominant trait, or carries an X-linked recessive trait. In addition, IVF may be used in conjunction with a surrogate mother if a hysterectomy has been performed. Also women who cannot ovulate, such as those with Turner's syndrome, may wish to opt for an egg donor and IVF if they can be hormonally prepared for pregnancy.

The use of IVF, however, may entail numerous legal problems. On a general level, there are many questions about the extent to which it can be regulated or even prohibited by state and federal agencies (21). These issues, however, are beyond the scope of this discussion. Nevertheless, if the technology becomes readily available, then the law of informed consent would require that prospective parents be told that long-term effects of IVF on the conceptus are unknown. Physicians should also screen ovum donors for genetic risks and should keep the donor's genealogic history. Surrogate mothers should be examined for previous problems with pregnancy, possible Rh incompatibility, and the use of drugs, alcohol, tobacco, and even caffeinated beverages (64). Moreover, once the woman has become pregnant, the physician should offer the full array of prenatal diagnostic techniques.

A doctor who negligently performed an IVF could be liable for a wide variety of damages. Any women's physical injuries suffered in the course of negligently performed ova retrieval or conceptus implantation would almost surely be compensable. Although damages probably will not be available if an IVF conceptus does not survive until birth, parents will be able to state a cause of action if children are born defective as a result of physician negligence.

The cognizability of the claims of such children who are born alive, however, will turn on the nature of the physician's tortious acts. Defects caused by mishandling of an ovum or a conceptus are analytically very similar to prototypical prenatal injuries since the child at least theoretically could have been born healthy. Hence, the child's claim would probably be compensable. By contrast, a defective child's assertion that the disorders were the result of inappropriate choice of ova or sperm that carried a deleterious trait is more like a cause of action for wrongful life since that child could not have been born without defects. Thus, the child's cause of action might well be dismissed in most states (*16, 21*).

Future Trends

The Impact of Abortion Laws

The state of the law regarding abortion has had a substantial impact on genetic counseling. In general, the Supreme Court has held that some right of access to abortion is protected by the Constitution. This is reflected in the decisions in which the Court struck down various restrictions that were passed by state legislatures not to promote the health of pregnant women but rather solely to make it more difficult to obtain abortions (*5, 55*). By contrast, in the most recent of a series of decisions regarding the rights of indigent women to federally or state-funded abortions (*3, 42*), the Court upheld the Hyde Amendment, which drastically restricts the availability of federal funding for these procedures (*27, 78*). The Hyde Amendment does not permit the use of such money even for selective abortion of defective fetuses, a fact that was not addressed by the Court (*33*). Although the Court's votes on decisions in this area have frequently been close, it is unlikely that its position on either the basic right of access or federal or state funding will change unless a right-to-life amendment to the Constitution is passed or unless there is a change in the composition of the Court. Of these two possible sources of change, it is the authors' view that the latter is far more likely.

Neither the Hyde Amendment nor the Court's decisions prohibit the states from using their own resources to provide abortions either to all indigent women or only to those women who are at genetic risk. Currently, however, most states have chosen not to provide these services. Moreover, in this time of fiscal conservatism and the strengthening of the right-to-life movement, it is probable that more and more states will refuse to fund abortions. Thus, selective abortion essentially is not an option for indigent women unless physicians or hospitals simply choose to absorb the costs of second-trimester abortions themselves or unless private funding is available. The post-Roe court decisions have been silent on abortion for genetic indications.

Self-Determination in Reproductive Decisions

In contrast to the pressure to limit or eliminate reproductive options, there is a general tendency to increase both the involvement of and the range of choices available to patients in their own medical care. This is reflected first in the emerging requirement that physicians' disclosures of risks and alternative treatments be measured against the informational needs of patients, not the practice of other physicians (*9, 14, 77*). Moreover, the law is giving greater protection to the rights of patients in some circumstances at least to refuse treatment. For example, adult Jehovah's Witnesses who do not have dependent children may refuse blood transfusions (*34*) and, in many instances, terminally ill patients may reject extraordinary medical care (*63*).

Those developments will doubtless cause significant changes in the traditional physician–patient relationships. In addition, the risk of liability may grow. A physician's omissions may increasingly be viewed as negligence if the law requires them not only to transmit genetic information but also to ensure that patients understand the information sufficiently to make informed reproductive decisions. Moreover, the requirements of proximate causation may become easier for plaintiffs to meet if the law recognizes that a subjective patient standard is necessary in order to protect parents' rights to choose.

There are, however, limits on the foreseeable expansion of the patient's role. The law does recognize a person's right in some cases to refuse extraordinary treatment in favor of maintenance care (*63*). Yet so long as treatment conforms to the appropriate standard of care, it is unlikely that the physician will be required against his/her will to provide a different course of medical care solely in response to a patient's demand. For example, a physician probably will not be forced to provide prenatal diagnosis to a young woman who has an empirically unfounded fear of chromosome anomalies, even though counseling should be provided. Indeed, the courts will be especially reluctant to impose affirmative duties on the physician in excess of the standard of the care triggered by their patients commands simply because the result of such procedures, on occasion, is abortion. Thus societal pressures against abortion may well limit the future growth of patient participation in genetic counseling (52).

If the decision whether or not to carry a knowingly defective child to term is left entirely with the parents, they may find themselves with a legal obligation of responsible parenthood that they heretofore have not had to face. In a 1960 decision by the Supreme Court of New Jersey the Court noted: "Justice requires that the principle be recognized that a child has a legal right to begin life with a sound mind and body" (73). This concept was carried even further in a comment made in a recent decision by an appellate court in California (18):

> If a case arose where . . . parents made a conscious choice to proceed with a pregnancy, with full knowledge that a seriously impaired infant would be born . . . we see no sound public policy which should protect those parents from being answerable for the pain, suffering and misery which they have wrought upon their offspring

Surely, if physicians can be liable for the birth of genetically defective children then it would seem reasonable to assume that once they have discharged their duties of disclosure of risks, diagnosis, and counseling, the burden would shift to the parents (23).

Conclusion

The physician who delivers good medical care in genetic counseling and screening need have little fear of legal liability. However, standard operating procedures frequently leave much to be desired. At the very least, clinicians who work with prospective parents should pursue continuing education courses in genetics, take genealogic histories of their patients, and offer heterozygote screening and prenatal testing so that they will be able to detect genetic risks. In addition, all physicians should know the location of the nearest genetic counseling center if they are unable or unwilling to provide the appropriate counseling themselves.

Financial support from the Institute for the Interprofessional Study of Health Law, an affiliation of The University of Houston Law School and The University of Texas Health Science Center at Houston, is greatly appreciated.

References

1. Anonymous v. Physician, 6 Fam L Rep 2565 (Conn. Supr. Ct. 1980)
2. Baldor v. Rogers, 81 So. 2d 658 (Fla. 1955)
3. Beal v. Doe, 432 U.S. 438 (1977)
4. Becker v. Schwartz, 46 N.Y. 2d 401, 386 N.E. 2d 807, 413 N.Y.S. 2d 895 (1978)
5. Bellotti v. Baird, 433 U.S. 622 (1979)
6. Berman v. Allen, 80 N.H. 421, 404 A. 2d 8 (1979)
7. BOTSTEIN D, WHITE RL, SKOLNICK M, DAVIS RW: Construction of a genetic linkage map in man using restriction fragment length polymorphisms. Am J Hum Genet 32:314, 1980
8. BROCK DJH, SCRIMGEOUR JB, NELSON MM: Amniotic fluid alpha-fetoprotein measurements in the early prenatal diagnosis of central nervous system disorders. Clin Genet 7:163, 1975
9. Canterbury v. Spence, 464 F. 2d 772 (D.C. Dir.) *cert. denied,* 409 U.S. 1064 (1972)
10. CAPRON AM: Tort liability in genetic counseling. Columbia Law Rev 79:618, 1979
11. Chrisaforgeorgis v. Brandenberg, 55 Ill. 2d 368, 304 N.E. 2d 88 (1973)
12. CHUBB JW, PILOWSKY PM, SPRINGELL HG, POLLARD AC: Acetylcholinesterase in human amniotic fluid: An index of fetal neural development? Lancet 1:688, 1979
13. Church Amendment, 42 U.S.C. §300a-7 (1977)
14. Cobbs v. Grant, 8 Cal. 3d 229, 502 P. 2d 1, 104 Cal Rptr 505 (1972)
15. COHEN ME: Park v. Chessin: The judicial development of the theory of wrongful life. Am J Law Med 4:211, 1978
16. Comment: Lawmaking and science: A practical look at in vitro fertilization and embryo transfer. Det Coll Law Rev 1979:429
17. Cox V. Stretton, 77 Misc. 2d 155, 352 N.Y. 2d 834 (Sup. Ct. 1974)
18. Curlender v. Bio-Science Laboratories, 165 Cal Rptr 477 (Cal. App. 1980)
19. Elliot v. Brown, 361 So. 2d 546 (Ala. 1978)
20. Endresz v. Friedberg, 24 N.Y. 2d 478, 248 N.E. 2d 901, 301 N.Y. S. 2d 65 (1969)
21. FLANNERY DM, WEISMAN CD, LIPSETT CR, BRAVERMAN AN: Test tube babies: legal issues raised by *in vitro* fertilization. Geo Law J 67:1295, 1979

22. FLETCHER JC: Ethics and amniocentesis for fetal sex identification. Hastings Center Rep 10:15, 1980
23. FLETCHER JF: Knowledge, risk and the right to reproduce. In Milunsky A, Annas GJ (eds): Genetics and The Law II. New York, Plenum Press, 1980
24. Gildiner v. Thomas Jefferson Univ. Hosp., 451 F. Supp. 692 (E.D. Pa. 1978)
25. Gleitman v. Cosgrove, 49 N.J. 22, 227 A. 2d 689 (1967), modified, Berman v. Allan, 80 N.J. 421, 404, A. 2d 8 (1979)
26. Hackworth v. Hart, 474 S.W. 2d 377 (Ky. 1971)
27. Harris v. McRae, 100 S.Ct. 2671 (1980)
28. Hawkins v. McGee, 84 N.H. 114, 146 A. 641 (1929)
29. Hays v. Hall, 488 S.W. 2d 412 (Tex. 1972)
30. Helling v. Carey, 83 Wash. 2d 514, 519 P. 2d 981 (1974)
31. Hood v. Phillips, 537 S.W. 2d 291 (Tex. 1976)
32. Howard v. Lecher, 42 N.Y. 2d 109, 366 N.E. 2d 64, 397 N.Y.S. 2d 363 (1977)
33. Hyde Amendment, Pub. L. No. 96–213, 93 Stat. 926 (Version effective in 1980)
34. In re Brooks Estate, 32 Ill. 2d 361, 205 N.E. 2d 435 (1965)
35. Jacobs v. Theimer, 519 S.W. 2d 846 (Tex. 1975)
36. Johnson v. Yeshiva Univ. 53 App. Div. 2d 523, 384 N.Y.S. 2d 455 (1976) (mem.), *aff'd on other grounds,* 42 N.Y. 2d 818, 364 N.E. 2d 1340, 396 N.Y.S. 2d 647 (1977)
37. Justus v. Atchison, 19 Cal. 3d 564, 565 P. 2d 122, 139 Cal Rptr 97 (1977)
38. KAN Y, DOZY A: Antenatal diagnosis of sickle-cell anemia by DNA analysis of amniotic-fluid cells. Lancet 2:910, 1978
39. Karlsons v. Guerinot, 57 App. Div. 2d 73, 394 N.Y.S. 2d 933 (1977)
40. KATZ J: Informed consent—a fairy tale? Law's vision. Univ Pitt Law Rev 39:137, 1977
41. Lipari v. Sears, Roebuck & Co., 49 U.S.L.W. 2120 (D.C. Neb. 1980)
42. Maher v. Roe, 432 U.S. 464 (1977)
43. Manion v. Tweedy, 257 Minn. 59, 100 N.W. 2d 124 (1959)
44. McIntosh v. Milano, 168 N.J. Super. 466, 403 A. 2d 500 (1979)
45. MEDICAL RESEARCH COUNCIL: Prenatal diagnosis of genetic disease in Canada: Report of a collaborative study. Can Med Assoc J 115:739, 1976
46. MILUNSKY A, REILLY P: The "new" genetics: Emerging medicolegal issues in prenatal diagnosis of hereditary disorders. Am J Law Med: 1:71, 1975
47. Mone v. Greyhound Lines, Inc., 368 Mass. 354 331 N.E. 2d 916 (1975)

48. Naccarato v. Grob, 384 Mich. 248, 180 N.W. 2d 788 (1970)
49. NICHD AMNIOCENTESIS REGISTRY: The safety and accuracy of mid-trimester of pregnancy. DHEW Publ. No. (NIH) 78–190 (1978)
50. N.J. Stat. Ann. 26:4–15 (1979)
51. N.Y. Civ. Prac. Law § 244–a (McKinney 1979)
52. Note: Father and mother know best: Defining the liability of physicians for inadequate genetic counseling. Yale Law J 87:1488, 1978
53. Park v. Chessin, 88 Misc. 2d 222. 387 N.Y.S. 2d 204 (Sup. Ct. 1976) *modified*, 60 App. Div. 2d 80, 400 N.Y.S. 2d 110 (1977), *Modified sub nom.* Becker v. Schwartz, 46 N.Y. 2d 401, 386 N.E. 2d 807, 413 N.Y.S. 2d 895 (1978)
54. Pearson v. Boines, 386 A. 2d 651 (Del. 1978)
55. Planned Parenthood of Missouri v. Danforth, 428 U.S. 52 (1976)
56. Porter v. Lassiter, 91 Ga. App. 712, 87 S.E. 2d 100 (1955)
57. Presley v. Newport Hosp., 117 R.I. 177, 365 A. 2d 748 (1976)
58. PROSSER WL: Handbook on the Law of Torts, 4th ed. St. Paul, Minn: West Publishing Co., 1971, § 36, pp. 190–204 (negligence per se); § 42, pp. 244–250 (proximate cause)
59. Report to the Medical Research Council by their working party on amniocentesis: An assessment of the hazards of amniocentesis. Br J Obstet Gynaec, vol 85, suppl 2, 1978
60. Robbins v. Footer, 553 F. 2d 123 (D.C. Cir. 1977)
61. ROBERTSON HB: Toward rational boundaries of tort liability for injury to the unborn: Prenatal injuries, preconception injuries and wrongful life. Duke Law J 1978:1401 (1978)
62. Roe v. Wade, 410 U.S. 113 (1973)
63. Satz v. Perlmutter, 379 So. 2d 359 (Fla. 1980)
64. SCHWARZ RH, YAFFE SJ (EDS): Drugs and chemical risks to the fetus and newborn. Prog Chem Biol Res, vol 36, 1980
65. Shaheen v. Knight, 11 D.&C. 41 (Lycoming Cty, Pa. C.P. 1957)
66. SHAW MW: Review of published studies of genetic counseling: a critique. In Lubs HA, DeLa Cruz F (eds): Genetic Counseling, New York, Raven Press, 1977
67. SHAW, MW: In vitro fertilization: For married couples only? Hastings Center Rep 10:4, 1980
68. Shilkret v. Annapolis Emergency Hosp. Ass'n, 276 Md. 187, 349 A. 2d 245 (1975)
69. Siirila v. Varrios, 58 Mich. App. 721, 228 N.W. 2d 801 (1975), *aff'd on other grounds*, 398 Mich. 576, 248 N.W. 2d 171 (1976)
70. Simonsen v. Swenson, 104 Neb. 224, 177 N.W. 831 (1920) (per curiam)
71. Sindell v. Abbott Laboratories, 607 P. 2d 524, 163 Cal Rptr 132 (Sup. Ct. 1980)

72. SMITH AD, WALD NJ, CICKLE HS, STIRRAT GM, BOBROW M, LAGERCRANTZ H: Amniotic-fluid acetylcholinesterase as a possible diagnostic test for neural-tube defects in early pregnancy. Lancet 1:685, 1979
73. Smith v. Brennan, 157 A. 2d 497 (N.J., 1960)
74. Speck v. Finegold, 408 A. 2d 496 (Pa. Super. 1979)
75. Tarasoff v. Regents of the Univ. of Cal., 17 Cal. 3d 425, 551 P. 2d 334, 131 Cal Rptr 14 (1976)
76. WALTZ JR, INBAU FE: Medical Jurisprudence. New York: MacMillan, 1971, pp 17–28, 234–53, 274–75
77. Wilkinson v. Vesey, 110 R.I. 606, 295 A. 2d 676 (1972)
78. Williams v. Zbaraz, 100 S. Ct. 2694 (1980)
79. WRIGHT EE: The legal implications of refusing to provide prenatal diagnosis in low-risk pregnancies or solely for sex selection. Am J Med Genet 5:391, 1980
80. Zoterell v. Repp, 187 Mich. 319, 153 N.W. 692 (1915)

Discussion[1]

Q: At what time in the pregnancy is the fetus considered viable?

DR. SHAW: The specific day in gestation has not been decided. A footnote in Roe v Wade (62) says the period of viability is generally recognized as the time between 24 and 28 weeks of gestation, but that the time must be left up to the discretion of the physician. You might recall the case where after a vasectomy and an abortion, the issues revolved around that particular point. Was the fetus viable at the time of the abortion, or was it not? There, just as in anything that must be proved in medicine, you have expert witnesses who will testify in one direction or another.

Q: To what extent are persons other than the physician responsible for errors?

DR. SHAW: As I said before, anyone can be sued for negligence, not just licensed physicians but any health-care provider at any level, including the registrar at the hospital or the information person who leads the person in the wrong direction. The negligence is determined by the reasonable, prudent information that would be given by a genetic counselor in the same situation as the one under question. In other words, the actions an M.A. or a Ph.D. genetic counselor would be compared with the level of

---

[1] This question-and-answer session followed Dr. Shaw's presentation in Monterey.

competence of others with the same degree and level of competence and skill. So, one is always compared with one's peers in determining whether the duty was kept or whether negligence occurred.

Q: If a couple seeking counseling is told that their expected child is most apt to be born defective and then decide they are willing to have the baby and the baby is born deformed, there is no reason for suit?

Dr. Shaw: That is correct.

Q: Recently a suit was brought in Washington, DC, against a hospital that did not have a CAT scanner available and the patient, who had been in a traumatic accident, developed severe brain defects as a result. Could also a hospital be sued for not providing genetic testing if the family was unable to go to a medical center for such testing or could not afford it or, for some reason, was not able to go elsewhere? Would a hospital be liable for not having that service available?

Dr. Shaw: Hospitals and physicians are not required to offer all to all, everything to everybody. The hospital must make decisions as to whether, for example, it will have an emergency room or not. If an emergency room is available, the hospital is then required to take in any and all people who come to the emergency room—at least for the emergency part of the treatment, not for continuing treatment.

Obviously, unique genetic services may sometimes be found in only one laboratory in the country and it may not be feasible to send the patient there. Reasonableness is the standard. If a hospital has, say, 3000 births a year, is a large city hospital, and is taking care of many pregnancies in the year, and if a significant percentage of those births is to older mothers, the hospital then has a duty to have some services to provide to those older mothers. Different alternatives are available: amniotic fluid can be withdrawn and mailed or taken to another place for testing; the hospital can set up its own testing center; or it may send the patient to another center where the test is done. The hospital should provide care consistent with its population of patients. In general, no one is required to offer services, and hospitals and physicians should know where the closest reference places are.

Q: Because there is a great deal of controversy, would you please define what constitutes informed consent?

DR. SHAW: Informed consent is the requirement that the courts have made in medical settings for the health-care provider to disclose to the patient or to the prospective counselee the risks possible in any procedure. This can involve a diagnostic procedure, or a treatment, or risks of side effects of drugs that would be necessary for the patient to be able to weigh in making a decision whether or not to undergo the diagnostic procedure, whether or not to undergo the treatment, or whether or not to swallow the drugs. These disclosures must be made. In addition, alternatives to the recommended procedure must be disclosed to the patient so that the patient can make an informed decision. This is particularly important in genetics, in which there are a number of reproductive alternatives: practicing contraception; deciding never to have children and adopting children, or never to have children and not adopting children; using artificial insemination; deciding to go ahead and have a pregnancy and have it tested before term by amniocentesis; or refusing all other options and having the baby. The courts, in general, have held physicians to the standard of disclosure that other physicians make. But this is rapidly changing; about 13 states now require physicians to make disclosures that patients would want to know, whether or not other physicians disclose them. This is called the patient's standard of disclosure rather than the physician's.

Cytogenetic Abnormalities Related to Mental Retardation

Park S. Gerald

The importance of cytogenetic abnormalities in the etiology of mental retardation is manifested by the fact that the first cytogenetic disorder demonstrated in humans was the presence of trisomy 21 in Down's syndrome (1). Since that time, the abnormalities found to be associated with mental retardation have become so numerous as to make even listing them lengthy. For that reason, I will focus primarily on some recent discoveries that appear to demonstrate new categories of cytogenetic abnormalities related to mental retardation.

First, however, let me present a brief overview of the frequency of cytogenetic abnormalities in general. The earliest time of life at which cytogenetic abnormalities could appear would be during gametogenesis. As yet, there are no data available for this period, although a method for studying the cytogenetics of sperm has been developed (2). On the other hand, much information is available from the examination of abortuses. Such data indicate that more than 60% of spontaneous, first-trimester abortuses have a chromosomal abnormality (3). The majority of these are trisomies for various chromosomes. Most of these abnormalities are lost during gestation, as indicated by the frequency of abnormalities even among stillbirths and neonatal deaths (see Table 1).

The neonatal surveys performed during the early 1970s gave us firm data on the frequency with which abnormalities of chromosome numbers occur (5). The discoveries of the late '70s and the '80s are pointing our attention in new directions. Instead of concentrating on gross, numerical changes, we are becoming aware of the importance of subtle lesions, the analysis of which requires

Table 1. **The Fate of 1000 Pregnancies**[a]

Outcomes	No. of pregnancies	No. with chromosome abnormalities	
Spontaneous abortion	150	75.00	(50%)
Macerated stillbirth	5	0.59	(12%)
Nonmacerated stillbirth	5	0.19	(3.7%)
Neonatal death	10	0.56	(5.6%)
Living	830	4.22	(0.5%)
	1000	80.56	(8%)

[a] Modified from the data of Alberman and Creasy (4).

greater technical skills, an increased understanding of the structure of chromosomes, and the use of sophisticated instruments and technologies with which the cytogeneticist has often not had previous experience.

Chromosomal Fragile Sites

The first category of these newly encountered cytogenetic lesions I will discuss is the fragile site. Cytogeneticists are quite familiar with the usual variety of chromosomal breakage events, which for the most part occur randomly. The term "fragile site" is intended to describe a specific chromosomal region that breaks frequently and nonrandomly, and several such fragile sites are now recognized. In each case, the fragile site has proven to be inherited. Therefore, they are considered likely to represent alterations in the DNA, although no information on the DNA sequence of these region is yet available. Several different categories of fragile sites exist and are distinguishable largely on the basis of the conditions required for their demonstration. The conditions required for demonstration of the currently known sites and their specific locations have been summarized by Sutherland and Hinton (6) (see Table 2).

Of all the fragile sites now known, only the one on the X chromosome is definitely associated with disease (Figure 1). (It is possible, of course, that the other fragile sites, which affect autosomes, will be found to produce symptoms when homozygous.) The first description of a family affected with the fragile-X disorder was in 1969 by Dr. Herbert Lubs (7). Males from several generations of this family were affected with mental retardation and were related in the fashion expected for an X-linked

Table 2. **Fragile Sites on Human Chromosomes** (6)

Fragile site	Folate, thymidine sensitive	pH sensitive	BrdU[a] required
2q11	yes	yes	no
20q11	yes	yes	no
Xq27	yes	yes	no
10q23	yes	no	no
11q13	yes	no	no
12q13	yes	no	no
16p12	yes	no	no
10q25	no	no	yes
16q22	no	no	no

[a] BrdU, 5-bromodeoxyuridine.

disorder. Further, the mothers of several of the affected males exhibited fragility of one X chromosome in some of their cells. No additional instances of this condition were reported for seven years. This lapse of time now appears to be the consequence of the technique required for the demonstration of the fragile site. At the time of Dr. Lubs' original study, the medium used by most cytogeneticists for culturing peripheral leukocytes was medium 199. Beginning in the early 1970s, the use of more enriched media became popular in cytogenetics. In 1977, Sutherland reported in a landmark paper (8) that enriched media suppressed the appearance of the fragile site on the X chromosome. Further

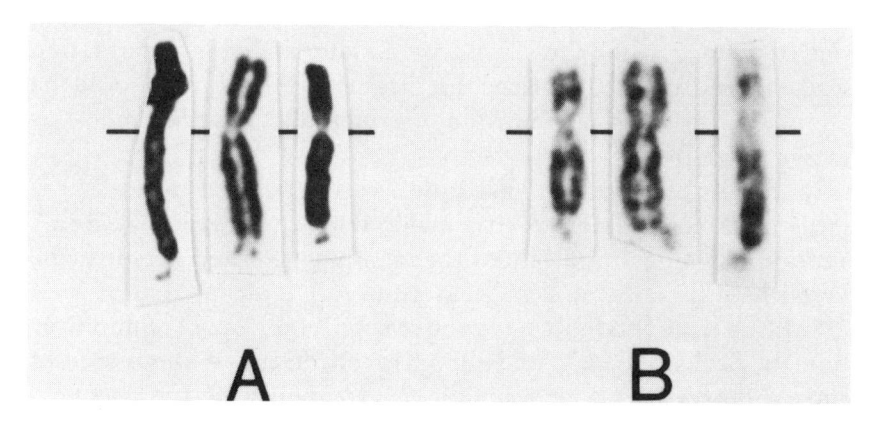

Fig. 1. The X chromosomes from six different metaphases from a male with the fragile X syndrome

The metaphases were stained with Giemsa either without (A) or with (B) prior treatment with Giemsa

studies have shown that folate and thymidine are the factors responsible for this effect (*8, 9*).

Once it became cytogenetically possible to diagnose this abnormality, numerous reports of the condition have been published and reveal that about one-third of families with X-linked mental retardation have the fragile-X abnormality. The affected males in these families have a phenotype sufficiently constant that the diagnosis could be suspected in some instances on clinical grounds alone. The clinical features I have found most useful for suggesting this diagnosis are a family history of an X-linked disorder, a normal to enlarged head circumference, prominent mandibular symphysis, and significant to marked testicular enlargement.

What proportion of mentally retarded males have the fragile-X syndrome? This point is particularly important because often there are many more males than females residing at institutions caring for the mentally retarded (*10*). In a large population survey of mentally retarded individuals, including both institutionalized and noninstitutionalized individuals, Turner and Turner (*10*) found the expected excess of males. This excess is therefore a part of the biology of mental retardation and is not simply the consequence of social factors related to institutionalization. Those same authors concluded that the male excess could very likely result from the presence of one or more X-linked diseases causing mental retardation, and estimated that the frequency of X-linked mental retardation among these males was about the same as the frequency of Down's syndrome. The available information leads to the prediction that the fragile-X syndrome should be about one-third as common among mentally retarded males as Down's syndrome.

In 203 residents of an institution caring for the mentally retarded, Sutherland found five males with the fragile X (*11*). A survey in progress at a school for mentally retarded persons (the Wrentham State School in Massachusetts) confirms that at least 2% of the male residents have the fragile X (personal communication: B. Sachs, I. Lukk, and D. Meryash). Both of these studies thus support the prediction that the frequency of the fragile X may approach one-third that of Down's syndrome among males with mental retardation.

Although the fragile-X syndrome, as initially described, is a disease of males, many investigators have noted a possibly increased frequency of mild mental retardation among female relatives of males with the fragile-X disorder. That some females who are heterozygous for this condition are significantly affected is clearly evident from the recent study of Turner et al. (*12*). A survey of females residing in special schools disclosed that five of 128 examined possessed the fragile X in some of their cells. The female relatives of these girls were also examined, and one-third of those genetically predicted to carry the abnormal X chromosome had significant mental deficit.

The factors affecting the expression of the fragile X in females are very poorly understood. Only about one-third of the female genetically obligate carriers exhibit the fragile X in their metaphases. The ability to detect the fragile site may possibly correlate with clinical expression, mentally retarded females being thought more likely to exhibit the abnormal X in their metaphases. It is tempting to assume that the variation in clinical symptomatology in the female is the result of Lyonization of the X chromosome (according to which theory only one of the two X chromosomes in every female cell is functional, the other being inactive). If the X chromosome with the fragile site were inactivated in a given cell, conceivably the cell would not be affected by whatever the fragile X does (or does not do). Examination of the inactivation process in peripheral leukocytes, however, suggests that the fragile X is randomly inactivated in carrier women (*13*). Because presumably it is the brain cells that are affected in mentally retarded individuals, I am uncertain what conclusions should be drawn from these studies of peripheral leukocytes.

The expression of the fragile X in cultured cells is an enigmatic phenomenon. Even when the folate and thymidine content of the medium is severely limited, not all of the metaphases in a peripheral blood culture from an affected male exhibit an abnormal X. Indeed, the proportion of cells with an abnormal X is rarely more than 50% and is often less than 15%. When cultured fibroblasts are used, no abnormality of the X can be detected at all, although the addition of fluorouracil to the medium may possibly facilitate the expression of the fragile site in these cells (*14*). Because of this limitation in detection, the practicality of antenatal diagnosis is still under study.

Not only do we not know why the abnormality of the X is not expressed in every metaphase, we cannot rationally explain the connection between the cytogenetic finding and the clinical symptomatology. Although I have referred to a fragile site on the X chromosome, actually most abnormal X chromosomes have only a constriction, rather than a point of breakage. The constriction is believed to produce a weak point in the chromosome structure, making it susceptible to breakage: hence its designation as a fragile site. We have no information on the molecular factors causing the constriction on the X chromosome. On the other hand, there is a small amount of experimental information concerning the fragile site on chromosome 16. Unlike the fragile site on the X, the site on chromosome 16 is independent of the medium used. About one person in several thousand exhibits this fragile site spontaneously (15), and in each case it has been inherited. By chance it was discovered that treatment with distamycin A during the culture period produces an apparently identical site on one chromosome 16 in metaphases from some individuals (16), but the individuals whose chromosome 16 responds in this fashion usually do not exhibit the fragile site spontaneously. As suggested by the confinement of the response to only one member of the chromosome 16 pair, the response to distamycin is inherited. These results support the notion that the chromosome 16 fragile site is the result of a change in the DNA. Perhaps further study of this effect will give insights applicable to the understanding of fragile sites in general.

Prader–Willi Syndrome

The newly discovered cytogenetic basis for the Prader–Willi syndrome typifies a second category of cytogenetic advancement. In childhood and adulthood this syndrome is characterized by mental retardation, neonatal hypotonia, hypogonadism, obesity, short stature, and small hands and feet. The obesity is accompanied by a voracious appetite, which is the more remarkable because, during early infancy, patients with this condition exhibit difficulty in feeding and have severe failure to thrive. So excessive are the eating habits of some patients that measures are necessary to prevent the child from stealing food or from eating food set out for the family pet! The syndrome was first described in 1956 (17) and, until recently, there was no suspicion that a cytogenetic lesion was present. The story of how this lesion was detected is representative of our new-found appreciation of the importance of (dimensionally) small cytogenetic abnormalities.

Conventional cytogenetic studies were performed on several patients with this syndrome as soon as this tool became available. A few patients, perhaps 10%, were found to have various gross chromosomal changes, but it did not at first seem likely that these chromosomal changes were causally related to the syndrome. In the first place, the occurrence of these abnormalities in only a small fraction of patients decreased the likelihood that they were relevant. Secondly, the changes were often of a type not expected to produce a gain or loss of genetic material. Only after it became apparent that rearrangements of chromosome 15 were particularly common among the reported abnormalities was attention concentrated on this chromosome. Ledbetter et al. (*18*) showed that a very small deletion could be detected in one chromosome 15 in many patients with this syndrome. Because of the small size of the deletion, it cannot be detected unless elongated chromosomes from early metaphases or late prophase cells are examined. Cytogeneticists in general are indebted to Dr. Yunis for providing the technology and for demonstrating the importance of examining such elongated chromosomes (*19, 20*).

Although the role of deletions of chromosome 15 in the etiology of the Prader–Willi syndrome is unquestionable, it is still not clear how certain rearrangements, such as the Robertsonian-type translocations found in a few patients, produce the syndrome. Robertsonian translocations are believed to affect only the short arms of the chromosomes involved. If a Robertsonian translocation can be the etiology of this syndrome, it may demonstrate that loss of genetic material from the short arm of chromosome 15 may cause the same phenotype as loss from the long arm; otherwise, we must believe that rearrangements of this type are far more complicated than we can demonstrate, even with our improved technology. The picture becomes still more complicated when it is noted (*21*) that some patients diagnosed as having Prader–Willi syndrome have a small, extra chromosome (possibly derived from chromosome 15)! One can only conclude that abnormalities of chromosome 15 appear to be present in many patients with this syndrome but that the precise relationship between the chromosomal abnormality and the clinical findings is often obscure.

What Conclusions Can We Draw?

The foregoing example demonstrates that an extra, small chromosome may cause clinical abnormalities. Yet some normal individuals have a small extra chromosome in their karyotype (22). How can we differentiate the supposedly innocent variety of small extra chromosomes from that which causes phenotypic changes? Abnormal chromosomes derived from chromosome 15 are apparently likely to cause difficulty, as supported by the growing number of reports of patients with a small extra chromosome known as an inverted duplicated 15. Such a chromosome is presumably produced by the joining together of the short arm, centromere, and proximal long-arm portion of two chromosomes 15. With only a small amount of chromosomal material present, we can not prove that it is derived from chromosome 15 by simple banding studies, even when greatly elongated chromosomes are analyzed. Fortunately, the short arm–centromeric region of this chromosome stains distinctively because of its content of 5-methylcytosine, a relatively unusual DNA base (23). Clinically, patients with this chromosomal disorder have been characterized by mental retardation and seizures (23, 24). It is probable that the length of the long-arm segment that is included determines the clinical symptomatology: one patient with minimal amounts of chromosome 15 long-arm material in the extra chromosome has a normal intellect (25).

Forthcoming Developments

These few selected examples demonstrate that cytogenetics is no longer a strictly morphologic discipline but is developing a molecular orientation. When our knowledge of the gene content of chromosomes is sufficiently complete, we should be able to predict the phenotype of a given cytogenetic abnormality. The first steps towards realizing this ultimate goal are already underway. For example, several laboratories have isolated DNA segments from the human X chromosome. Several different methods have been used, but all have depended on the use of recombinant DNA techniques. The most successful approaches have separated the X chromosome from the rest of the chromosome complement in the initial step—either by chromosome sorting with a fluorescence-activated sorter or by selecting a human–rodent hybrid cell line whose human chromosome content includes essentially only the desired chromosome. DNA is prepared from the isolated chromosome or hybrid cell line, digested with an endonuclease, and ligated into a vector that is capable of multiplying within a bacterial host. Colonies of bacteria containing the recombinant DNA are then grown from single bacterium, resulting in purification and amplification of the recombinant DNA, including the inserted human DNA segment.

In the procedures used so far, segments from a particular chromosome are randomly isolated. Consequently, it takes considerable effort to find a DNA piece derived from a specific region, such as the fragile-X site, but it is nonetheless possible. Once this has been accomplished, we will be able to study the molecular basis of the fragile-X disorder. With luck, this could be a single-gene defect whose product can be therapeutically replaced.

The chromosome-sorting approach should be particularly applicable to the analysis of the small extra chromosome. The instrument used for chromosome sorting examines the contents of a very small stream of fluid containing a dilute suspension of chromosomes. The dilution is sufficient to ensure that the individual chromosomes are well separated from one another. The stream is illuminated by a fluorescent light source, and the amount of DNA in each chromosome is measured by the intensity of the emitted fluorescence. The stream is then broken into individual droplets, which are selectively charged, and the charged droplets are deflected from the main stream by an electrical field. The presence of the charge, and hence the deflection, is determined by the fluorescent signal. The net result is that a droplet containing a chromosome with the desired DNA content can be diverted into a test tube, and quantities of that chromosome obtained with reasonable purity. If the inverted duplicated chromosome 15 can be isolated by this means, it can then be examined for its DNA content. These new and powerful techniques should provide answers to some of the questions I have presented.

This work is supported in part by a program project grant from the National Institution of Child Health Human and Development (HD-04807) and by the Mental Retardation Research Program (HD 06276).

References

1. Lejeune, J., Gantier, M., and Turpin, R., Etude des chromosomes somatiques de neuf enfants mongoliens. *Compt. Rend.* **248**, 1721–1722 (1959).
2. Rudale, E., Jacobs, P. A., and Yanagimachi, R., Direct analysis of the chromosome constitution of human spermatozoa. *Nature* **274**, 911–913 (1978).
3. Carr, C. H., and Gedeon, M., Population cytogenetics of human abortuses. In *Population Cytogenetics,* E. B. Hook and I. H. Porter, Eds., Academic Press, New York, NY, 1977, pp 1–9.
4. Alberman, E. D., and Creasy, M. R., Frequency of chromosomal abnormalities in miscarriages and perinatal deaths. *J. Med. Genet.* **14**, 313–315 (1977).
5. Hook, E. B., and Hamerton, J. L., The frequency of chromosome abnormalities detected in consecutive newborn studies—differences between studies—results by sex and by severity of phenotypic involvment. In *Population Cytogenetics* (see ref. *3*), p 353.
6. Sutherland, G. R., and Hinton, L., Heritable fragile sites on human chromosomes VI. Characterization of the fragile site at 12q, 13. *Hum. Genet.* **57**, 217–219 (1981).
7. Lubs, H. A., A marker X chromosome. *Am. J. Hum. Genet.* **21**, 231–244 (1969).
8. Sutherland, G. R., Fragile sites on human chromosomes: Demonstration of their dependence on the type of tissue culture medium. *Science* **197**, 265–266 (1977).
9. Sutherland, G. R., Heritable fragile sites on human chromosomes I. Factors affecting expression in lymphocyte culture. *Am. J. Hum. Genet.* **31**, 125–135 (1979).
10. Turner, G., and Turner, B., X-linked mental retardation. *J. Med. Genet.* **11**, 109–113 (1974).
11. Sutherland, G. R., Heritable fragile sites on human chromosomes II. Distribution, phenotypic effects, and cytogenetics. *Am. J. Hum. Genet.* **32**, 136–148 (1980).
12. Turner, G., Brookwell, R., Daniel, A., Selikowitz, M., and Zilibowitz, M., Heterozygous expression of X-linked mental retardation and X-chromosomes marker fra(X)(q27). *N. Engl. J. Med.* **303**, 662–664 (1980).
13. Jacobs, P. A., Glover, T. W., Mayer, M., Fox, P., Gerrard, J. W., Dunn, H. G., and Herbst, D. S., X-linked mental retardation: A study of 7 families. *Am. J. Med. Genet.* **7**, 471–489 (1980).
14. Glover, T. W., FUDr induction of the X chromosome fragile site:

Evidence for the mechanism of folic acid and thymidine inhibition. *Am. J. Hum. Genet.* **33**, 234–242 (1981).
15. Magenis, R. E., Hecht, F., and Lovrien, E. W., Probable localization of haptoglobin locus in man. *Science* **170**, 85–87 (1970).
16. Schmid, M., Klett, C., and Niederhofer, A., Demonstration of a heritable fragile site in human chromosome 16 with distamycin A. *Cytogenet. Cell Genet.* **28**, 87–94 (1980).
17. Prader, A., Labhart, A., and Willi, H., Ein Syndrom von Adipositas, Kleinwachs, Kryptorchismus und Oligophrenie nach Myatonieartigem Zustand im Neugeborenenalter. *Schwiez. Med. Wochenschr.* **86**, 1260–1261 (1956).
18. Ledbetter, D. H., Riccardi, V. M., Airhart, S. D., Strobel, R. J., Keenan, B. S., and Crawford, J. D., Deletions of chromosome 15 as a cause of the Prader–Willi syndrome. *N. Engl. J. Med.* **304**, 325–329 (1981).
19. Yunis, J. J., Sawyer, J. R., and Ball, D. W., The characterization of high-resolution G-banded chromosomes of man. *Chromosome* **67**, 239 (1978).
20. Yunis, J. J., and Ramsay, N., Retinoblastoma and subband deletion of chromosome 13. *Am. J. Dis. Child.* **132**, 161 (1978).
21. Wisniewski, L. P., Witt, M. R., Ginsberg-Fellner, F., Wilner, J., and Desnick, R., Prader–Willi syndrome and bisatellited derivative of chromosome 15. *Clin. Genet.* **18**, 42–47 (1980).
22. Walzer, S., and Gerald, P. S., A chromosome survey of 13,751 male newborns. In *Population Cytogenetics* (see ref. *3*).
23. Schreck, R., Berg, W. R., Erlanger, B. F., and Miller, O. J., Preferential derivation of abnormal G-like chromosome from chromosome 15. *Hum. Genet.* **36**, 1–12 (1977).
24. Wisniewski, L., Hassold, T., Heffelfinger, J., and Higgins, J. V., Cytogenetic and clinical studies in five cases of inv dup (15). *Hum. Genet.* **50**, 259–270 (1979).
25. Stetten, G., Sroka-Zaczek, B., and Corson, V. L., Prenatal detection of an accessory chromosome identified as an inversion duplication (15). *Hum. Genet.* **57**, 357–359 (1981).

Discussion

Q: Is there a connection between the phenotype that resembles acromegalia and the disorder acromegalia itself?

DR. GERALD: I do not have information on that point. Assays for hormones in these individuals have not shown abnormalities.

Tests to see if something would stimulate the testes have given no information, and biopsies of the testes do not show anything remarkable—only more tissue, with a little more fluid.

Q: What is the incidence of this disease?

DR. GERALD: Sutherland looked at 203 males in institutions for the mentally retarded, and found five, two of them brothers, to be affected, a 2–3% incidence. We looked at about 100 individuals with a family history or with increased testicular size. We found 11 cases in this group but the base population was not completely surveyed. This is 2% of the population, but we suspect it will be closer to 3% if completely studied. The data I cited from Australia indicated that the frequency of X-linked mental retardation should be about the same as that of Down's syndrome among males, which has a frequency of about 15% in institutions. Thus we should have 5% in the male population, considering that in families with X-linked mental retardation, ignoring the testicular story, about one-third have fragile X. Somewhere between 2 and 5% is the probable final figure for males who are institutionalized—not among all retarded. There are, therefore, multiple causes, X-linked in nature, for mental retardation. They produce a similar picture in that the patients do not have other malformations to suggest a different syndrome, nor do they have behavioral characteristics to suggest Lesch–Nyhan syndrome.

Q: What is the probable incidence of Down's syndrome and fragile-X disease occurring together?

DR. GERALD: Based on the number of individuals with Down's syndrome but assayed for fragile-X disease, by chance we should find it with a frequency of about 1 in 3000 patients examined. I do not think there have been 3000 examined, let alone 3000 with Down's syndrome, but we have already found two. On a statistical basis alone, this would seem to be a meaningful association, but I am not trying to assert that, because it is also true that the real common denominator is how many curiosities have you wondered about, and if you focus on just one curiosity, you are getting an incorrect assessment.

DR. GATTI: What is abnormal about the gait and speech in the fragile-X chromosome patients?

DR. GERALD: I do not have it in sufficient detail at the moment, so it is a subject to be investigated.

Dr. Gatti: Is there any possibility that they could be mistaken for an ataxia telangiectasia type of syndrome?

Dr. Gerald: I do not think so because these patients have none of the other features, and they are old enough to have shown telangiectasia of the eye and related symptoms.

II

CLINICAL DIAGNOSIS

Tay–Sachs Disease:
A Model for Genetic Disease Control

Michael M. Kaback

The control of human genetic disease is not equivalent to the control of human genes. The latter would be considered eugenics, whereas disease control is the fulfillment of what medicine always has been about. Three general strategies could be used to achieve some degree of control of any given hereditary disease: effective prevention, effective therapy, or, ideally, cure. Although the possibilities for "genetic" cures of certain disorders are foreseeable, these are not realistic considerations now and probably won't be for at least a decade. Therefore, in this discussion I will not focus on such approaches.

Because effective therapy of genetic disease is addressed by others in this conference, I will direct my comments primarily to the prevention of human genetic disease. This notion is not a new one. Passages from the oldest books of the Talmud suggest that a man not marry a woman if there are two or more generations of epilepsy in her family—perhaps the earliest written example of genetic counselling and the prevention of genetic disease through selective reproduction or selective mating. Genetic counselling of this type (leading to altered reproductive patterns or mating choices) has been the major way, historically, by which genetic disease has been prevented. But exciting and impressive technological breakthroughs in the relatively recent past, on a wide variety of scientific fronts, have brought us to a new situation where we can begin to address some additional and innovative concepts of prevention.

In concert with the dramatic recent explosion of new technology, important social and ethical changes in Western society have created an atmosphere in which such technological advances might be used for the prevention of certain genetic disorders. Considerations of family size, informed participation in health-related decision-making on the part of the public, changing attitudes toward abortion and the quality of human life—all have contributed to creating a more receptive environment for the application of many of these technological breakthroughs.

A Strategy for Prevention of Recessive Genetic Disease

If three prerequisites are met, a strategy for the prospective prevention of a recessive genetic disease might be considered. First, the disease is most amenable to control if it occurs in a defined population. Second, there must be a simple, accurate, and inexpensive way to identify carriers of the gene in question. Through screening reproductive-age individuals in the defined population for carriers of the recessive trait, one can thereby find individuals, and in turn couples, at risk for the disease before the birth of index cases. From a disease control perspective, this is important because in the great majority (about 80%) of autosomal recessive diseases—when a child is identified with such a disorder and a careful family history is taken—there is no known history of the disease in either side of the family before the index case. Waiting for the first affected child to be born in the family to identify the family as being at risk will not have much impact on the overall incidence of the disease.

The third requirement for prospective disease control is that there be an acceptable and available reproductive alternative that can be offered to those families discovered to be at risk through carrier screening. For example, if the disease can be detected in the fetus in early pregnancy through amniocentesis, then prenatal monitoring of each pregnancy in a couple found to be at risk could assure the couple of being able to have only unaffected children and, at the same time, enable them to prevent the birth of children afflicted with the disease in question. Prevention in this sense is secondary, i.e., prevention of the birth of affected children by termination of pregnancy where the fetus is found to be afflicted. For recessive disorders, the odds are 75% that each pregnancy will be unaffected. Although clearly an imperfect alternative, such an approach can provide an important option for many families: it enables them to have children who will not suffer with disease and also provides a means to prevent the birth of those who are afflicted with the disease for which they are at risk.

Tay–Sachs Disease: The Prototype

Tay–Sachs disease was the first recessive disorder to meet these criteria for prospective prevention. This autosomal recessive condition is a progressive and uniformly fatal neurodegenerative disease of infancy. It is the result of intralysosomal accumulation of the cerebral sphingolipid, GM_2 ganglioside, in neurons throughout the central nervous system. Since its original description (1, 2), it has become well established that this disorder occurs approximately 100 times more frequently in infants born of European Jewish extraction than in non-Jewish populations. This history and the fundamental clinical, pathological, and biochemical advances that contributed to our current understanding of this disorder have been reviewed recently (3).

Not until 1969 was the fundamental biochemical deficiency underlying this disease identified—a complete deficiency of the specific lysosomal acid hydrolase hexosaminidase A (Hex A). This glycoprotein specifically catalyzes the hydrolytic cleavage of the terminal N-acetylgalactosamine from GM_2 ganglioside. The inability to cleave this amino sugar moiety from the parent molecule results in the progressive accumulation of this sphingolipid. This in turn leads to lysosomal engorgement, cytoplasmic "ballooning," and ultimately neuronal cell disruption and cell loss. The development and utilization of synthetic chromogenic or fluorogenic substrates greatly facilitated the biochemical study of Tay–Sachs disease and other lysosomal storage disorders. In 1969, three groups working independently, using synthetic substrates as well as radiolabeled GM_2 ganglioside, conclusively demonstrated the absence of Hex A activity in tissues and body fluids from patients with Tay–Sachs disease (4–6).

These discoveries were followed closely by the demonstration of intermediate activities of Hex A in obligatory carriers of the Tay–Sachs disease gene—parents of infants with Tay–Sachs disease (7). With important modifications of the assay method and subsequent automation, methods were developed for applying these preliminary discoveries to screening for Tay–Sachs disease carriers in large populations (*8, 9*).

The third major criterion was satisfied with the demonstration of applicability of similar biochemical methodology to cultured amniotic fluid cells obtained by amniocentesis at 16 to 18 weeks of pregnancy (*10–12*). This provided a capability for accurate and relatively safe prenatal diagnosis of Tay–Sachs disease and thereby the critical reproductive option for at-risk families. Through prenatal monitoring of all pregnancies in at-risk couples (determined to be at risk either by the prior birth of an affected child or by virtue of both parents having been found to be carriers by heterozygote screening) such couples could be aided, if they so chose, selectively to have children without Tay–Sachs disease. Given that each pregnancy has a 75% chance of leading to an unaffected offspring, families could thus be helped (assuming they would elect to terminate those pregnancies in which the fetus was found to be affected) to achieve their family goals without the fear of giving birth to a child who would suffer and die in infancy from Tay–Sachs disease.

The complexities and methodologies of carrier detection and prenatal diagnosis have been reported elsewhere (*13, 14*). Let me point out, however, that extensive studies were carried out before the population screening to assure maximal accuracy of the screening (with serum) and backup test (with leukocytes), and the feasibility of achieving program goals.

Setting up a Genetic Screening Program

With these technical and laboratory considerations established, we then addressed the issues of mass screening in the defined population. First we elected to go into the community to find out whether the community would support such a genetic disease prevention program or not. For us to assume that we know the dynamics of a defined community is probably a great error. It is obviously important, if such a program is to be delivered on a voluntary basis, that people have some understanding of what's at stake. To screen people without first educating them creates more problems than it's going to solve. Second, to screen people without counselling those found to be positive is also going to lead to sizeable problems. If only one message has emerged from our experience with Tay–Sachs disease programs, it is that genetic screening cannot be done in a "vacuum": all three components—education, screening, and counselling—must be involved.

After developing the methodology, we needed to have support from the medical community and from the religious community, because ethical, moral, and social questions as well as reproductive ones are addressed by this kind of an approach. Human reproduction in our society is heavily imbued with issues of ethics and morality. In every area where Tay–Sachs disease programs have emerged, the rabbinate have been enthusiastic in their support and have participated actively in bringing these programs to their communities. They consistently have supported the concept that this kind of information be available to individuals so that they can make the most informed reproductive decisions for themselves. *That is the goal:* to give individuals maximum information in making their own reproductive decisions.

In the delivery of such a program, we try to educate young, reproductive-age people. We try to do this in a number of ways, not knowing which will be the most effective: through the medical community, the religious sector, community organizations, the media, trained volunteers, and open forums in the community. Such approaches are not unique to Tay–Sachs disease programs, but should be relevant to any outreach voluntary health program. Most recently, this educational effort is beginning to make its impact in the schools. In many junior and senior high schools and in colleges, youngsters are coming to know that not just peas and frogs have genes, but also that people have genes, and sometimes these genes can create problems.

Interestingly, from our early experience, we found that it was not the physicians or religious leaders who had the major educational impact. Rather, television and other media appeared most to motivate people to come for testing. More recently, perhaps influenced by several successful litigations—the alleged result of physician omissions—doctors have been much more active in discussing carrier testing with their patients.

Impact of Tay–Sachs Disease Screening Programs

Since the initial pilot program began in Baltimore–Washington in 1970, more than 100 cities in 15 countries throughout the world have initiated Tay–Sachs disease education–screening–counselling programs. From that time through June 1981, more than 350 000

Jewish individuals have been screened voluntarily, over 14 000 carriers identified, and nearly 350 couples found to be at risk for this disease in their offspring (Table 1). None of these couples previously had had an affected child. In America alone, about one in 29 Jewish individuals tested is a carrier for the Tay–Sachs gene, a figure very close to that which was predicted earlier from disease incidence data, e.g., about one in 30.

Seventy-seven centers throughout the world have now reported experience with the prenatal diagnosis of Tay–Sachs disease (Table 2). By 1981, nearly 1000 pregnancies had been monitored for this disease. Before prenatal diagnosis was available, families who had had a child with Tay–Sachs disease, in almost every instance stopped having children. They were unwilling to risk other chil-

Table 1. **Tay–Sachs Disease: Heterozygote Screening, 1971–1981**

Country	No. tested	Carriers identified[a]	At-risk couples identified
United States	291 798	11 220	272
Canada	35 662	1 889	30
Israel	18 116	585	18
South Africa	2 225	215	4
Europe	1 799	118	4
Brazil	503	15	8
Mexico	315	13	1
Total	350 418	14 055	337

[a] Includes individuals with Tay–Sachs disease probands or known carriers in their families.

Table 2. **Prenatal Diagnosis of Tay–Sachs Disease (TSD) in 77 Worldwide Centers, 1969–1981**

	Pregnancies determined to be at risk by		
	Carrier screening	Previous child	Total
Pregnancies monitored	295	617	912
TSD fetuses identified	56	146	202
Elective abortions	51	138	189[a]
Diagnoses confirmed	45	135	180[b]
Unaffected offspring born	238[c]	470[d]	708

[a] Six identified after 26 weeks of pregnancy; abortion refused for seven; 13 infants affected as predicted.
[b] Materials unusable or unavailable for confirmation in nine cases.
[c] One child diagnosed with TSD at nine months, identified as unaffected fetus by amniocentesis.
[d] One pregnancy "spontaneously" aborted one week after amniocentesis.

dren because of the 25% recurrence rate with each pregnancy. Not only did they stop having children, but also divorce, separation, alcohol abuse, and suicide were more common in such families. Now, however, because of the availability of prenatal monitoring, there have been 617 pregnancies in that group of couples who had had one or more previous children with Tay–Sachs disease. Of these, 470 pregnancies resulted in healthy, unaffected children, as predicted by fetal testing. Almost all of these 470 children would never had been conceived or born had not this technology been available to these families.

In addition, 295 pregnancies were monitored in couples found to be at risk through screening. Fifty-six of these fetuses were identified as having Tay–Sachs disease. In almost every instance, the family elected to abort the pregnancy. In almost all instances where the pregnancy was not terminated, it was because the diagnosis was made too late in pregnancy for the option of abortion to be a legal consideration.

What, if any, has been the impact of these activities on the incidence of Tay–Sachs disease? In 1970, it was estimated that between 50 and 100 infants with Tay–Sachs disease were born each year in North America, about 80–85% of whom were of European Jewish extraction. In 1980, amongst the Jewish population of the United States and Canada, there were only 13 children newly diagnosed with Tay–Sachs disease. Perhaps a few cases might have been missed, but through our Tay–Sachs Disease Data Collection Center, it is highly likely that this is very close to the actual number. This represents between a 65 and 85% decrease in the incidence of Tay–Sachs disease in the Jewish population of North America since 1970. This may not be completely due to screening and prenatal diagnosis, but, certainly, a very substantial part of it must be.

Other Considerations in Genetic Screening Programs

A number of other critical issues must be addressed when considering voluntary carrier screening in adult populations. Such issues apply to any such program, not just to our experience with Tay–Sachs disease. Methodology must be solid. Manpower must be available. The community, if testing is to be done voluntarily, must participate at all stages—from planning to delivery. Pre-testing education and post-testing counselling are absolutely vital and cannot be minimized. Important legal issues such as protection of privacy and confidentiality must be kept in mind. There must be follow-up to assess the impact of such an effort.

The methodologies of carrier detection and prenatal diagnosis should be standardized. Interlaboratory quality control should be established, and continuing surveillance maintained. Such a program provides people with information, relevant not to themselves, but about their reproduction. There is no way of knowing immediately if testing results are right or wrong. Rather, one may have to wait many years to observe reproductive outcomes (if at all), to validate testing results. A call from a lawyer may be the first warning of inaccurate testing.

Manpower cannot be underestimated. It must be built into the system to be sure that appropriate education and counselling services are available and a predefined part of such a program. A related issue is the training and licensure of laboratory and counselling personnel. There now is an American Board of Medical Genetics, which sponsors certification examinations for individuals at various levels of medical genetic service delivery systems. There will probably be a comparable laboratory certification process in the near future as well. People involved in reproductive or genetic testing probably need to have special training to do these kinds of tests because of the unique implications of test results.

Our center has established an International Quality Control Program for Tay–Sachs disease carrier testing. We sponsor, under the auspices of the National Tay–Sachs Disease and Allied Disorders Association an annual "blinded" quality assessment of all testing centers throughout the world. In 1981, we carried out an assessment of 41 laboratories in 12 countries involved in serum screening for Tay–Sachs carriers by the heat- or pH-inactivation assay. Thirty-nine of these laboratories made no errors in diagnosis (each receiving six to 10 obligate carrier samples and an equal number of noncarriers). Labs that had difficulties were consulted with and not "certified" until 100% accuracy on blinded testing was achieved. This program now conducts both serum and leukocyte quality assessment studies annually in all testing laboratories. Community physicians and the public are encouraged to utilize only laboratories that have been so certified by the Quality Control Subcommittee of the National Tay–Sachs Disease and Allied Disorders Association.

Legal Issues in Genetic Testing

Litigations involving Tay–Sachs disease carrier identification and prenatal testing already have arisen. With regard to carrier screening, suits have been brought against physicians and laboratories for failure to recommend testing, for advice not to be tested, for mislabeling of blood samples, and for incorrect counselling derived from such errors. In each instance, litigation was initiated by the diagnosis of an affected child. Other actions have been brought against laboratories for errors in the identification of carriers or against private laboratories that had no mechanism to ensure that the test results were communicated to patients. Prenatal diagnosis also has been the basis of litigation because of laboratory errors, and because of laboratories conducting these determinations with insufficient controls so that they weren't able to interpret their data accurately.

Other Genetic Disorders

About one in 12 black Americans carries the gene for sickle cell anemia, which means that about one in 150 black couples is at risk for having children with homozygous sickle cell disease, and therefore that about one in 600 black American children are born with this serious disorder. Sickle cell disease is very different from Tay–Sachs. It does not affect the nervous system primarily; it can be compatible with a long, fruitful, and productive life; and it is much more variable in its clinical picture. But it does occur in a defined population and we certainly can identify carriers. For families that want the information, prenatal diagnosis for sickle cell anemia, although still relatively new, is an available option at this time. The recombinant DNA methods for detecting fetal sickle cell are no longer experimental methods in those centers with expertise (*15, 16*). I do not necessarily advocate prenatal diagnosis for sickle cell anemia or beta-thalassemia, but I do advocate informing people of the availability of this option so that they can make their own decisions. Such reproductive decisions should be the families', based on knowledge, rather than that of the "well-meaning physician," making such decisions for his or her patients.

The one-in-30 carrier frequency in American Jews for Tay–Sachs disease is about the same as the frequency of beta-thalassemia heterozygosity in Americans of Greek and Italian extraction. Again, one in 900 couples will be at risk, and the risk with each pregnancy is one in four, which results in a one-in-3600 birth incidence.

Other relatively "common" recessive traits occurring in defined populations in the U.S. include alpha-thalassemia in Southeast Asians and Chinese, and cystic fibrosis in Caucasian Americans. Both of these disorders occur about once in 2500 births in the respective populations, thereby indicating a carrier frequency of about one in 25 persons of such background. Carrier detection and prenatal diagnosis is available currently for sickle cell and alpha- and beta-thalassemia, but has not yet been demonstrated conclusively for cystic fibrosis. Such developments are anticipated in the near future, thereby providing the basis for potential programs of population screening and disease control similar to those with Tay–Sachs disease.

Unquestionably, such efforts are likely to expand in the future. Contingent with the practical and scientific issues raised by such programs, critical social, legal, and ethical questions similarly are involved. In one sense, prospective carrier screening and prenatal diagnosis can be seen as a "positive" approach to the control of serious genetic disease. Perhaps this is best seen as an interim strategy; awaiting the development of a simple and totally effective therapy, or even a more primary form of prevention (preconception). Ultimately, we can hope that advances in the molecular genetics of humans will provide a means of "correcting" or replacing the defective genes and thereby curing such disorders completely.

References

1. Tay, W., Symmetrical changes in the region of the yellow spot in each eye of an infant. *Trans. Opthal. Soc. UK* **1**, 55–57 (1881).
2. Sachs, B., A family form of idiocy, generally fatal, associated with early blindness. *J. Nerv. Ment. Dis.* **21**, 475–479 (1896).
3. O'Brien, J. S., The gangliosidoses. In *The Metabolic Basis of Inherited*

Disease, J. B. Stanbury, J. B. Wyngaarden, and D. S. Fredrickson, Eds., 4th ed., McGraw-Hill, New York, NY, 1978.
4. Okada, S., and O'Brien, J. S., Tay–Sachs disease: Generalised absence of a beta-D-N-acetylhexosaminidase component. *Science* **165,** 698–700 (1969).
5. Sandhoff, K., Variation of beta-N-acetylhexosaminidase pattern in Tay–Sachs disease. *FEBS Lett.* **4,** 351 (1969).
6. Kolodny, E. H., Brady, R. O., and Volk, B. W., Demonstration of an alteration of ganglioside metabolism in Tay–Sachs disease. *Biochem. Biophys. Res. Commun.* **37,** 526–531 (1969).
7. O'Brien, J. S., Okada, S., Chen, A., and Fillerup, D. L., Tay–Sachs disease: Detection of heterozygotes and homozygotes by serum hexosaminidase assay. *N. Engl. J. Med.* **283,** 15–20 (1970).
8. Kaback, M. M., Thermal fractionation of serum hexosaminidase: Applications to heterozygote detection and diagnosis of Tay–Sachs disease. *Methods Enzymol.* **28,** 862–867 (1973).
9. Lowden, J. A., Skomorowski, M. A., Henderson, F., and Kaback, M. M., The automated assay of hexosaminidases in serum. *Clin. Chem.* **19,** 1345–1349 (1973).
10. Schneck, L., Friedland, J., Valenti, C., Adachi, M., Amsterdam, D., and Volk, B. W., Prenatal diagnosis of Tay–Sachs disease. *Lancet* **i,** 582–583 (1970).
11. Navon, R., and Padeh, B., Prenatal diagnosis of Tay–Sachs genotypes. *Br. Med. J.* **iv,** 17–20 (1971).
12. O'Brien, J. S., Okada, S., Fillerup, D. L., Veat, M. L., Adornato, B., Brenner, P. H., and Leroy, J. G., Tay–Sachs disease: Prenatal diagnosis. *Science* **172,** 61–64 (1971).
13. Kaback, M. M., Zeiger, R. S., Reynolds, L. W., and Sonneborn, M., Approaches to the control and prevention of Tay–Sachs disease. *Prog. Med. Genet.* **10,** 103–134 (1974).
14. Kaback, M. M., Tay–Sachs disease: Screening and prevention. *Prog. Clin. Biol. Res.* **18** (1977).
15. Kan, Y. W., Trecartin, R. F., Golbus, M. S., and Filly, R. A., Prenatal diagnosis of β-thalassemia and sickle cell anemia. *Lancet* **i,** 269 (1977).
16. Kan, Y. W., and Dozy, A. M., Antenatal diagnosis of sickle-cell anemia by DNA analysis of amniotic fluid cells. *Lancet* **ii,** 910 (1978).

Discussion

Q: Are there screening programs for other sphingolipid-storage diseases—Niemann–Pick disease, Gaucher's disease, Krabbe's disease, and so forth?

DR. KABACK: Although there are fairly well-defined populations for several of them, the control of such diseases is not as clearcut as Tay–Sachs. The major problem is carrier detection. None of these diseases is amenable to an inexpensive, simple, and accurate method of carrier detection, thus making mass screening impractical at this time. All of them can be detected prenatally, and carrier detection (with lymphocytes or cultured skin fibroblasts) is available for close family members where such diseases have occurred.

Q: What is the role of hexosaminidase B?

DR. KABACK: Hexosaminidase B does not act on GM_2 ganglioside. Hex B will cleave the terminal N-acetylhexosamine, but only after the neuraminic acid group is first removed. The biological role of hexosaminidase B is not known at this time.

Q: Is there a theoretical advantage of carriers for Tay–Sachs, similar to the protection that sickle cell trait affords against malaria?

DR. KABACK: Some epidemiological data suggest that individuals who are heterozygotes for Tay–Sachs disease may have a selective resistance to pulmonary tuberculosis. If you reflect on the Middle Ages in Central-Eastern Europe, in the small ghetto communities where the Jews lived, epidemics of tuberculosis occurred. Hence, there may have been selective forces at that time which made it biologically advantageous to be a carrier for the Tay–Sachs gene. If so, this would have increased the likelihood of survival and reproduction, thereby enriching the next generation for this gene. Other geneticists argue that this is less likely than simply "founder effect" and genetic drift. These are associated with inbreeding within populations such that, by chance, the frequency of a gene becomes enriched over multiple generations in a relatively isolated population. So geneticists still disagree as to how to account for the high frequency of this gene in Jewish populations.

Q: What chromosome is specific for the hexosaminidases?

DR. KABACK: The hexosaminidase genes are on human chromosomes number 15 and 5. Hex A is composed of alpha and beta subunits. The gene for the alpha subunit is on chromosome number 15. Hex B is composed only of beta subunits, the gene for which is on chromosome number 5.

Q: Are there any experimental models for sphingolipid-storage diseases?

DR. KABACK: Yes. One of the most interesting is a cat colony with GM_2 gangliosidosis. The disorder is actually the equivalent of Sandhoff's disease in humans, because the cat is lacking both hexosaminidase A and B, and it accumulates GM_2 as well as other oligosaccharides. There are also animal models for several other sphingolipid storage diseases. There is a dog with GM_1 gangliosidosis, and there is a cat with a Krabbe's-disease equivalent. A number of other animal models for lysosomal storage disorders have been reported. The task is to identify them and inbreed them. Several probands have been picked up serendipitously but, unfortunately, the mother or father had been run over by a car or wasn't in a breeding colony, and the lines therefore were lost. Another important model is that of mannosidosis in cattle, which has been studied extensively in New Zealand.

DR. DIETZ: You indicated that very young children did not show symptoms of the disease. Is that because they have some enzyme from their mother, or did they initially synthesize it—which would be similar to children who, in many cases, synthesize disaccharidase?

DR. KABACK: The explanation is probably a reflection of our limited ability to assess the nervous system of very young children. The disease is already present at birth. The infants do not get hexosaminidase A from their mother. They do not have differential metabolism as fetuses or newborns. The GM_2 is there and building up in their brain cells from early in pregnancy. Either a threshold of build-up has to be reached before symptoms are evident, or we simply are not good enough to pick up the abnormality clinically.

DR. IBBOTT: Why isn't the fetus protected if the mother has hexosaminidase A?

DR. KABACK: The enzyme doesn't appear to cross the placenta.

Cancer Susceptibility as a Birth Defect

Richard A. Gatti

Certain strains of inbred mice are genetically susceptible (or resistant) to induction of leukemia with specific viruses (*1–3*). The classic example of this is the experiment in which the Gross leukemia virus is injected into animals of two strains, C3H and C57BL. After several weeks, the C3H mice begin to develop leukemia until virtually all of them die with the disease. Few of the C57BL mice, if any, develop leukemia and then only after a much longer incubation (sometimes more than one year). This susceptibility is not controlled by a single genetic locus, but one important locus, Rgv-1 (i.e., resistance to Gross virus), maps to the major histocompatibility complex (MHC)[1] on chromosome 17. Rgv-2 maps elsewhere. Other genes for susceptibility to viral-induced leukemia in mice also map to within or near the MHC, such as those for resistance to Friend and Moloney virus-induced leukemias (Figure 1). What is unclear at this writing is how these genes produce these effects and how these genotypes are translated into cancer-susceptible phenotypes.

In humans, perhaps the most convincing evidence that cancer susceptibility can be inherited is the large list on inherited disorders that are associated with an increased risk of cancer (Table 1). Analyzing these human models of cancer susceptibility has proven to be an arduous task. Cancer-affected individuals in such families usually do not differ in any apparent way from other members of the family who manifest the inherited syndrome but do not develop cancer. In some families the type of cancer varies within a certain pattern; in others it is always the same type of cancer.

---
[1] Abbreviations used: MHC, major histocompatibility complex; LOD, log odds determination; AT, ataxia-telangietasia; IGH, immunoglobulin heavy chains.

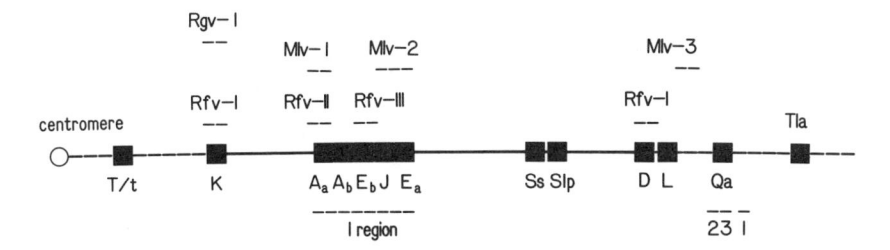

Fig. 1. Location of genes conferring resistance or susceptibility to viral-induced leukemias in mice

This genetic area is located on chromosome 17 and includes the major histocompatibility complex or H2

One can argue that some cancers in high-risk cancer families could arise from environmental causes that affect all members of that family; and in some families this argument may be valid. In other pedigrees, however, individuals who develop cancer often live in different cities or countries, in different generations, and have totally different life-styles. Further, one can argue that, although most people are exposed to those environmental factors

Table 1. **Cancer-Associated Genetic Syndromes**

	Inheritance pattern[a]
Xeroderma pigmentosum	AR
Ataxia-telangiectasia	AR
Fanconi's anemia	AR
Bloom's syndrome	AR
Werner's syndrome	AR
Basal cell nevus carcinoma syndrome	AD
Cowden's syndrome	AD
Multiple endocrine neoplasia—I, II, III	AD
Familial polyposis—I, II, III	AD
Neurofibromatosis	AD
Tuberous sclerosis	AD
Tylosis	AD
Wiskott–Aldrich syndrome	XL
Lymphoproliferative syndrome	XL
Congenital agammaglobulinemia	XL
Severe combined immunodeficiency	AR, XL
Retinoblastoma	AD

[a] AR = autosomal recessive, AD = autosomal dominant, XL = X-linked.

at one time or another, most people do not develop cancer. Thus, the concept of a genetic susceptibility to cancer must be considered seriously. Major issues that need resolution are: (*a*) to what extent does a genetic predisposition influence the incidence of cancer in the general population and in specific families, and (*b*) what are the mechanisms by which a genetic susceptibility would interact with environmental factors such as carcinogens to produce malignancy?

Identifying Cancer-Susceptible Individuals

An initial step in such analyses must be to identify and characterize cancer-susceptible individuals. Two approaches can be adopted: (*a*) test many different parameters to identify what abnormal factors or functions may influence the expression of cancers in those persons; and (*b*) characterize the genomes of these individuals as fully as possible to localize or map the area or areas that link to cancer expression in their pedigree.

One important limitation to both of these approaches is that not all cancer-susceptible individuals develop or express cancer. Expression depends on many factors, some of which are less obvious than others:

1. *Age of onset.* If a cancer-susceptible newborn dies in infancy of other causes, cancer will not have been expressed. Many families have a mean age of onset for cancer well after 50 years of age. Thus, those persons dying well before 50 from other causes will not be relevant for analysis. Another feature of this may be that an immunodeficiency that leads to cancer expression in later life also leads to overwhelming infection in some family members at a much earlier age. For example, if those individuals of former generations who died in childhood of tuberculosis were to represent the same cohort as those who are now developing cancer in old age, an increased incidence of cancer in this family would follow the introduction of effective treatment for tuberculosis after a lag-time of perhaps four or five decades.

2. *Sex.* In families where breast cancer is prevalent, it is not uncommon to see it skip a father and be expressed in his three daughters. Having mature breast tissue may be a prerequisite for attack by some carcinogen(s). Similarly, if six sons and no daughters are born to a family prone to breast cancer, it is not difficult

to appreciate why an inherited susceptibility would not be expressed in that generation.

3. *Iatrogenic effects.* (*a*) Hysterectomy was commonly performed in the United States during the 1940s and '50s. In families susceptible to uterine or cervical cancer, expression would be distorted by this treatment in family studies involving those generations. (*b*) The use of estrogens for menopausal symptoms might also affect this expression. (*c*) Long-term immunosuppressive therapy, e.g., for renal transplants, is associated with a 10- to 100-fold increase in cancer (4). This could be partly due to an unmasking of cancer-susceptibles in the general population. (*d*) Agents used in the treatment of one cancer may induce the development of a second primary in some patients; could those individuals be genetically susceptible? (*e*) Some industrial carcinogens may also be dangerous primarily to a few persons who are genetically susceptible, yet produce little or no cancer in the majority of the population. The latter situation represents an important challenge to both biologists and industry, one that could simplify the handling of certain ubiquitous carcinogens.

4. *"Homeostatic cures."* A much more difficult factor to evaluate in cancer expression is the body's ability to compensate for cancer susceptibility by using other defense mechanisms such as immunosurveillance to identify and destroy an early cancer, thereby masking the expression of a cancer-susceptibility gene. This mechanism may explain the fact that most viral-induced leukemias in mice develop under the influence of more than one gene.

Family Studies

Despite these problems with cancer expression, most of which can be handled by computerized algorithms for "incomplete penetrance," numerous cancer-associated inherited disorders and familial cancer syndromes have been identified in which the pattern of cancer is compatible with mendelian inheritance of one type or another (Table 1). Our laboratory is working primarily with families in whom the pattern of cancer expression is compatible with an autosomal dominant inheritance. This is accomplished with the assistance of a computer program called GENPED. Once such cancer families are identified, we use a panel of more than

Table 2. **Markers Analyzed**

Erythrocyte antigens:
ABO, Lewis, Rhesus, MNSs, Duffy, Lutheran, Kell, Kp, Kidd, P
Erythrocyte enzymes:
adenylate kinase 1 (AK1), 6-phosphogluconate dehydrogenase (6-PGD), adenosine deaminase (ADA), phosphoglycolate phosphatase (PGP), acid phosphatase (AcP), galactose-1-phosphate uridylyltransferase (GALT), glutamic pyruvate transaminase (GPT), esterase D (EsD), glyoxalase 1 (GLO-1), phosphoglucomutase 1 subtyping by immunoelectrophoresis (PGM-1 by IEP)
Serum proteins:
haptoglobin (Hp), vitamin D-binding protein (Gc), pseudocholinesterase (E2), amylase 2 (AMY2), properdin B factor (Bf), immunoglobulin Gm (IGH)
Leukocyte antigens:
HLA-A, HLA-B, HLA-C

30 genetic markers to characterize as much of the genome as possible (Table 2). We then attempt to see whether any part of that genome co-segregates with (i.e., is linked to) the cancer expression in that family.

Family Pi (Figure 2) demonstrates this type of approach and has yielded evidence compatible with the hypothesis of a possible cancer-susceptibility gene in or near the MHC area on the short arm of chromosome 6 (5), the area homologous with the mouse MHC on chromosome 17 (Figure 1).

Family Pi can be described either as a cancer-syndrome family in which several different kinds of cancer are manifested—in this family they included primarily breast, endometrial, and gastrointestinal cancers—or as a breast-cancer family, breast cancer having been seen in two sisters and their first-degree relatives. As indicated in Figure 2, half of the members of generation II and III had cancer. Ovarian cancer has not been observed in this family, nor have brain tumors. One member had multiple myeloma. The age of onset of cancer is interesting in that no one younger than 46 years of age has developed cancer, despite the high incidence of cancer in the two oldest living generations and the extensive size of the two younger generations. The family is Jewish, originating from Eastern Europe. All members of the second generation lived most of their adult lives in the United States. The bulk of the family's remaining generations have resided in California.

HLA marker studies clearly delineated four ancestral haplotypes, A26 B39 and A28 B14 in one spouse and A2 B38 and A3 B39 in the other; each of these haplotypes was observed in

FAMILY P

□ Male
II' Spouses of II generation
■ Deceased

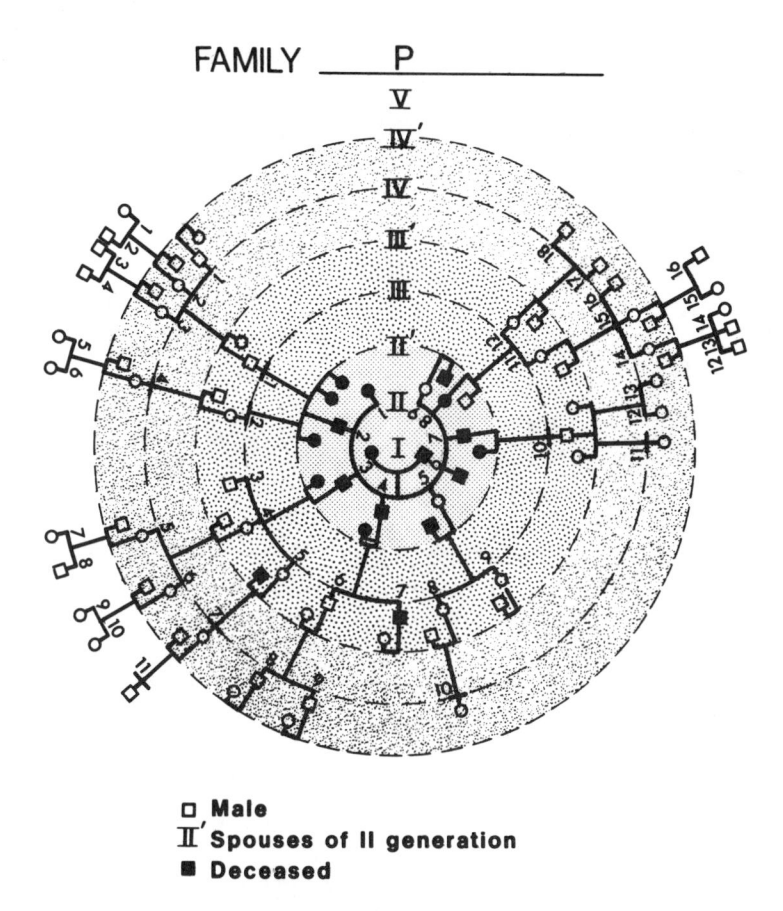

Fig. 2. Pedigree of Family Pi, a high-risk cancer family
II', spouses of generation II; *filled* (*black*) shapes indicate deceased

at least three family members. The segregation of these haplotypes could also be followed by the Bf and GLO-1 markers. HLA-C typing was not generally informative. We observed that the A3 B39 haplotype (Figure 3) was absent from the two branches of the family that are free of cancer. Of the eight affected members who could be genotyped for HLA, seven shared the same "3-39" haplotype. The one discordant member (i.e., she had cancer but did not have this haplotype) could have inherited a recombinant chromosome carrying a cancer-susceptibility gene located to either side of the HLA-A or -B loci—this is possible because her father had the "3-39" haplotype—but the data for GLO-1

HIGH-RISK CANCER FAMILY Pi

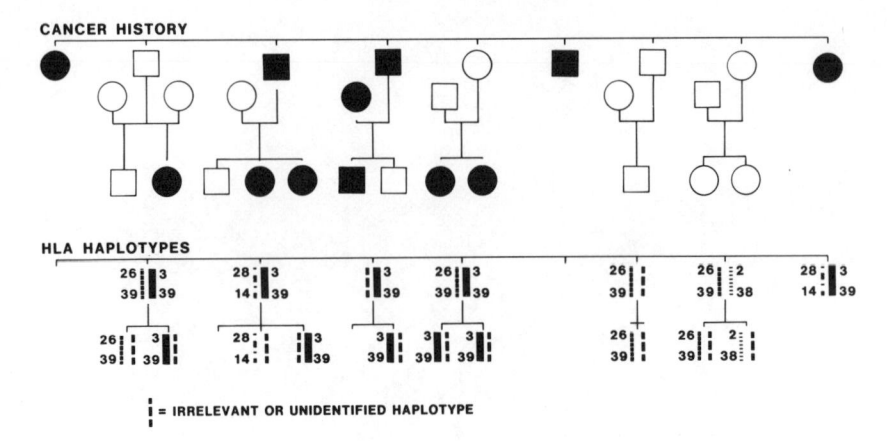

Fig. 3. Comparison of cancer-affected individuals with segregation of the HLA haplotypes in Family Pi

Note co-segregation of cancer with haplotype A3 Bw39

typing (not shown in the Figure) indicated that this haplotype was inherited intact on the HLA-B end, which did not support such a crossover hypothesis. Crossover on the HLA-A end could not be ruled out. It is also possible that this discordant individual developed breast cancer for reasons unrelated to the postulated MHC-related cancer-susceptibility gene.

To look at these data another way, in generation II we expected to find the parental haplotype, "3–39", in 50% of the members; we found it in *all* members with cancer. In generation III, where 25% might be expected to carry the "3–39" haplotype, 80% of members were observed to have cancer. Statistical evaluation of these relationships is rather complex: consider, for example, that the actual haplotypes of generation III depend on the haplotypes of generation II. There are many other such considerations, and most of them have been incorporated into another computer program, LIPED, which we used for analysis of genetic linkage (6). The program considers, for example, age of onset of disease and the degree of penetrance or expression of a particular gene. We believe the latter to be extremely important when the expression of cancer as a phenotype is equated with the presence of a cancer-susceptibility gene.

Table 3 summarizes the highest LOD (log odds determination)

Table 3. **Highest LOD Scores for Each Marker in Family Pi**

Marker[a] (and chromosome assignment)	LOD score, cancer vs other loci
ABO (9)	0.038
Lewis	−0.002
Rhesus (1)	0.147
MNSs (4)	0.449
Duffy (1)	0.089
Kp	0.017
Kidd	0.182
P	0.025
AK1 (9)	−0.001
6PGD (1)	−0.006
ADA (20)	0.018
PGP (16)	0.232
AcP (2)	0.566
GALT (9)	0.013
GPT	0.097
EsD (13)	0.013
GLO-1 (6)	0.166
PGM-1 (IEP) (1)	0.079
Haptoglobin (16)	0.039
Gc (4)	0.026
Pseudocholinesterase	−0.003
AMY2 (1)	−0.013
IGH (14)	−0.012
Bf (6)	0.162
HLA (6)	0.638[b]

[a] Markers identified in Table 2.
[b] $\theta_m, \theta_f = 0.30, 0.01$.

scores from the LIPED analysis, for each potential linkage pair. A confident statement of linkage between two loci can only be made with a LOD score of three or greater. However, one is extremely unlikely to achieve such a level of confidence from analyzing a single pedigree. As can be seen in Table 3, although the LOD score for HLA is higher than any of the others, it is far from significant when it stands alone. A LOD score of 0.638 corresponds to greater than four-to-one odds in favor of linkage over no-linkage. More families will have to be studied before a more definite conclusion can be reached. Specifically, if four more similar families showed this level of LOD scores, linkage between HLA and a cancer-susceptibility gene could be confirmed. We also noted higher LOD scores for acid phosphatase (0.566) and for blood group MNSs (0.449). It is difficult at present, however, to discern the potential biological significance of such findings.

Family N was described by Lynch et al. (7) over 10 years ago as a family containing multiple cancers in many persons. Again, there was evidence suggesting that the cancer expression might be co-segregating with the MHC, as identified by HLA typing. In one branch, 20 of 21 members with cancer have the same HLA haplotype. Three problems have arisen in the analysis of this enormous pedigree (n=450):

1. In one branch of the family, the 2–12 haplotype associated with cancer may not derive in all cases from the same ancestor because one parent of a large branch may be homozygous for the 2–12 haplotype; thus, this branch may not be informative for co-segregation.

2. Another branch of the family has some cancer-affected members but the pattern of cancer is not comparable with that of the rest of the family, making it difficult to know how these members should be scored in the genetic analysis: are they cancer-susceptibles or unaffecteds?

3. Very few branches of this family are free from cancer, thereby making it difficult to find negative controls for linkage studies. Further efforts to extend the HLA typing in Family N are underway in our laboratories in collaboration with Lynch and co-workers.

Braun and co-workers (8) have described yet another cancer pedigree, in which colon cancer appears to co-segregate with the HLA of one haplotype in six of nine members with cancer, suggesting linkage (LOD score = 1.06). In this family (n = 66), all but one member with cancer had adenocarcinoma of the colon; one-fourth of them had multiple primaries. The mean age of diagnosis was 38 years. On the other hand, age-of-onset corrections do not appear to have been included in those analyses.

King et al. (9) analyzed a panel of genetic markers in 11 families with breast cancer. Five of the families also manifested ovarian cancer. From this analysis, a "combined LOD" from six of those families was 1.84 for linkage with the GPT (glutamate pyruvate transaminase, or alanine aminotransferase) locus. It is unclear in this report, however, what the justifications were for excluding the other five families from the "combined LOD score."

Nongenetic Parameters

Let us return for a moment to the approach of trying to identify cancer-susceptibles by characterizing various nongenetic parameters in members of high-risk cancer families. When another marker, such as a clinical syndrome, also identifies members as "premalignant" or cancer susceptible, we can study even autosomal recessive disorders. An example of this is ataxia-telangiectasia (AT), a disorder of children and young adults characterized by progressive cerebellar ataxia, oculocutaneous telangiectases, frequent sinopulmonary infections, numerous immunological abnormalities, and an increased risk of malignancy. Roughly 15% of such patients develop cancer, despite their early demise. From this we can assume that roughly one of six of these patients is premalignant and might manifest some laboratory aberration that could then be correlated with cancer susceptibility.

Over a decade ago, our report of cancer among immunodeficiency patients (10) lent strong support to the theory that immunosurveillance might play a key role in the development of cancer. Since then, many attempts have been made to characterize the immune status of premalignant or cancer-susceptible persons. Thus far, however, a reliable immunologic indicator of cancer susceptibility or genetic risk has not been identified, and the role of immunosurveillance in oncogenesis remains unclear.

Prodded by the above considerations, we have tried to analyze both the immune status and the genetics of patients with AT and of their family members. Linkage of the gene for AT to HLA was ruled out in our study of nine multiplex families (11). Documentation of a tandem translocation of chromosome 14q in some patients with this disorder (12) has focused our followup genetic studies on the possibility of a cancer-susceptibility gene on the long arm of chromosome 14, where the IGH genes for immunoglobulin heavy chains also map (13–15). In the interim, we attempted to analyze further the type and extent of the immunodeficiency in this group of cancer-susceptible patients (16), keeping in mind that their parents, the obligate heterozygotes, may also be susceptible to cancer (17) and may express intermediate states of the immunological defects seen in their children.

Our investigations confirmed earlier reports of (a) reduced proportions of T cells, perhaps T helper cells; (b) weak responses to in vitro stimulation of lymphocytes by mitogens, such as phytohemagglutinin; (c) IgA deficiency; and (d) increased concentrations of α-fetoprotein in serum (16). In addition, we found: increased concanavalin capping on lymphocytes; increased concentrations of cyclic nucleotides in T lymphocytes; a correlation between the increased capping and concentrations of cAMP; decreased neutrophil chemotaxis; and an IgG$_2$ deficiency in eight of 10 patients (16). Some parents had intermediate values for T cells, capping, cGMP, and neutrophil chemotaxis. These findings suggested to us that an underlying defect might involve the cytoskeletal structure of the patients' cells, either primarily or secondarily to a biochemical defect, although other hypotheses could also be proposed. Further studies of microtubular integrity are in progress.

As yet, none of the parameters we measured can identify the heterozygotes among parents or siblings. This is not surprising when one considers that even the profile for the homozygotes, the patients, is far from uniform (Table 4). Even when many parameters were taken together in a weighted average, no clear profile for the heterozygote could be derived. This can be appreciated by comparing the putative "heterozygote index" in the next-to-last line of Table 5 with the data in Table 6. All of the individuals listed in Table 6 are parents of AT patients and, thus, obligate

Table 4. **Frequency of Abnormal Parameters in 12 Patients with Ataxia-Telangiectasia**

Parameter	% of patients abnormal
Alkaline phosphatase increased	87
T cells (En) decreased	83
IgG$_2$ decreased	78
α-Fetoprotein (AFP) increased	75
Lactate dehydrogenase increased	75
Neutrophil chemotaxis decreased	73
IgA decreased	67
cAMP/cGMP (T cells) increased	60
Capping (concanavalin A) increased	58
B cells surface membrane Ig (SmIg) increased	58
B cells (α-p23,30) increased	50
Phytohemagglutinin (PHA) response decreased	50
T cells α-naphthyl acid esterase (ANAE) decreased	50
DNA repair (γ-radiation damage) decreased	45
T cells (α-T MoAb) decreased	36
T suppressor activity (concanavalin A-induced) decreased	25

Table 5. **Multiparameter Analysis of Six Siblings of Ataxia-Telangiectasia Patients**[a]

	Siblings[b]					
	1	2	3	4	5	6
En	*[c]		*			
α-T			*			
ANAE	*		NT	NT	*	*
PHA	*					
Tsupp			*		*	
Capping	?					?
cAMP			*	*		*
cGMP	*		?	*		
A/G ratio					?	?
SmIg		?	*	*		
α-B				*		
IgA	*	*	*	*	*	*
IgG₂			*			
AFP						
DNA repair	*	*		*		
"Index"[d]	30	9	32	23	13	14
Heterozygote	?		?	?		

[a] Parameters as in Table 4.
[b] Not all siblings were from the same family.
[c] * denotes an abnormality of that parameter; NT = not tested; ? = borderline results.
[d] Weighted average based on percentages shown in Table 4.

Table 6. **Putative Heterozygote "Index" for Obligate AT Heterozygotes**[a]

Family	Mo/Fa	Index
A	Mo	5
	Fa	5
B	Mo	8
	Fa	6
C	Mo	16
	Fa	13
D	Mo	8
	Fa	29
E	Mo	39
F	Mo	21
G	Mo	0
H	Mo	8
	Fa	9

[a] Weighted average based on Table 4. Mo, mother; Fa, Father.

heterozygotes. As can be seen, the putative "index" has high values in only some of the parents (a normal person should have an index of zero). One mother had a zero index. Also, it is unlikely that all six siblings studied were heterozygotes, as indicated by the putative "index" (three would be the expected frequency). Thus, while a weighted index *might* prove useful in identifying AT heterozygotes, we do not feel that the index used in Tables 5 and 6 is a reliable indicator of heterozygosity.

A drawback to immunologic studies of this kind is that, even if they were to help us appreciate a common pathogenetic mechanism in this disorder, a great deal more information would be necessary to elucidate how this defect relates to the genetic defect or to the clinical expression of cancer. We remain, in the case of AT patients, without a genetic location for the cancer-susceptibility gene and without a means of evaluating the degree of influence the genetics of this situation has upon the expression or "penetrance" of cancer.

Genetic mechanisms must play a relatively minor role for oncogenesis in children with primary immunodeficiencies, because these patients develop primarily lymphoid malignancies and not the full spectrum of cancers seen in either the "nonimmunodeficient" pediatric population or in the adult population (*18*). Were their immunodeficiency a key factor, one would expect to see the full spectrum of pediatric cancers among these immunodeficient children.

Summary

The term "cancer diathesis," as used in the old literature, has a direct modern translation into "inherited cancer susceptibility," but this concept still requires further documentation in humans. Inherited cancer susceptibility is well documented in mouse models. Linkage analyses with extensive panels of genetic markers, including probes for DNA polymorphisms (*19*), may link cancer-susceptibility genes to distinct parts of the human genome in the near future; however, the difficulties of distinguishing cancer "affected" from "nonaffected" individuals by clinical phenotypes will remain a major limitation in family analyses. The three genetic areas that appear, at present, to be the most likely candidates for immune-related cancer susceptibility genes are the X chromosome (see Table 1), chromosome 6p (HLA-related), and chromosome 14q (IGH and AT-related).

Finally, we must also consider that once we succeed in developing means by which we can reliably identify cancer-susceptible members of families and in the general population, we will have to learn how such information can best be utilized. If *you* were susceptible to cancer, either in general or to a specific cancer, would you really want to know? If we could identify cancer susceptibility as a "birth defect," would this and should this alter medical and personal decisions? These are difficult ethical questions, which will require careful consideration.

This work was partially supported by USPHS grant no. GM 29788.

References

1. Klein, J., Genetic control of virus susceptibility. In *Biology of the Mouse Histocompatability-2 Complex,* Springer-Verlag, New York, NY, 1975, pp 389–410.
2. Lilly, F., The role of genetics in Gross virus leukemogenesis. *Bibl. Haematol. (Basel)* **36,** 213–200 (1970).
3. Devre, P., Gisselbrecht, S., Pozo, P., and Levy, J. P., Genetic control of sensitivity to Moloney leukemia virus in mice. II. Mapping of three resistant genes within the H-2 complex. *J. Immunol.* **123,** 1806–1812 (1979).
4. Penn, I., The incidence of malignancies in transplant recipients. *Transplant Proc.* **7,** 323 (1975).
5. Gatti, R. A., Sparkes, R. S., Field, L. L., Spence, M. A., Harris, N. S., and Freidin, M., Genetic linkage analysis in a high-risk cancer family: HLA and 24 other markers. *Cancer Genet. Cytogenet.,* in press.
6. Hodge, S. E., Morton, L. A., Tideman, S., Kidd, K. K., and Spence, M. A., Age-of-onset correction available for linkage analysis (LIPED). *Am. J. Hum. Genet.* **31,** 761–762 (1979).
7. Lynch, H. T., Thomas, R. J., Terasaki, P. I., Ting, A., Guirgis, H. A., Kaplan, A. R., Magee, H., Lynch, J., Kraft, C., and Chaperon, E., HL-A in cancer family "N." *Cancer* **36,** 1315–1320 (1975).
8. Sivak, M. V., Schleutermann-Sivak, D., Braun, W. A., and Sullivan, B. H., A linkage study of HLA and inherited adenocarcinoma of the colon. *Cancer* **48,** 76–81 (1981).
9. King, M. C., Go, R. C. P., Elston, R. C., Lynch, H. T., and Petrakis, N. L., Allele increasing susceptibility to human breast cancer may be linked to the glutamate–pyruvate transaminase locus. *Science* **208,** 406–408 (1980).

10. Gatti, R. A., and Good, R. A., Occurrence of malignancy in immunodeficiency disease. *Cancer* **28,** 89–98 (1971).
11. Hodge, S., Berkel, I., Gatti, R. A., Boder, E., and Spence, M. A., Ataxia-telangiectasia and xeroderma pigmentosum: No evidence of linkage to HLA. *Tissue Antigens* **15,** 313–317 (1980).
12. McCaw, B., Hecht, F., Harnden, D. G., and Teplitz, R. L., Somatic rearrangement of chromosome 14 in human lymphocytes. *Proc. Natl. Acad. Sci. USA* **72,** 2071–2075 (1975).
13. Croce, C. M., Shander, M., Martinis, J., Cicurel, L., D'Ancona, G. G., and Koprowski, H., Preferential retention of human chromosome 14 in mouse × human B cell hybrids. *Eur. J. Immunol.* **10,** 486–488 (1980).
14. Smith, M., Krinsky, A. M., Arredondo-Vega, F., Wang, A. L., and Hirschhorn, K., Confirmation of the assignment of genes for human immunoglobulin heavy chains to chromosome 14. *Cancer Genet. Cytogenet.* **32,** 318 (1982).
15. Solomon, E., Goodfellow, P., Chambers, S., Spurr, N., Hobart, M. J., Rabbits, T. H., and Povey, S., Confirmation of the assignment of immunoglobulin heavy chain genes to chromosome 14, using cloned DNA as molecular probes. *Cancer Genet. Cytogenet.* **32,** 319 (1982).
16. Gatti, R. A., Bick, M., Tam, C. F., Medici, M. A., Oxelius, V., Holland, M., Goldstein, A. L., and Boder, E., Ataxia-telangiectasia: A multiparameter analysis of eight families. *Clin. Immunol. Immunopathol.* **23,** 501–516 (1982).
17. Swift, M., Sholman, L., Perry, M., and Chase, C., Malignant neoplasms in the families of patients with ataxia-telangiectasia. *Cancer Res.* **36,** 209–215 (1976).
18. Spector, B., Perry, G., and Kersey, J., Genetically-determined immunodeficiency diseases (GDID) and malignancy. Report from the Immunodeficiency-Cancer registry. *Clin. Immunol. Immunopathol.* **11,** 12–29 (1978).
19. Wyman, A. R., and White, R., A highly polymorphic locus in human DNA. *Proc. Natl. Acad. Sci. USA* **77,** 6754–6758 (1980).

Discussion

Q: Rather than reflecting an underlying disorder, such as a cytoskeletal disorder, might not the increased capping simply be reflecting the relationships of disordered subpopulations of lymphocytes being seen in this disease?

DR. GATTI: Yes, it's very possible. In fact, we are just preparing to investigate that now. We want to see whether different subsets of T cells and of course B cells too cap differently. Of course, that wouldn't relate to the neutrophil chemotaxis or the cAMP abnormality.

Q: What is the status of research on cancer as related to autoimmunity and antibody isolation? Is immunosuppressive therapy tied in with this?

Dr. Gatti: It probably is tied in, although I don't have any pertinent answers to your questions at the moment. More and more information indicates that patients on immunosuppression, not only for renal transplants but also for other long-term immunosuppressive therapy and even some short-term therapy, have developed malignancies with a 10- to 100-fold increase over the general population. The malignancies are mainly lymphoid, but not totally.

Dr. Good: When we first showed that the thymus was abnormal in patients with ataxia-telangiectasia, we found it to be small, about one-third to a quarter of normal size in most patients. It has an abnormal morphology and does not seem to be directing the development of the T lymphocytes very well. We were not surprised when two functional assays demonstrated that the concentrations of thymic hormones were very low. However, our observations contradict your studies with the radioimmunoassay for thymosin alpha 1. That radioimmunoassay is not very accurate at low concentrations—it shows considerable thymic hormone in thymectomized patients. I think the functional assays are more reliable, giving results that fit very well with the immunoglobulin abnormalities, the antibody production abnormalities, and the abnormality of functional development of the T cells: in other words, the deficiency of the thymus should be decreased.

Dr. Gatti: I agree with you. We were surprised to find normal thymosin levels.

Dr. Good: The radioimmunoassay may be much more useful at high concentrations, but the functional assays are extremely reliable at low hormone concentrations.

Dr. Gatti: The drawback is that there's been a lot of controversy over standardizing the functional assays between laboratories.

Genetic Disorders of the Endocrine Glands

David L. Rimoin

Genetic disorders of the endocrine glands provide an excellent model for the study of the mechanisms of gene action in clinical disease and illustrate the diversity of pathogenetic mechanisms that result in genetic heterogeneity. All types of genetic disturbances, including point mutations, chromosomal aberrations, and polygenic factors have been demonstrated to be operative in endocrine disorders. The recent explosion of knowledge in the fields of endocrinology and genetics has allowed for the delineation of specific pathogenetic mechanisms in many of these disorders. Endocrine disorders are expressed primarily by excess or reduced action of one or more hormones, and a wide variety of distinct pathogenetic mechanisms may result in the same endocrine deficiency or hyperfunctional syndrome (Table 1).

In those genetic disorders in which the mutation directly alters hormonal structure or synthesis, the endocrine glands can be divided into two major classes: those that produce peptide hormones (pituitary, parathyroid, pancreas, and thyroid parafollicular cells) and those that produce nonpeptide hormones (thyroid follicular cells, adrenal cortex, adrenal medulla, and gonads). Similarly, for those disorders that involve peripheral resistance to hormonal action, disorders can be classified on the basis of whether they involve lipid-soluble or water-soluble hormones, because the lipid-soluble hormones exert their effect via an intracellular protein receptor, whereas the water-soluble hormones act at the cell membrane via the cyclic nucleotides.

In this paper, I will discuss the various possible genetic mechanisms that can result in endocrine dysfunction.

Table 1. **Pathogenetic Mechanisms in the Genetic Disorders of the Endocrine Glands**

Hormonal Insufficiency Syndrome
A. Active hormone does not reach target cell
  1. Decreased synthesis or secretion of hormone
     a) Structural mutation of gene
     b) Gene deletion
     c) "Regulatory" mutation
     d) Neurostimulatory defect
     e) Tropic hormone deficiency
     f) Inborn error of hormonal biosynthesis
     g) Defect in cleavage of active peptide from prohormone
     h) Developmental malfunction of gland—aplasia, hypoplasia, or dysplasia
     i) Degenerative disorders—toxic, autoimmune, infarction, or generalized metabolic defect
     j) Defect in secretory mechanism
  2. Hormone inactivation
     a) Hormonal antagonist
     b) Rapid degradation or excretion
B. Target-cell insensitivity
  1. Water-soluble hormones
     a) Decrease in receptor number
     b) Decreased receptor affinity
     c) Competition for binding site (e.g., antibody to receptor)
     d) Abnormalities in generating second messenger
     e) Post-receptor defects
  2. Lipid-soluble hormones
     a) Decreased concentration of cytoplasmic receptor
     b) Decreased affinity of cytoplasmic receptor
     c) Instability or degradation of hormone-receptor complex
     d) Defect in delivery or binding to nuclear acceptor

Carrier Protein Abnormality
A. Carrier protein deficiency
B. Carrier protein excess

Glandular Hyperplasia
A. Direct effect of mutation on glandular function
B. Effect secondary to increased glandular stimulant
C. Result of feedback system stimulation due to primary hormonal deficiency

Glandular Neoplasia
A. With hormonal hypersecretion
B. With no change in glandular function
C. With destruction of gland and resulting hormonal deficiency

Endocrine-Deficiency Disorders

A wide variety of distinct pathogenetic mechanisms can result in the same endocrine-deficiency state (*1*). The clinical features of hormonal deficiency may result from (*a*) decreased synthesis or secretion of biologically active hormone, (b) inactivation or degradation of the hormone before reaching the target cell, and (c) target-cell insensitivity to hormonal action.

Decreased Synthesis or Secretion of Active Hormone

Several different genetic mechanisms can result in the decreased synthesis or secretion of active hormone. In considering those genetic disorders in which the mutation directly alters hormonal structure or synthesis, the endocrine glands should be divided into two major classes: those that produce polypeptide hormones (pituitary, parathyroid, pancreas, and thyroid parafollicular cells) and those that produce nonpeptide hormones (thyroid follicular cells, adrenal cortex, adrenal medulla, and gonads). A structural gene mutation could directly alter the structure and function of a peptide hormone, whereas nonpeptide structure could only be indirectly influenced by the genome through mutations affecting the enzymes that govern their biosynthesis.

Structural mutations of a gene coding for a polypeptide hormone may result in a hormone that is structurally altered but still capable of normal function, a hormone whose function is markedly reduced, or a hormone that has been so altered as to be completely incapable of performing its biological activity. The degree of functional inactivation of the hormone would depend on how the amino acid substitution affected the active site of the molecule. A point mutation could also have various effects on the immunological activity of the hormone, depending on the resulting tertiary structure of the molecule. In the evaluation of endocrine dysfunction, assays measuring both the biological and immunological properties of the molecule should be available. Structural mutations could thus result in altered peptides in which (a) biological function is decreased but antigenic activity is preserved [cross-reactive material(CRM)-positive mutations], or (b) both biological and antigenic activities are lost (CRM-negative mutations). Because radioimmunoassays are based entirely on the immunological properties of the molecule, they are incapable of distinguishing between a normal polypeptide hormone and a CRM-positive mutant molecule. Clinical evidence of hormonal deficiency and a bioassay would be required to make this distinction. A bioassay, on the other hand, would not be capable of distinguishing between a CRM-negative structural mutation and a mutation resulting in decreased synthesis of the normal protein. Further information could also be gleaned from radioreceptor assays, in which the ability of the hormone to bind to its receptor would be one index of the hormone's biological activity.

Several structural mutations affecting peptide hormone function have now been described. These include point mutations in the pro-insulin gene that interfere with the cleavage of the C-peptide, resulting in decreased production of active insulin molecules, and point mutations in which an amino acid substitution occurs in the biologically important part of the insulin molecule, resulting in decreased ability to bind to insulin receptors and even more defective ability to stimulate its biological response at the cellular level (2, 3). In addition to point mutations, the gene coding for a peptide hormone could be deleted, in whole or in part, resulting in decreased synthesis of active hormone. This has been described in an unusual type of isolated growth-hormone deficiency (type A), in which restriction endonuclease techniques have delineated an approximately 7.5 kilobase deletion in the growth hormone gene (4). These individuals secrete no recognizable somatotropin, either biologically or immunologically, and they develop antibodies against the somatotropin molecule when treated with exogenous growth hormone. The recent explosion in DNA technology should lead to the recognition of more and more such structural defects in the genes coding for peptide hormones. In addition, "regulatory" mutations, resulting in decreased synthesis of the normal gene product, should come to light.

Genetic errors may result in peptide hormone deficiency states by various mechanisms that do not directly involve the gene coding for the hormone. Control of hormonal secretion often involves a complex feedback system, abnormalities in any part of which may result in decreased hormonal secretion. For example, it is now apparent that the pituitary hormones are under the direct control of releasing (-liberin) and inhibitory (-statin) hormones liberated by the hypothalamus. A developmental abnormality of the hypothalamus, or a mutation in the genes controlling the synthesis of a releasing factor in the hypothalamus, may result in the same endocrine-deficiency state as a structural or regulatory mutation of the gene coding for the hormone. Approximately two-thirds of the cases of multitropic or panhypopituitary dwarfism involve a hypothalamic rather than a pituitary defect, because the administration of thyroliberin (thyrotropin-releasing hormone) can result in pituitary secretion of thyrotropin in these individuals. In addition, the autosomal recessive form of isolated somatotropin deficiency appears to be a hypothalamic, rather than a pituitary, defect because autopsy studies of at least three individuals with this syndrome have revealed normal pituitary somatotropic cells (5).

The nonpeptide hormones, such as thyroxin, the catecholamines, and the steroids, are produced by a sequence of metabolic reactions governed by a series of enzymes. Each of the enzymes is under the direct control of a specific gene (1). Mutation of any of these genes may alter hormonal synthesis, usually without a change in hormone structure. Thus a hormonal-deficiency state may result from a mutation in any one of the genes coding for any of the enzymes involved in the biosynthesis of the hormone. Such a metabolic block can result in clinical symptoms by: (a) deficiency of the end product of the pathway (e.g., hypothyroidism in congenital goitrous cretinism); (b) the accumulation of intermediary products proximal to the block (e.g., hypertension in the adrenogenital syndromes, resulting from excess desoxycorticosterone); (c) the production of byproducts that are usually not present in large quantities and normally are not of great metabolic significance (e.g., virilization in the adrenogenital syndromes, caused by androgen excess); or (d) the inhibition or stimulation of other metabolic pathways (e.g., increases in corticotropin secretion, because of the stimulation of the negative feedback system in the adrenogenital syndromes). An enzyme deficiency could also account for a peptide hormone deficiency if the active peptide hormone arose by cleavage of a larger inactive peptide (e.g., insulin from pro-insulin, parathyrin from proparathyrin, etc.), or if the peptide hormone has a nonpeptide component (e.g., glycoproteins, such as the gonadotropins).

Hormonal-deficiency states also result from developmental anomalies. Aplasia or hypoplasia of an endocrine gland may result in complete or partial functional insufficiency or the organ (1). These anomalies may directly involve the specific endocrine gland (such as congenital absence of the pituitary or agoitrous cretinism) or a specific anomaly of a hypothalamic regulatory center (such as supraoptic neuronal hypoplasia in diabetes insipidus), or may be part of a complex congenital malformation syndrome (such as anencephaly or holoprosencephaly). In congenital malformations of the pituitary, the tropic hormone deficiencies may also result in secondary atrophy and deficiency of the target endocrine organs (e.g., adrenal cortex, thyroid, gonads).

The genetic degenerative disorders may result in hormonal-deficiency states by disrupting the functional capabilities of an endocrine gland (1). This may arise through an accumulation of a toxic compound within the gland (e.g., hemochromatosis, Wolman's disease), infarction of the gland (e.g., hemoglobinopathies), cellular infiltration (e.g., histiocytosis X), or an autoimmune process (e.g., thyroiditis). In many of these complex genetic disorders, however, the pathogenetic mechanism resulting in the hormonal deficiency is unknown. Several glands may be affected simultaneously in these degenerative disorders, such as in the pluriglandular deficiency syndromes, in which the hereditary abnormality appears to result in a general autoimmune disease, or in hemochromatosis, where iron deposition may damage the pancreas and pituitary and may secondarily lead to atrophy of the gonads by gonadotropin deficiency.

Genetic defects might also exist in the secretory mechanism of the cell, perhaps because of a defect in the glandular sensor to the normal stimulus or a defect in the mechanism by which a hormone is released from the gland.

In addition to single-gene mutations, the endocrine glands may be affected by chromosomal aberrations or aneuploidy. Development of the fetal gonad depends on the sex chromosomal constitution, especially on the presence or absence of a Y chromosome and the balance between the number of X's and the Y. A disturbance of this chromosomal balance will lead to gonadal maldevelopment or degeneration. Various abnormalities in endocrine function have also been described in several of the autosomal cytogenetic syndromes, such as pituitary hypoplasia in trisomy 13. But these endocrine abnormalities are for the most part infrequent and nonspecific, and are part of generalized malformation syndromes.

Hormonal Antagonists

An endocrine-deficiency state could also result from the presence of compounds antagonistic to the action of the hormone. For example, antihormonal antibodies can bind a hormone and render it inactive, thus preventing the effective action of the hormone at the target organ. On the other hand, antibodies directed against the hormonal receptor on the target cell could result in the inability of the active hormone to bind to the target cell. The latter is one of the documented mechanisms of target-cell insensitivity in diabetes mellitus (2). An abnormality in the metabolism or excretion of the hormone could also result in a normally secreted hormone's being rapidly inactivated or excreted.

Target-Cell Insensitivity

A clinically apparent hormonal-deficiency state may be the result of end-organ unresponsiveness to the hormone. Depending on whether or not a feedback system exists between the effector organ and the endocrine gland, concentrations of the hormone in the serum may be normal or above-normal. The target-organ insensitivity syndrome can be suspected in an individual who has a clinical syndrome of hormonal deficiency, with normal or above-normal plasma concentrations of the hormone. Target-organ insensitivity can be documented by the demonstration of a lack of metabolic response to the exogenous administration of the hormone in question. Documentation of such a defect can now be approached at the cellular level by studying the binding of the hormone to the patient's isolated cells or the concentration of hormonal receptors in such cells, or by studying the in vitro metabolic activity of the hormone (2).

The syndromes of target-organ insensitivity should be divided into those associated with water-soluble hormones vs those associated with lipid-soluble hormones. The lipid-soluble hormones—the iodothyronines, the steroids, and 1,25-dihydroxy vitamin D—traverse the lipid-rich membrane of the target cell and first interact with intracellular components. The specific receptors for steroids and vitamin D are soluble cytoplasmic components that complex with hormone. These hormone–receptor complexes undergo a variety of transformations and move to the nucleus, where they regulate gene expression. The thyroid hormones regulate gene expression, but appear to have their receptors in the nucleus rather than in the cytoplasm. Thus various potential genetic defects could result in a peripheral insensitivity to steroid hormones (e.g., deficiency of the cytoplasmic receptor, reduced affinity of the cytoplasmic receptor, instability of the receptor–hormone complex, reduced binding of the steroid–receptor complex to the nuclear acceptors). Several such defects have already been described in the testicular feminization syndromes (6).

On the other hand, the water-soluble hormones—the peptide hormones and the catecholamines—do not traverse the plasma membrane, but interact directly with cell-surface receptors. The combination of the hormone and the receptor initiates a transmembrane message, which for most hormones results in the activation of adenylate cyclase (EC 4.6.1.1) at the inner surface of the membrane. This catalyzes the conversion of ATP to cyclic AMP, a soluble "second messenger" that diffuses through the cell and activates a protein kinase enzyme that phosphorylates intracellular proteins, especially enzymes, and thus regulates their activity. Insulin, prolactin, somatotropin, and alpha-adrenergic catecholamines, however, do not act through adenylate cyclase, but through other intracellular messengers. One can thus postulate a variety of defects that could interfere with the action of the water-soluble hormones at the cellular level, for example, an absence or deficiency of the receptors, abnormal affinity of the receptor for the hormone, competitive binders of the hormone receptor that deplete the receptor sites available for the hormone, abnormalities in the generation of the second messenger, or various post-receptor defects. Indeed, many of these mechanisms have already been described (2). For example, insulin-receptor defects have been described in which there are abnormalities in receptor number (e.g., acanthosis nigricans syndrome–type A), defects in receptor affinity (e.g., myotonic dystrophy), and antireceptor antibodies (e.g., acanthosis nigricans syndrome–type B, ataxia telangiectasia), and defects associated with normal receptor binding but having a post-receptor defect (e.g., acanthosis nigricans syndrome–type C, leprechaunism) (7). Similar heterogeneity has been described in pseudohypoparathyroidism, in which target-organ insensitivity to parathyrin can exist because of a defect in the regulatory component of adenylate cyclase, as well as various post-receptor defects (8).

One must be careful to differentiate the various forms of target-cell insensitivity to hormonal action from those disorders of hormonal biosynthesis that can mimic their clinical features. For example, the pseudovaginal–perineal–scrotal hypospadias (PPSH) syndrome, an autosomal recessive disorder now known to be due to a deficiency of 5-alpha-reductase, results in congenital malformations of the urogenital tract that resemble target-organ insensitivity to testosterone (9). This insensitivity was appreciated only after it was determined that conversion of testosterone to dihydrotestosterone was required for testosterone to exert its action on certain tissues. Similarly, vitamin D-resistant rickets (hypophosphatemic rickets), which appears to be secondary to target-organ insensitivity to vitamin D, can be confused with vitamin D-responsive rickets, in which there appears to be a metabolic defect in the biosynthesis of 1,25-dihydroxy vitamin D (10).

Thus many different pathogenetic mechanisms can result in the same clinical phenotype—apparent hormonal insufficiency. Recognition of the specific genetic defect involved for each individual patient is important to be able to provide the appropriate therapy and genetic counseling.

Abnormalities in Transport of Hormone to Target Organ

Abnormal values for laboratory tests of endocrine function may be the result of genetic defects in carrier proteins. Whereas polypeptide hormones as a rule circulate free in plasma, all lipid-soluble hormones are bound reversibly to one or more proteins in the plasma. Genetic defects in the structure or function of these proteins may lead to altered hormone concentrations in blood. The concentration of the biologically active free hormone is usually within normal limits in such individuals, however, and thus there is no clinical evidence of endocrine dysfunction. Genetic defects in thyroxin-binding globulins, for example, can result in abnormally low or high concentrations of total plasma thyroxin in individuals who are clinically euthyroid (1).

Glandular Hyperplasia or Neoplasia

Genetic factors may also result in hyperplasia or neoplasia of an endocrine gland. Glandular hyperplasia may occur as a primary phenomenon (e.g., chief cell hyperplasia in familial hyperparathyroidism), or be secondary to a primary hormonal deficiency and the resulting increased stimulation via a feedback system (e.g., adrenal hyperplasia in the adrenogenital syndromes or goiter in the inborn errors of thyroxin synthesis). Glandular hyperplasia could also be the result of an abnormal signal to the target cell (e.g., immunoglobulins from patients with Grave's disease can simulate the effects of thyrotropin on the thyroid). When not ascribable to a primary hormonal deficiency, the glandular hyperplasia is usually associated with overproduction of the hormone or hormones in question and the resulting clinical syndrome of hormone excess.

Although there may be hereditary neoplasms affecting only one endocrine gland, the most common forms of glandular neoplasia involve multiple endocrine organs, an example being the various multiple endocrine adenomatosis syndromes. Glandular neoplasia can result in hormonal hypersecretion, or there may be no change in glandular function, or there may be a hormonal-deficiency state following the destruction of the gland by the neoplasm. As in other heritable neoplasias, the pathogenetic mechanism involved in these disorders is unknown but in certain instances appears to follow directly upon glandular hyperplasia.

Modes of Inheritance

All types of simple mendelian inheritance (autosomal dominant and recessive, X-linked dominant and recessive) have been demonstrated in the heritable disorders of the endocrine glands. Dominantly inherited traits are those that can be seen in the presence of only one mutant gene, whereas recessive traits are expressed clinically only in the absence of a normal allele. It must be stressed, however, that dominance and recessivity usually refer to the phenotype and not the genotype—a mutant may express itself clinically only in the homozygous state (recessive) but may be detected biochemically in the heterozygous state (dominant).

Several generalizations can be made concerning the mode of inheritance of traits that result from specific pathogenetic mechanisms. Recessively inherited traits usually involve an enzyme deficiency, whereas dominantly inherited conditions are often associated with an abnormal structural protein. With minor modification, these generalizations hold true for the heritable disorders of the endocrine glands. Hormonal-deficiency states are usually recessively inherited, while those resulting in glandular hyperplasia or neoplasia are almost always dominantly inherited.

The inborn errors of metabolism associated with enzyme deficiencies are probably recessive in their inheritance, because enzymes ordinarily are required in such small quantities. One normal structural gene coding for the enzyme (in the heterozygous state) can probably produce enough of the normal enzyme to suffice for average metabolic function. Thus, at the clinical level, these traits are recessive; that is, the presence of one normal gene in the heterozygote will result in a normal phenotype, and the abnormal clinical state occurs only in the absence of a normal allele. The mutant gene, however, can often be detected in the heterozygous state by enzyme assays or provocative tests. Thus the chemical abnormality is inherited in a dominant or co-dominant fashion. This is true of the inborn errors of thyroxin and corticosteroid metabolism that are inherited as autosomal recessive traits.

This same principle holds true for the polypeptide hormone deficiencies, which are also usually inherited as autosomal recessive traits. Polypeptide hormones, like enzymes, ordinarily are present in minute quantities in the circulation, so the presence of one normal structural gene in the heterozygote may allow for the synthesis of sufficient hormone to meet everyday needs, resulting in a normal phenotype. In the absence of a normal gene coding for the peptide hormone, none or markedly subnormal amounts of functional hormone are synthesized, resulting in a clinical deficiency syndrome. Recognition of the effects of the mutant gene in heterozygote carriers of the peptide-hormone deficiency disorders has thus far been unsuccessful. A reduced amount of the normal human somatotropin gene, however, has been demonstrated in heterozygotes for the somatotropin deletion type A isolated somatotropin deficiency syndrome (4).

Exceptions to this rule of recessivity may be expected, because both a "regulatory" type of mutation leading to diminished synthesis of peptide hormones and mutations resulting in developmental anomalies of the endocrine glands may be inherited as dominant traits. Indeed, in the dominantly inherited vasopressin-sensitive form of diabetes insipidus, a disorder involving deficiency of the antidiuretic hormone vasopressin, absence of secretory neurons in the supraoptic nucleus of the hypothalamus has been documented (11). But in spite of these exceptions, structural mutations affecting the amino acid sequence of a hormone should be suspected in recessively inherited peptide-hormone deficiency diseases, whereas in the recessively inherited nonpeptide-hormone deficiency disorders, defects in the enzymes controlling their biosynthesis should be suspected.

Genetic forms of neoplasia are usually inherited as autosomal dominant traits (for example, the colonic polyposes, the basal cell nevus syndrome, and the phakomatoses). Many of the hereditary lymphoproliferative disorders and those neoplasms associated with a recognized enzyme deficiency (e.g., xeroderma pigmentosum), however, are inherited as autosomal recessive traits. In addition, several neoplasms have been shown to be associated with a small chromosomal deletion. The heritable neoplastic disorders of the endocrine glands, such as multiple endocrine adenomatosis and the medullary thyroid carcinoma–pheochromocytoma syndrome, as well as the non-neoplastic hormonal hypersecretion syndromes, are all inherited as dominant traits. Exceptions to these generalizations certainly exist, but knowledge of the mode of inheritance of a genetic disorder may indicate the specific pathogenetic mechanism.

Genetic Heterogeneity

Recognition of genetic heterogeneity is a major concern in the diagnosis, counseling, treatment, and investigation of hereditary diseases. Similar phenotypes may be produced by mutations at several different gene loci (genocopies), by chromosomal aberrations, or by environmental agents (phenocopies). For example, male hypogonadism may result from several simply inherited disorders such as isolated gonadotropin deficiency, the Reifenstein syndrome, or the Kallmann syndrome; from chromosomal aberrations such as the Klinefelter syndrome; or from various environmental insults such as mumps or radiation (1). The recognition of such heterogeneity has important implications in genetic counseling and hormonal replacement therapy. For example, the parents and siblings of individuals with Klinefelter syndrome or mumps orchitis are unlikely to have other affected children, whereas the risk of recurrence may be as high as 50% of males for the sibs of patients with the Kallmann or Reifenstein syndromes. Gonadotropin preparations may restore fertility and secondary sexual characteristics in individuals with isolated gonadotropin deficiency, whereas they would be ineffective in patients with Klinefelter syndrome. Heterogeneity not only exists in relatively common disorders such as hypogonadism, but may also be found in rare, apparently distinct endocrine diseases. For example, there are several different genetic forms of isolated somatotropin deficiency, and both autosomal recessive and X-linked forms of congenital adrenal hypoplasia have been described.

Heterogeneity in genetic disease can be demonstrated by the recognition of variability in the clinical features, genetic modes of transmission, genetic linkage relationships, biochemical defects, or metabolic errors of a syndrome. If the affected members of two families have a similar phenotype but differ in their modes of inheritance or in specific biochemical or metabolic abnormalities, an attempt should be made to delineate further the differences between these kindreds or to explain the differences as secondary phenomena, rather than to simply pass them off as "variants" of the same disorder. It is through the demonstration of such heterogeneity that the basic pathogenetic mechanisms involved in these disorders will be recognized.

References

1. Rimoin, D. L., and Schimke, R. N., *Genetic Disorders of the Endocrine Glands*, C. V. Mosby, St. Louis, MO, 1971.
2. Roth, J., and Grunfeld, C., Endocrine systems: Mechanisms of disease, target cells and receptors. In *Textbook of Endocrinology*, 6th ed., R. H. Williams, Ed., W. B. Saunders, Philadelphia, PA, 1981, pp 15–72.
3. Given, B. D., Mako, M. E., Tager, H. S., Baldwin, D., Markese, J., Rubenstein, A. H., Olefsky, J., Kobayashi, M., Kolterman, O., and Poucher, R., Diabetes due to secretion of an abnormal insulin. *N. Engl. J. Med.* **302**, 129–135 (1980).
4. Phillips, J. A., Hjelle, B. L., Seeburg, P. H., and Zachman, M., Molecular basis for familial isolated growth hormone deficiency. *Proc. Natl. Acad. Sci. USA* **78**, 6372–6375 (1981).
5. Rimoin, D. L., The pituitary gland. In *Principles and Practice of Medical Genetics*, A. E. H. Emery and D. L. Rimoin, Eds., Churchill Livingstone, Edinburgh, in press (1983).
6. Gritten, J. E., and Wilson, J. D., The syndromes of androgen resistance. *N. Engl. J. Med.* **302**, 198–209 (1980).
7. Flier, J. A., Kahn, C. R., and Roth, J., Receptors, anti-receptor antibodies and mechanisms of insulin resistance. *N. Engl. J. Med.* **300**, 413–419 (1979).

8. Farfel, Z., Brickman, A. S., Kazlow, H. R., et al., Defect of receptor–cyclase coupling in pseudohypoparathyroidism. *N. Engl. J. Med.* **303**, 237–242 (1980).
9. Imperato-McGinley, J., Peterson, R. E., and Gautier, T., Male pseudohermaphroditism secondary to 5α-reductase deficiency: A review. In *Fetal Endocrinology,* J. J. Novy and J. A. Resko, Eds., Academic Press, New York, NY, 1981, pp 359–382.
10. Rasmussen, H., and Anast, C., Familial hypophosphatemic (vitamin D resistant) rickets and vitamin D-dependent rickets. In *Metabolic Basis of Inherited Disease,* 4th ed., J. B. Stanbury et al., Eds., McGraw Hill, New York, NY, 1978, p 1537.
11. Braverman, C. E., Mancian, J. P., and McGoldrick, D. M., Hereditary idiopathic diabetes insipidus. A case report with autopsy findings. *Ann. Intern. Med.* **63,** 503–508 (1965).

III

NEW DIAGNOSTIC PROCEDURES

Most Cancers May Have a Chromosomal Defect

Jorge J. Yunis

There are at least 200 basically different types of nonfamilial neoplasias in humans (1). About 40 of these disorders have known counterparts with a familial dominant pattern (2). Given this basic one-to-one relationship, it has been proposed that there are some 200 human cancer genes; when a gene is defective (e.g., by point mutation or deletion), the individual is born with a predisposition to a given type of neoplasia. Alternatively, a carcinogen may affect a basically normal gene, and nonfamilial cancer ensues.

Given increasing numbers of neoplasias found to have a consistent chromosome defect (3), chromosomal rearrangement may be a common pathway to the development of nonfamilial neoplasia, regardless of the type of carcinogen involved. Although the neoplastic process must ultimately be explained at the molecular level, a substantial fraction of neoplasias show a cytogenetic abnormality: in a structural chromosomal rearrangement, for example, an event may be molecular and yet still be "visible" under the microscope, because of the unusually large size of the accompanying chromosome segment often involved in the deletion or translocation process.

Already more than 25 neoplasias have been found to have a specific chromosome defect (Table 1). In most instances, the defects were either a deletion of a specific chromosome band or bands or a reciprocal translocation with consistent sub-band breakpoints. In some malignancies, such as the acute leukemias and lymphomas, different subgroups with consistent chromosome defects and markedly different prognoses have been described. For example, seven consistent defects have been defined in sub-

Table 1. **Neoplasms with a Known Consistent Chromosomal Defect**[a]

Type	Cytogenetic category	Critical[b] chromosome breakpoint or deletion	References
Leukemias			
Chronic myelogenous leukemia	t(9;22)	22q11.21	3–6
Acute nonlymphocytic leukemia			
M1, M2, M4–M6	del 5q		7,8
	del 7q		9
M1	t(9;22)	22q11.2	10–12
M2	t(8;21)		13–14
M3	t(15;17)		15,16
M4, M5[d]	t(9[c];11)	11q23	17
M1, M2, M4–M6	+8		18
Chronic lymphocytic leukemia	+12		19,20
	t(11;14)[c]	11q13.5	
Acute lymphocytic leukemia			
L1–L3	t(4;11)		21,22
L3	t(9;22)	22q11.2	10,11,23
L3	t(8;14)	8q24.1	24,25
Lymphomas			
Burkitt's, small non-cleaved cell (non-Burkitt's),[d] large cell immunoblastic[d]	t(8;14)	8q24.13	26–31
Follicular small cleaved,[d] follicular mixed,[d] and follicular large cell[d]	t(14;18)	18q21.3	26
Small lymphocytic[d]	+12		
	del 11q[c]	q13.5	26
Solid tumors			
Neuroblastoma	del 1p	1p31p36	32,33
Small cell carcinoma of lung	del 3p	3p14p23	34
Mixed parotid gland tumor	t(3;8)[c]		35
Papillary cystoadenocarcinoma of ovary	t(6;14)		36
Constitutional retinoblastoma[d]	del 13q[e]	13q14.13	37
Retinoblastoma[c]	del 13q	13q14	38
Aniridia–Wilms' tumor[d]	del 11p[e]	11p13	39,40
Wilms' tumor[c]	del 11p	11p13	41
Meningioma	del 22q		42–44

[a] Modified from Yunis (*3*).
[b] Sub-band definition with high-resolution chromosomes.
[c] Not well established.
[d] Analyzed with high-resolution chromosomes.
[e] Found in all cells of the body.

groups of acute nonlymphocytic leukemia (ANLL), three in acute lymphocytic leukemia, and four in non-Hodgkin's lymphoma (Table 1). In some groups of patients, such as in the ANLL-M1 subgroup (4, 5), patients may have either a deletion 5q, deletion 7q, or a translocation 9;22 (3, 46); in M2 many patients have a t(8;21) (46); in M3 most patients have a t(15;17) (46); and in M4 and M5 we have found a translocation involving band 11q23 (17). Also, in non-Hodgkin's lymphoma, three high-grade malignancies [Burkitt's, small noncleaved cell (non-Burkitt's), and large-cell immunoblastic lymphoma] have the same chromosome translocation t(8;14) (q24.1;q32.3), and three related lower-grade malignancies (follicular small cleaved, follicular mixed, and follicular large-cell lymphoma) have a t(14;18) (q32.3;q21.3) (26).

Until recently, solid-tumor research was hampered by limitations in the ability to disaggregate solid-tumor cells and stimulate them to proliferate preferentially in short-term cell cultures. In spite of this, seven different types of solid tumors have been discovered to have a consistent chromosome defect in their tumor cells: a small-cell carcinoma of the lung, ovarian papillary cystoadenocarcinoma, neuroblastoma, nonfamilial retinoblastoma and Wilms' tumor, mixed parotid gland tumor, and meningioma (Table 1). Also, in constitutional neoplasias (constitutional retinoblastoma and the aniridia–Wilms' tumor syndrome), a specific chromosome-band deletion is found in all cells of the body.

Mechanisms of Carcinogenesis

The well-characterized human malignancies fall into two general categories: those with a deletion of a specific chromosome band or bands, and those with a reciprocal translocation with consistent sub-band breakpoints. Because of the common occurrence of two major chromosomal mechanisms and the unusually high frequency of deletions in carcinomas and translocations in leukemias and lymphomas, these two types of rearrangements probably play a crucial role in carcinogenesis.

Regarding neoplasias with a chromosome deletion, of special significance is the finding that in both the constitutional (1% of cases) (37) and the more common types of retinoblastoma (hereditary and sporadic forms) (2), the same chromosome defect is found, involving a deletion of band 13q14 (37, 38). These observations suggest the possibility that a critical DNA sequence is lost during the process of chromosomal rearrangement. In each patient the deleted segment may vary considerably in size at both ends of band 13q14 (37) and the deletion is associated with a 50% loss of esterase D activity (the genes for retinoblastoma and esterase D are linked); even though duplication of band 13q14 shows no tumor and 150% esterase D activity (47), there apparently is an actual loss of function rather than a direct activation or inactivation of a genetic site. A similar situation exists for the Wilms' tumor "site" because a loss of band 11p13 predisposes to Wilms' tumor (39, 40) and is accompanied by a 50% loss of catalase activity (48), whereas duplication of band 11p13 shows 150% enzyme activity with no tumor development (the gene for catalase is located in 11p13). Furthermore, the missing chromosome segment in the aniridia–Wilms' tumor syndrome may again vary in length at both ends of band p13 (39).

The number of consistent chromosomal deletions found in association with specific human neoplasias is growing very rapidly, particularly among the carcinomas. As shown in Table 1, of the neoplasias known to have a consistent chromosome defect, most of the carcinomas carry a deletion, whereas the majority of leukemias and lymphomas have a reciprocal translocation. Recently, a deletion 11p13 has been found in a few cases of nonconstitutional Wilms' tumor (41). All these findings together strongly suggest that a loss of genetic function (regulatory sequence?) is central to the development of some types of neoplasia.

The mechanism of carcinogenesis involved in malignancies with a reciprocal translocation may or may not basically differ from those for chromosomal deletion. The consistency of the breakpoints involved suggests that a given DNA-site ("cancer gene") may be altered during the translocation process (3). As mentioned earlier, in the high-grade malignancy known as Burkitt's lymphoma, most cases have a translocation 8;14 with breakpoints at sub-bands q24.1 and q32.3, respectively (31). In follicular small cleaved cell lymphoma, a low-grade malignancy, most cases show a translocation 18;14 with breakpoints at sub-bands q21.3 and 32.3, respectively (26). The finding of different donor chromosomes (chromosome 8 or 18) and a common receptor chromosome (chromosome 14) in these two completely different lymphomas suggests that the donor chromosome site is critical to the development of a specific type of neoplasia (*3, 26*). Yet, the consistency of the breakpoint (sub-band q32.3) in the receptor chromosome 14 (14q+ marker chromosome) suggests that such a site may have a functional advantage (*49*). The very recent localization of the heavy-chain genes to this same band (*50*) raises the intriguing possibility that the 14q+ marker chromosome is related to the rearrangement of DNA coding for immunoglobulin heavy chain that occurs during normal differentiation of lymphoid cells (*51, 52*).

Presumably, a donor chromosome may carry a cancer gene sequence at its breakpoint site and, when placed next to a promotor (such as the ones involved in immunoglobulin production), may initiate a given type of lymphoma. Alternatively, a cancer gene may become inactivated when translocated to certain specific sites in the genome, as could happen when a transposon moves to a new site and turns off a neighboring gene (*53*).

Techniques for Studying Chromosomes

The use of standard chromosome banding techniques (150–300 bands per haploid set) has shown that approximately 50% of the patients with ANLL and acute lymphocytic leukemia (*46, 54, 55*), 95% of the patients with chronic myelogenous leukemia (*56*), 95% of the patients with non-Hodgkin's lymphomas (*57*), and approximately 70% of all carcinomas (*54, 55*) have a chromosomal defect. Using our high-resolution chromosome techniques (400–1000 bands per haploid set) (*17, 26, 58*), we have found that 98% of all patients studied with either newly diagnosed or previously treated malignancy have a chromosome defect; this includes 24 cases of chronic myelogenous leukemia, 44 of ANLL, 13 of acute lymphocytic leukemia, 45 with non-Hodgkin's non-Burkitt's lymphoma, and 23 with solid tumors, including cancer of the vulva, cervix, ovary, breast, colon, esophagus, and lung (*3, 17, 26, 58*).

With our technique, we use a very short-term culture of tumor cells (3–5 h for leukemias and lymphomas, seven days for solid tumors), synchronizing cells with methotrexate (10^{-7} mol/L) for 17 h, and briefly exposing the culture to Colcemid (demecolcine), 50 ng/mL, for 10 min (*17, 26, 58*). Because of the increased chromosome resolution and partial selectivity for dividing tumor cells

(*59*), the methotrexate cell synchronization allows identification of previously undetectable chromosomal defects and a much better definition of the breakpoints involved in the observed chromosomal rearrangements. The new chromosome defects found in the subgroups of leukemia and lymphoma, as well as in the constitutional neoplasias listed in Table 1, which includes approximately one-third of all disorders to date, were obtained with the use of the new chromosome technology.

In addition, the sub-band breakpoints in various malignancies have been defined. For example, using prophasic and prometaphasic chromosomes (1200- and 850-band stages, respectively), we have defined the breakpoint in 11 patients of chronic myelogenous leukemia at the level of the Giemsa-negative sub-band 22q11.21 (*3*). Also, in two patients with Burkitt's lymphoma, the breakpoint in the donor chromosome 8 was found to be at sub-band q24.13 (*3*). In neither disease was evidence found for position effect, chromosomal loss, or amplification of chromosomal material, and the translocations were found to be reciprocal (*70*).

Thus far, all neoplasias studied at diagnosis with the high-resolution technology have a chromosome defect; among leukemias and lymphomas, two-thirds of the cases have one of the recurrent abnormalities shown in Table 1 (*17, 26, 59,* and unpublished data). One of the important problems remaining is the lack of direct evidence that the consistent chromosomal defects found in a given neoplasia precede the development of the malignancy and are indeed the initiating event of the neoplastic process. The finding of consistent chromosomal defects preceding the development of neoplasia should favor the concept of causation. Thus far, a deletion of 5q and (or) 7q has been found in some preleukemic patients who later developed ANLL (*60,* and unpublished data). Also, a few patients have had a t(9;22) before the development of a clear clinical picture of chronic myelogenous leukemia (*61–63*), suggesting that perhaps this alteration allows the precancerous stem cell to divide without restraint and eventually colonize most of the marrow.

A second problem relates to the lack of information of what percentage of neoplasias have a *consistent* chromosomal defect rather than just *some* type of chromosome defect. For example, although most cases of chronic myelogenous leukemia and Burkitt's lymphoma have a t(9;22) and t(8;14), respectively, most ANLL-M2 patients have chromosomal abnormalities but do not show a t(8;21). There are several possible explanations for this: (a) the same gene loci may be affected but not visible under the microscope or with currently available techniques; (b) new chromosomal subgroups may emerge when refined large-scale studies are performed; and (c) some neoplasias may arise by different mechanisms, including multiple "permissive" chromosomal sites.

With regard to the first possibility, recent findings indicate that when the standard direct bone marrow technique is used, non-leukemic cells may be found dividing preferentially so that some leukemias may falsely show a "normal" chromosome constitution. In the ANLL-M3 subgroup, for example, only about half of all reported cases show a t(15;17), and there is a differential geographic distribution for t(15;17)-positive and -negative cases (3, 64). With a short-term culture and cell synchronization we found that seven out of seven cases were t(15;17)-positive, while direct preparations showed three cases to have normal chromosomes (3, 59, and unpublished data). This may result from a preferential division of erythroblasts in direct preparations, whereas leukemic granulocytes could be the major dividing population in culture (65). Also, because of the tendency of M3 chromosomes to be contracted and poorly banded with standard techniques, the translocation t(15;17) may go unnoticed without the use of cell synchronization and high-resolution chromosome analysis.

It has been generally assumed that some, if not most, neoplasias should not show a primary chromosome defect, because a carcinogen may act at the submicroscopic level. Although this still remains a possibility, growing evidence indicates that a sizeable fraction of human neoplasias have a clonal and stable proliferation of a consistent chromosome defect (often a deletion or translocation); it is equally possible that carcinogens may initiate neoplasia through reorganization of genetic material rather than through point mutation (53, 66).

The very recent application of high-resolution chromosome analysis to the study of neoplasia has already uncovered subtle defects not previously detected (17). Also, with the aid of careful histopathologic and immunologic studies, several previously unrecognized chromosomal-histopathologic subgroups have been uncovered in non-Hodgkin's non-Burkitt's lymphoma (26) (Table 1). This strongly suggests that new, chromosomally distinct subgroups of neoplasias will continue to emerge.

Secondary Chromosomal Defects

Besides a few dozen "cancer-gene" sites suggested by the study of cancer families (2) and by chromosome studies (3), there may be additional multiple "permissive" sites in the genome that could potentiate, if not initiate, a malignant process. This idea gains credence from the existence of nonrandom yet "nonspecific" chromosomal changes often found in various malignancies, which may confer a general proliferative advantage to the tumor cell. For example, a trisomy 8 can be found singly or in association with other chromosomal abnormalities in the various subgroups of ANLL (M1, M2, M4–M6); an isochromosome 17q or a trisomy 8 is often found during the terminal or blast crisis of chronic myelogenous leukemia (55); singly or in combination, a del 6q or 17p, and trisomy 3, 7, and 12 are found associated with a t(14;18) in patients with "transformed" follicular small-cell lymphoma, and in follicular mixed and follicular large-cell lymphoma (26); a del 6q is not uncommon in various types of lymphoma (57); and finally, a duplication 1q25q32 is often seen among patients with preleukemia, ANLL, non-Hodgkin's lymphoma, breast carcinoma, cancer of the colon, melanoma, cervical carcinoma, and myeloma (67–69).

Prognosis and Treatment

Aside from its increasing importance in understanding neoplasia, the study of chromosomes is proving to be of value in determining prognosis and in selecting therapy for patients with hemato- and lymphopoietic neoplasias. For example, we recently found that most patients with follicular small cleaved-cell lymphoma have a balanced translocation t(14;18) (26). If this is the only chromosome defect demonstrable, the prognosis is much better than if there are associated chromosome defects (5–7 years' survival vs 1–2 years). Also, chromosome analysis is particularly important in patients with acute lymphocytic leukemia because, although many of these patients can be cured, those with a translocation 4;11, 8;14, or 9;22 generally live only a few months unless they are treated by bone marrow transplantation (3).

Supported in part by grants GM-26800, CA 31024, and CA 33314 from the National Institutes of Health.

References

1. Knudson, A. G., Genetics and cancer. In *Cancer: Achievements, Challenges and Prospects for the 1980's*, **1**, J. H. Burchenal and H. F. Oettgen, Eds., Grune and Stratton, New York, NY, 1981, pp 381–396.
2. Mulvihill, J. J., Miller, R. W., and Fraumeni, J. F., *Genetics of Human Cancer*, Raven Press, New York, NY, 1977.
3. Yunis, J. J., Specific fine chromosomal defects in cancer: An overview. *Hum. Pathol.* **12**, 503–514 (1981).
4. Rowley, J. D., A new consistent chromosomal abnormality in chronic myelogenous leukemia identified by quinacrine fluorescence and Giemsa staining. *Nature* **243**, 290–293 (1973).
5. Gahrton, G., Zech, L., and Lindsten, J., A new variant translocation (19q+,22q−) in chronic myelocytic leukemia. *Exp. Cell Res.* **86**, 214–216 (1976).
6. Bottura, C., and Coutinho, V., G/G translocation and chronic myelocytic leukaemia. *Blut* **29**, 216–218 (1974).
7. van den Berghe, H., David, G., Michaux, J. L., Sokal, G., and Verwilghen, R., 5q-acute myelogenous leukemia. *Blood* **48**, 624–626 (1976).
8. Oshimura, M., Freeman, A. J., and Sandburg, A. A., Chromosomes and causation of human cancer and leukemia. XXVI. Banding studies in acute lymphoblastic leukemia (ALL). *Cancer* **40**, 1161–1172 (1977).
9. Borgström, G. H., Teerenhovi, L., Vuopio, P., de la Chapelle, A., van den Berghe, H., Brandt, L., Golomb, H., Lauwagie, A., Mitelman, F., Rowley, J., and Sandberg, A. A., Clinical implications of 7 monosomy in acute non-lymphocytic leukemia: A cytogenetical and clinical study. *Cancer Genet. Cytogenet.* **2**, 115–126 (1980).
10. Bloomfield, C. D., Peterson, L. C., Yunis, J. J., and Brunning, R. D., The Philadelphia chromosome (Ph¹) in adults presenting with acute leukemia: A comparison of Ph¹+ and Ph¹− patients. *Br. J. Haematol.* **36**, 347–358 (1977).
11. Bloomfield, C. D., Lindquist, L. L., Brunning, R. D., Yunis, J. J., and Coccia, P. F., The Philadelphia chromosome in acute leukemia. *Virchows Arch. Cell Pathol.* **29**, 81–91 (1978).
12. Whang-Peng, J., Henderson, E. S., Knutsen, T., Freireich, E. J., and Gart, J. S., Cytogenetic stain in acute myelocytic leukemia with spe-

cial emphasis on the occurrence of the Ph[1] chromosome. *Blood* **36**, 448–457 (1970).
13. Rowley, J. D., Identification of a translocation with quinacrine fluorescence in a patient with acute leukemia. *Ann. Genet. (Paris)* **16**, 109–112 (1973).
14. Kamada, N., Okada, K., Oguma, N., Tanaka, R., Mikami, J., and Uchino, H., C–G translocation in acute myelocytic leukemia with low neutrophil alkaline phosphatase activity. *Cancer* **37**, 2380–2387 (1976).
15. Golomb, H. M., Rowley, J. D., Vardiman, J., Baron, J., Locker, G., and Krasnow, S., Partial deletion of the long arm of chromosome 17. *Arch. Intern. Med.* **136**, 825–828 (1976).
16. Rowley, J. D., Golomb, H. M., Vardiman, J., Fukuhara, S., Dougherty, C., and Potter, D., Further evidence for a nonrandom chromosomal abnormality in acute promyelocytic leukemia. *Int. J. Cancer* **20**, 869–872 (1977).
17. Yunis, J. J., Bloomfield, C. D., and Ensrud, K., All patients with acute nonlymphocytic leukemia may have a chromosomal defect. *N. Engl. J. Med.* **305**, 135–139 (1981).
18. Rowley, J. D., and Potter, D., Chromosomal banding patterns in acute lymphocytic leukemia. *Blood* **47**, 705–721 (1976).
19. Autio, K., Turunen, O., Penttilä, O., Eramma, E., de la Chappelle, A., and Schröer, J., Human chronic lymphocytic leukemia: Karyotypes in different lymphocyte populations. *Cancer Genet. Cytogenet.* **1**, 147–155 (1979).
20. Gharton, G., Robert, K. H., Friberg, K., Zech, L., and Bird, A. G., Extra chromosome 12 in chronic lymphocytic leukaemia. *Lancet* **i**, 146–147 (1980).
21. van den Berghe, H., David, G., Broeckaert-van Orshoven, A., Louwagie, A., Verwilghen, R., and Casteels, R., A new chromosome anomaly in acute lymphoblastic leukemia (ALL). *Hum. Genet.* **46**, 173–180 (1979).
22. Prigogina, E. L., Fleischman, E. W., Puchkova, G. P., Kulagina, O. E., Majakova, S. A., Salakirev, S. A., Frenkel, M. A., Khvatova, N. V., and Peterson, I. S., Chromosomes in acute leukemia. *Hum. Genet.* **53**, 5–16 (1979).
23. Propp, S., and Lizzi, F. A., Philadelphia chromosome in acute lymphocytic leukemia. *Blood* **36**, 353–360 (1970).
24. Berger, R., Bernheim, A., Brouet, J. C., Daniel, M. T., and Flandrin, G., t(8;14) translocation in a Burkitt's type of lymphoblastic leukemia (L3). *Br. J. Haematol.* **43**, 87–90 (1979).
25. Mitelman, F., Andersson-Anvret, M., Brandt, L., Catovsky, D., Klein, G., Manolov, G., Manolova, Y., Mark-Vendel, E., and Nilson,

P. G., Reciprocal 8;14 translocation in EBV-negative B-cell acute lymphocytic leukemia with Burkitt-type cells. *Int. J. Cancer* **24,** 27–33 (1979).
26. Yunis, J. J., Oken, M., Kaplan, M. E., Ensrud, K., Howe, R. R., and Theologides, A., Distinctive chromosomal abnormalities in histologic subtypes of non-Hodgkin's lymphoma. *N. Engl. J. Med.* **307,** 1231–1236 (1982).
27. Manolov, G., and Manolova, Y., Marker band in one chromosome 14 from Burkitt's lymphoma. *Nature* **237,** 33–34 (1972).
28. Zech, L., Haglund, U., Nilsson, K., and Klein, G., Characteristic chromosomal abnormalities in biopsies and lymphoid cell lines from patients with Burkitt and non-Burkitt lymphomas. *Int. J. Cancer* **17,** 47–56 (1976).
29 van de Berghe, H., Parloir, C., Gosseye, S., Englebienne, V., Cornu, G., and Sokal, G., Variant translocation in Burkitt lymphoma. *Cancer Genet. Cytogenet.* **1,** 9–14 (1979).
30. Berger, R., Bernheim, A., Bertrand, S., Fraisse, J., Frocrain, C., Tanzer, J., and Lenoir, G., Variant chromosomal t(8;22) translocation in four French cases with Burkitt lymphoma-leukemia. *Nouv. Rev. Fr. Hematol.* **23,** 39–41 (1981).
31. Manolova, Y., Manolov, G., Kieler, J., Levan, A., and Klein, G., Genesis of the 14q+ marker in Burkitt's lymphoma. *Hereditas* **90,** 5–10 (1979).
32. Brodeur, G. M., Sekhon, G. S., and Goldstein, M. N., Chromosomal aberrations in human neuroblastomas. *Cancer* **40,** 2256–2263 (1977).
33. Gilbert, F., and Balaban, G., The homogeneously staining region and double minutes in human neuroblastomas and retinoblastomas. In *Gene Amplification,* R. T. Schimke, Ed., Cold Spring Harbor Laboratory, NY, 1982, pp 185–191.
34. Wake, N., Hreshchyshyn, M. M., Piver, S. M., Matsui, S., and Sandberg, A. A., Specific cytogenetic changes in ovarian cancer involving chromosomes 6 and 14. *Cancer Res.* **40,** 4512–4518 (1980).
35. Mark, J., Dahlenfors, R., Ekedahl, C., and Stenman, G., The mixed salivary gland tumor—a normally benign human neoplasm frequently showing specific chromosomal abnormalities. *Cancer Genet. Cytogenet.* **2,** 231–241 (1980).
36. Whang-Peng, J., Kao-Shan, C. S., Lee, E. C., Bunn, P. A., Carney, D. N., Gazdar, A. F., and Minna, J. D., Specific chromosome defect associated with human small-cell lung cancer: Deletion 3p(14;23). *Science* **215,** 181–182 (1982).
37. Yunis, J. J., and Ramsay, N., Retinoblastoma and subband deletion of chromosome 13. *Am. J. Dis. Child.* **132,** 161–163 (1978).
38. Balaban-Malenbaum, G., Gilbert, F., Nichols, W. W., Hill, R.,

Shields, J., and Meadows, A. T., A deleted chromosome no. 13 in human retinoblastoma cells: Relevance to tumorigenesis. *Cancer Genet. Cytogenet.* **3**, 243–250 (1981).
39. Riccardi, V. M., Sujansky, E., Smith, A. C., and Francke, U., Chromosomal imbalance in the aniridia–Wilms' tumor association: 11p interstitial deletion. *Pediatrics* **61**, 604–610 (1978).
40. Yunis, J. J., and Ramsay, N., Familial occurrence of the aniridia–Wilms' tumor syndrome with deletion 11p13-14.1. *J. Pediatr.* **96**, 1027–1030 (1980).
41. Kaneko, Y., Egues, M. C., and Rowley, J. D., Interstitial deletion of short arm of chromosome 11 limited to Wilms' tumor cells in a patient without aniridia. *Cancer Res.* **41**, 4577–4578 (1981).
42. Zang, K. D., and Singer, H., Chromosomal constitution of meningiomas. *Nature* **216**, 84–85 (1967).
43. Mark, J., Karyotype patterns in human meningiomas. A comparison between studies with G- and Q-banding techniques. *Hereditas* **75**, 213–220 (1973).
44. Zankl, H., and Zang, K. D., Cytological and cytogenetical studies on brain tumors. IV. Identification of the missing G chromosome in human meningiomas as no. 22 by fluorescence technique. *Hum. Genet.* **14**, 167–169 (1972).
45. Bennett, J. M., Catovsky, D., Daniel, M. T., Flandrin, G., Galton, D. A. G., Gralnick, H. R., and Sultan, C., Proposals for the classification of acute leukemias. *Br. J. Haematol.* **33**, 451–458 (1976).
46. Rowley, J. D., Chromosome changes in acute leukemia. *Br. J. Haematol.* **44**, 339–346 (1980).
47. Sparkes, R. S., Sparkes, M. C., Wilson, M. G., Towner, J. W., Benedict, W., Murphree, A. L., and Yunis, J. J., Regional assignment of genes for human esterase D and retinoblastoma to chromosome band 13q14. *Science* **208**, 1042–1044 (1980).
48. Junien, C., Turleau, C., de Grouchy, J., Said, R., Rethoré, M. O., Tenconi, R., and Dufier, J. L., Regional assignment of catalase (CAT) gene to band 11p13. Association with the aniridia–Wilms' tumor–gonadoblastoma (WAGR) complex. *Ann. Genet.* **23**, 165–168 (1980).
49. Kaiser-McCaw, B., Hecht, F., Harnden, D. G., and Teplitz, R. L., Somatic rearrangement of chromosome 14 in human lymphocytes. *Proc. Natl. Acad. Sci. USA* **72**, 2071–2075 (1975).
50. Kirsch, I. R., Morton, C. C., Nakahara, K., and Leder, P., Human Ig heavy chain genes mapped to a region of translocations in malignant B-lymphocytes. *Science* **216**, 301–303 (1982).
51. Brack, C., Hirama, A., Lenhard-Schueller, R., and Tonegawa, S., A complete immunoglobulin gene is created by somatic recombination. *Cell* **15**, 1–14 (1978).

52. Davis, M. M., Kim, S. K., and Hood, L. E., DNA sequences mediating class switching in α-immunoglobulins. *Science* **209,** 1360–1365 (1980).
53. Cairns, J., The origin of human cancers. *Nature* **289,** 353–357 (1981).
54. Mitelman, F., and Levan, G., Clustering of aberrations to specific chromosomes in human neoplasms. IV. A survey of 1,871 cases. *Hereditas* **95,** 79–139 (1981).
55. Sandberg, A. A., *The Chromosomes in Human Cancer and Leukemia,* Elsevier/North Holland Biomedical Press, Amsterdam, Netherlands, 1980.
56. Rowley, J. D., Ph[1]-positive leukemia, including chronic myelogenous leukemia. In *Clinics in Haematology,* G. D. Pennington, Ed., Saunders Co. Ltd., London, U.K., 1980, pp 55–86.
57. Rowley, J. D., and Fukuhara, S., Chromosome studies in non-Hodgkin's lymphomas. *Sem. Oncol.* **7,** 255–265 (1980).
58. Yunis, J. J., New chromosome techniques in the study of human neoplasia. *Hum. Pathol.* **12,** 540–549 (1981).
59. Yunis, J., Comparative analysis of high resolution chromosome techniques of leukemic bone marrows. *Cancer Genet. Cytogenet.* **7,** 43–50 (1982).
60. Nowell, P. C., Preleukemias. *Hum. Pathol.* **12,** 522–530 (1981).
61. Canellos, G. P., and Whang-Peng, J., Philadelphia chromosome-positive preleukemic state. *Lancet* **ii,** 1227–1229 (1972).
62. Baccarani, M., Zaccaria, A., and Tura, S., Philadelphia chromosome-positive preleukemic state. *Lancet* **ii,** 1094 (1973).
63. Verhest, A., and van Schoubroeck, F., Philadelphia chromosome-positive preleukemic state. *Lancet* **ii,** 1386 (1973). Letter.
64. Second International Workshop on Chromosomes in Leukemia (1979): Chromosomes in acute promyelocytic leukemia. *Cancer Genet. Cytogenet.* **2,** 103–107 (1980).
65. Berger, R., Bernheim, A., and Flandrin, G., Absence of chromosome abnormalities and acute leukemia: Relationships with normal bone marrow cells. *C. R. Acad. Sci.* [D] (*Paris*) **290,** 1557–1559 (1980).
66. Klein, G., The role of gene dosage and genetic transpositions in carcinogenesis. *Nature* **294,** 313–318 (1981).
67. Najfeld, V., Singer, J. V., James, M. C., and Fialkow, P. J., Trisomy of 1q in preleukaemia with progression to acute leukaemia. *Scand. J. Haematol.* **21,** 24–28 (1978).
68. Rowley, J. D., Abnormalities of chromosome no. 1: Significance in malignant transformation. *Virchows Arch. B Cell Pathol.* **20,** 139–144 (1978).
69. Slavutsky, I., Labal de Vinuesa, J., Dupont, J., Mondini, N., and Brieux de Salum, S., Abnormalities of chromosome no. 1: Two cases

with lymphocytic lymphomas. *Cancer Genet. Cytogenet.* **3,** 341–346 (1981).
70. Yunis, J., Most cancers may have a chromosome defect. In *Gene Amplification* (see ref. *33*), pp 297–305.

Discussion

Q: When you find a consistent chromosome defect in leukemia, what percentage of the cells have such an abnormality?

DR. YUNIS: The percentage of cells with a given chromosome defect may vary between 5 and 100%. In acute leukemias the percentage is often between 50 and 100%. In chronic or subacute leukemias it could be lower.

Q: Have you looked for chromosome defects in the known familial carcinomas?

DR. YUNIS: We have only studied familial retinoblastoma and Wilms' tumor and do not generally find a chromosomal abnormality in the patient's blood cells. However, a consistent chromosome defect has been found in the tumor cells of patients with these hereditary conditions. This suggests that in familial neoplasias a gene in one chromosome may be defective at the submicroscopic level (point mutation, deletion?) and the patient is born with a neoplastic predisposition. For the tumor to be initiated, the second gene in the homologous chromosome needs to be affected, and this may often occur through chromosomal rearrangement (e.g., chromosomal band deletion).

Q: At the end of your presentation, you talked about the possibility of finding chromosomal defects in patients with colon cancer, breast cancer, etc. What evidence is there to indicate that there are such changes in patients with colon cancer and, if there is evidence, which chromosomes are involved?

DR. YUNIS: An extra chromosome 14 has been found in some patients with polyp of the colon and we have found several abnormalities, including homogeneous staining regions, in three carcinomas of the colon. Most of our work in the solid tumor is just beginning. Thus far, we have preliminary analysis in 23 carcinomas, including tumors of the breast, esophagus, colon, ovary, and cervix and all have chromosomal abnormalities.

Q: With certain chemical carcinogens you can produce changes of DNA that can be shown to be transferrable by transfection. Can you show those changes with these chromosomal analytical techniques?

DR. YUNIS: This is an interesting question, but we have not done such a study. We have been working exclusively with tumor cells from primary human neoplasias.

Q: Might you predict that chromosomal defects that are induced by chemical carcinogens could also be induced by oncogenic viruses?

DR. YUNIS: Yes, this is possible and there is such evidence in some experimental animal neoplasias. In humans, however, we know very little about specific carcinogens. Smoking has been linked to small-cell carcinoma of the lung and a partial deletion of the short arm of a chromosome 3 has been found. Also, some chemical solvents, insecticides, and pesticides have been implicated in the etiology of acute nonlymphocytic leukemias, particularly cases associated with a partial or complete deletion of a chromosome 5 and (or) 7. To my knowledge, there is no definitive evidence of a clear-cut and direct viral etiology of neoplasia in humans.

Q: Can you give us a reference and a brief description of your cytogenetic techniques for solid tumor?

DR. YUNIS: Information on these techniques can be found in *Human Pathology* [ref. *58,* above]. Essentially what we do is finely mince the tumor tissue, disaggregate the cells with collagenase and DNAse II, and grow them on a fibroblast feeder layer. The culture medium is supplemented with various growth factors to stimulate tumor-cell division; within three to seven days, one can obtain a large number of tumor cells for chromosomal analysis.

A Role for DNA Repair Mechanisms in the Genetics of Aging

Kathleen Y. Hall

Throughout evolution, cellular systems have been subject to various environmental stresses that have the capacity to alter the structural integrity of their DNA. Potential DNA-damaging agents include such forces as ionizing radiation, ultraviolet radiation, heat, and pH changes as well as a growing number of chemical compounds—various pesticides, aflatoxins, asbestos, combustion products, and, probably most important, free radicals produced in the metabolism of oxygen. To meet the challenges of these environmental stresses, biological systems have evolved various enzymic mechanisms that enable them to repair or eliminate the structural genetic damage induced. Because of the central role played by DNA in the organization and metabolic events of the cell, the capacity to repair such damage is basic to cellular and tissue function and, of course, to the ability of an organism to withstand the consequences of environmental stress. Correctly repaired genetic damage has little or no effect on the biological function of a system, whereas unrepaired or misrepaired DNA can result in changes in the physiological processes of cell growth, division, transcription, DNA replication, cell death, mutation, and malignant transformation. More recently, DNA damage has also been implicated in several disease processes, including cancer, aging, arteriosclerosis, arthritis, and hypertension.

Cells and organisms that are unable to repair DNA damage at a rate considered normal are more sensitive than normal cells to the effects of agents producing such damage. Several genetic syndromes are characterized by both a predisposition to various degenerative diseases, presumably mutagen based, and a deficiency in one or more facets of the DNA repair processes. Unrepaired or misrepaired DNA damage is now implicated as a causative factor in the manifestation of disease in such genetic syndromes as xeroderma pigmentosum, ataxia telangiectasia, Down's syndrome, systemic lupus erythematosus, Fanconi's anemia, and various progeroid syndromes. Affected individuals all show a predisposition to various degenerative diseases, such as malignancies, chromosomal aberrations, or premature aging.

Xeroderma pigmentosum is characterized by hypersensitivity of the skin to solar radiation and a high incidence of multiple carcinomas. The predisposition to cancer among these individuals is inversely proportional to their ability to repair DNA damage induced by ultraviolet irradiation (1). Fanconi's anemia is characterized by a high incidence of chromosome breaks and neoplasms. Cells from these patients are deficient in the excision repair of ultraviolet-induced pyrimidine dimers (2, 3). Ataxia telangiectasia is also characterized by an increased frequency of cellular mutation and an increase in spontaneous chromosome instability along with cerebellar ataxia (4, 5). Cells from these patients are extremely sensitive to ionizing irradiation and appear to be defective in recognizing gamma-radiation-induced damage (6). Although researchers disagree (7), cells from progeria patients, who exhibit characteristics of premature aging, are proficient in the repair of ultraviolet-induced DNA damage (8) but reportedly defective in the repair of single-strand breaks (9, 10). Down's syndrome and systemic lupus erythematosus similarly display facets of premature aging, increased malignancies, or immune dysfunction while being deficient in one or more steps of DNA repair (11). Other clinical defects—lympholytic leukemia (12), actinic keratasis, epidermal skin cancer (13), epidermodysplasia verruciformis (a form of multiple skin cancers) (14), and high blood pressure (15, 16)—have also been associated with abnormal excision of ultraviolet- or chemical-induced DNA damage in cells from patients who exhibit such defects.

Direct evidence for a role of DNA damage and its corollary repair or lack of repair in carcinogenesis came from the work of Hart and Setlow (17), who showed that the direct enzymic photoreactivation (a form of DNA repair) of ultraviolet-induced dimers in the gynogenetic teleost *Poecilia formosa* results in a corresponding decrease in the resulting number of tumors induced by ultraviolet light. Kakunaga (*18*) demonstrated that the cellular transformation frequency after treatment with the chemical carcinogens 4-nitroquinoline-1-oxide and 3-methylcholanthrene decreases with increasing time for excision repair, that is, the time allowed before DNA replication.

DNA Repair Processes

There are four general categories of DNA repair in mammalian cells: (*a*) excision or pre-replication; (*b*) strand-break repair; (*c*) post-replication repair; and (*d*) photoreactivation. Except for the latter, each of these is composed of multiple pathways, some of which are more error-prone than others. The *excision repair process* is usually specific for major distortions within the DNA, including the pyrimidine dimer induced by ultraviolet radiation and many types of chemical adducts formed by covalent bonds to one or more of the nucleic acids. In its simplest form, excision repair involves the removal of damaged parental DNA by a complex of enzymes. The general process involves four basic steps: incision, excision, polymerization, and ligation. The recognition of the damaged site in the DNA is accomplished by an endonuclease or an N-glycosidase (*19, 20*). The N-glycosidases catalyze the hydrolysis of the N-glycosidic bonds of the damaged nucleotide residues, leaving an apurinic site that is then recognized by a specific apurinic endonuclease (*21*). Similarly, other endonucleases are somewhat specific for the types of damage they act on (*20*). The second step in the excision process involves an exonuclease that degrades denatured but not native DNA (*22, 23*). This degradation releases the damaged region as well as several other nucleotides, the number depending on the nature of the damage. In the third step in the excision-repair process, a DNA repair polymerase provides for the insertion of the correct nucleotide in the remaining gap by using the opposite DNA strand as a template (*20*). In the final step of the repair process, the newly synthesized DNA is sealed to the parental DNA by the action of the enzyme ligase (*2*). This last step could lead to mutation if the nicked DNA is resealed by ligase before the damaged segment has been completely removed (*24*).

Direct *strand breaks* in the DNA may arise from exposure of cells to certain chemicals or ionizing radiation, including gamma and x-ray. The majority of strand breaks initiated in vivo appear to be mediated by the hydroxyl radical produced by the metabolism of oxygen (20). Radical scavengers are known to significantly influence the number of breaks occurring (25). There is a correlation between the capacity of agents such as 4-nitroquinoline-1-oxide derivatives to induce DNA strand breaks and their corresponding carcinogenicity (26). Similarly, there is a correlation between strand breaks and oncogenic transformation in SV40 virus (27). However, the mechanisms by which strand breakage might lead to oncogenic transformation are unknown. These lesions are thought to be repaired by simple ligase action unless single strands adjacent to one another on opposite DNA strands break (a double-strand break); this usually results in cell death (20).

In *postreplication* repair, DNA has to be newly synthesized from damaged templates. This system is important in cells actively synthesizing DNA and in cells unable to excise all the damage before DNA synthesis. Depending on the mechanism, this repair process is thought to consist of either an error-free or an error-prone repair process involving a gap opposite the damaged-strand template, a recombinational event, and the subsequent insertion of nucleotides into the gap across from the new template (20).

The last now-known repair system, a process referred to as *photoreactivation*, involves a group of enzymes that are specific for the monomerization of ultraviolet-induced pyrimidine dimers (28). A photoreactivation enzyme binds to irradiated DNA at a cyclobutane-type pyrimidine dimer. In the presence of photoreactivating light (300–600 nm), the enzyme is activated, converting the dimer into two monomers (28). Activity of photoreactivation enzymes has been demonstrated in several lower eukaryotic systems; only recently, however, has this type of enzymic activity been reported in human cells (29–31).

The ability of an organism to maintain the fidelity of the genetic apparatus through one of these repair systems would decree, of course, the accuracy of protein synthesis and DNA replication and the mutation rate of a cell. The amount of cellular damage that can accrue depends not only on the repair rate, but also on the state of cell differentiation and the condensation of the chromatin, the location of the damage (i.e., in an actively transcribed or a nontranscribed gene), the redundancy of the damaged allele, and the nature of the damage. Similarly, the ability of a cell to modify the damaging agent through radical scavengers or other enzymes will modulate the effects of agents having the capacity to damage DNA.

Unrepaired damage along a DNA strand as a cell enters replication will result in either the induction of a post-replication repair process (whether error-free or error-prone) or a chromosome aberration. Specific DNA-repair processes are known to alter the frequency of mutations and chromosomal aberrations induced in diploid human cells (*32, 33*). Cells defective in DNA-repair capacity to various degrees sustain a greater incidence of chromosomal aberrations (*34*). Any resulting aberration will be somewhat specific for the type of DNA damage and the position of the cell in the mitotic cycle at the time of damage (*34*). The results of such deviations in chromosomal structure will, of course, differ between the somatic cells and the gametes. Changes in the somatic cell population, through cell death or variations in the genetic program, will increase the susceptibility of the individuals to environmental stress. Genetic changes in the gametes will result in an increased proportion of birth defects and a resulting variation in the human gene pool (i.e., the sum total of genes available in the reproductive cells of the population that will be transmitted to the next generation). The total estimated number of deleterious genes, designated as the genetic load of a population, varies according to the degrees of cellular exposure to potential DNA-damaging agents, of activation and scavenging, and of genetic repair. New mutations increase the genetic load, and a large-scale introduction of new mutations may eventually result in a generalized decrease in the reproductive capacity and overall viability of a species (*35*). Although mutations are the evolutionary substrate for change, the change may not be necessarily beneficial; conversely, the same mutation that might reduce the viability of a species living under one set of environmental conditions might be advantageous under another set. Consequently, although a low mutation rate is probably essential for the survival of the human species, any rapid increase will almost certainly result in an increased genetic burden, and a subsequent decrease in viability and increase in health care (*35*).

Maximum Life Spans of Species

DNA-repair potential has also been implicated in the determination of the maximum life span of a species. Species maximum life span (MLS), defined as that age attained by the longest-living survivor of the species, does not vary greatly under diverse environmental conditions—which suggests that the aging process may be dictated by a specific genetic program sometimes referred to as "longevity genes." Such genes might involve those alleles capable of activation or deactivation of potentially harmful compounds, the alleles involved in free-radical scavenging, those regulating DNA repair, and certain alleles of the immune system (36).

A role for cellular maintenance of the genetic material as one causative factor in the determination of MLS was first suggested as part of the somatic mutation theory of aging (37). The central concept of this theory implied the accumulation of cellular mutations, presumably arising from unrepaired or misrepaired DNA damage. Correct genetic fidelity would be related to proper cellular, tissue, and system function and therefore to the rate of aging of an organism. Hart and Setlow (38) demonstrated in several mammalian species a correlation between MLS and repair of ultraviolet-induced DNA damage in fibroblasts. For seven species, including shrews, mice, elephants, and humans, they found a linear relationship between the logarithm of species MLS and the amount of DNA repair, as measured by unscheduled DNA synthesis.[1] A similar correlation between repair and MLS was found in rodents (36) and in both fibroblasts and lymphocytes from several species of primates (39). The relationship of lifespan potential to the integrity of the DNA was also displayed in paramecia (40), when photoreactivation repair of ultraviolet-induced pyrimidine dimers resulted in a prolongation of life span. In addition, DNA repair has been implicated in the age-related increase in sensitivity of human lymphocytes to bleomycin (41) and in an age-related decrease in the capacity to repair ultraviolet-induced lesions of human lymphocytes (42). However, decreases in repair capacity with age would likely also involve the replicative potential of the cell population.

Interestingly, many genetic syndromes that show an increased disposition to malignancies and an increased rate of aging, in addition to a repair defect, also are implicated in one or more immune

---

[1] Unscheduled DNA synthesis is measured by the amount of tritiated thymidine incorporated into the DNA after exposure to a damaging agent during periods of the cell cycle when the cell is not normally synthesizing DNA.

deficiencies. Moreover, susceptibility to systemic lupus erythematosus is known to be related to certain alleles of the main histocompatibility complex (MHC), a genetic regulatory complex located in chromosome 6 in humans and chromosome 17 in mice and known to serve as the master regulatory system for thymic-dependent immunity. Genes within or linked to the MHC have been shown to influence MLS in rodents (43), and the MHC may also regulate the activities of mitochondrial superoxide dismutase (EC 1.15.1.1) (44) and cAMP (45), both of which may be involved in or altered by the aging process. Several diseases in humans and mice, particularly autoimmune diseases, correlate with certain alleles of the MHC (46). Preliminary evidence in mice [H-2 typed (NZB × CBA)F_2 hybrid progeny] demonstrates that DNA-repair capacity but not gamma-induced damage correlates with MLS and segregates with parental haptolytes of the MHC (36). Thus one or more genes within or linked to the MHC apparently influence at least one step of the excision repair process. Portraying the MHC as a "master gene," serving in some sort of regulatory capacity over repair, immune function, and several other enzymic pathways, is attractive because relatively few gene rearrangements would be necessary to account for the relatively wide range (some 50-fold) of MLS seen in mammalian species (47, 48). Within the hominid subgroup, MLS has approximately doubled within the last three million years, much of this increase coming in the last 100 000–200 000 years. This rate of increase in life span within a short evolutionary time may indicate that the actual aging process is governed by the gene products of a small number of genes. For example, the MLS for humans is slightly more than twice as long as for chimpanzees, yet the similarity in protein and DNA structure between the two species is very high. Hybridization assays between the DNA of chimpanzees and humans demonstrate that less than 0.6% of the total DNA fails to hybridize (48). In rodents, too, mutations of a single gene or a small number of linked genes affect longevity (43).

Ed. note: For another discussion along these lines, the reader is referred to a chapter in a previous volume of the Beckman series: Hart, R. W., and Stephens, R. E., The comparative biology of longevity-assurance mechanisms. In *Aging—Its Chemistry*, Proceedings of the Third Arnold O. Beckman Conference in Clinical Chemistry, A. A. Dietz, Ed., Am. Assoc. Clin. Chem., Washington DC, 1980, pp 259–276.

References

1. Cleaver, J. E., Defective repair replication of DNA in xeroderma pigmentosum. *Nature* **218**, 652–656 (1968).
2. Poon, P. K., O'Brien, R. L., and Parker, J. W., Defective DNA repair in Fanconi's anemia. *Nature* **250**, 223–225 (1974).
3. Remsen, J. R., and Cerutti, P. A., Deficiency of gamma-ray excision repair in skin fibroblasts from patients with Fanconi's anemia. *Proc. Natl. Acad. Sci. USA* **73**, 2419–2423 (1976).
4. Webb, T., Harnden, D. G., and Harding, M., The chromosome analysis and susceptibility to transformation by simian virus 40 of fibroblasts from ataxia-telangiectasia. *Cancer Res.* **37**, 997–1002 (1977).
5. Vincent, R. A., Jr., Fink, A. J., and Huang, P. C., Unscheduled DNA synthesis in cultured ataxia telangiectasia fibroblast-like cells. *Mutat. Res.* **72**, 245–249 (1980).
6. Paterson, M. C., Smith, B. P., Lohman, P. H. M., Anderson, A. K., and Fishman, L., Defective excision repair of gamma-ray damaged DNA human ataxia telangiectasia fibroblasts. *Nature* **260**, 444–447 (1976).
7. Regan, J. D., and Setlow, R. B., DNA repair in human progeroid cells. *Biochem. Biophys. Res. Commun.* **59**, 858–864 (1974).
8. Cleaver, J. E., DNA repair and radiation sensitivity in human (xeroderma pigmentosum) cells. *Int. J. Radiat. Biol.* **18**, 557–565 (1970).
9. Epstein, J., Williams, J. R., and Little, J. B., Rate of DNA repair in progeria and normal human fibroblasts. *Biochem. Biophys. Res. Commun.* **59**, 850–857 (1974).
10. Rainbow, A. J., and Howes, M., Decreased repair of gamma-ray damaged DNA in progeria. *Biochem. Biophys. Res. Commun.* **74**, 714–719 (1977).
11. Hall, K. Y., Gatti, R., and Walford, R. L., Excision repair of UV and gamma induced DNA damage in Down's syndrome and systemic lupus erythematosus. *National Congr. Gerontol.* Toronto, Canada, 1981.
12. Pero, R. W., Bryngelsson, C., and Brandt, L., Carcinogen-induced repair and binding in the DNA of chronic lymphocytic leukemic lymphocytes. *Cancer Lett.* **2**, 311–317 (1977).
13. Lambert, B., Ringborg, U., and Swanbeck, G., Ultraviolet-induced DNA repair synthesis in lymphocytes from patients with actinic keratosis. *Invest. Dermatol.* **67**, 594–598 (1976).
14. Hammar, H., Hammar, L., Lambert, L., and Ringborg, U., A case report including EM and DNA repair investigations in a dermatosis associated with multiple skin cancers: Epidermodysplasia verruciformis. *Acta Med. Scand.* **200**, 441–446 (1976).
15. Pero, R. W., Bryngelsson, C., Mitelman, F., Thulin, T., and Nordén,

A., High blood pressure related to carcinogen-induced unscheduled DNA synthesis, DNA carcinogen binding, and chromosomal aberrations in human lymphocytes. *Proc. Natl. Acad. Sci. USA* **73**, 2496–2500 (1976).
16. Thulin, T., Pero, R. W., Bryngelsson, C., Mitelman, F., Nordén, A., and Scherstén, B., Deoxyribonucleic acid repair synthesis: A new factor for defining high blood pressure. *Clin. Sci. Mol. Med.* **51**, 695s–696s (1976).
17. Hart, R. W., and Setlow, R. B., Direct evidence that pyrimidine dimers in DNA result in neoplastic transformation. In *Molecular Mechanisms for Repair of DNA,* P. C. Hanawalt and R. B. Setlow, Eds., Plenum Press, New York, NY, 1975, p 719.
18. Kakunaga, T., The role of cell division in the malignant transformation of mouse cells treated with 3-methylcholanthrene. *Cancer Res.* **35**, 1637–1642 (1975).
19. Ishiwata, K., and Oikawa, A., Actions of human DNA glycosylases on uracil-containing DNA, methylated DNA and their reconstituted chromatins. *Biochim. Biophys. Acta* **563**, 375–384 (1979).
20. Friedberg, E. C., Bonura, T., Reynolds, R. J., and Radany E. H., Some aspects of the enzymology of DNA repair. In *Progress and Environmental Mutagenesis,* M. Alacevic, Ed., Elsevier–North Holland Biomedical Press, Amsterdam, 1980, p 175.
21. Haseltine, W. A., Gordon, L. K., Lindan, C. P., Grafstrom, R. H., Shaper, N. L., and Grossman, L., Cleavage of pyrimidine dimers in specific DNA sequences by a pyrimidine dimer DNA-glycosylase of *M. luteus. Nature* **285**, 634–641 (1980).
22. Doniger, J., and Grossman, L., Human correxonuclease purification and properties of a DNA repair exonuclease from placenta. *Biol. Chem.* **251**, 4579–4587 (1976).
23. Kaplan, J. C., Kushner, S. R., and Grossman, L., Enzymatic repair of DNA and purification of two enzymes involved in excision of thymine dimers from ultraviolet-irradiated DNA. *Proc. Natl. Acad. Sci. USA* **63**, 144–151 (1969).
24. Seebury, E., and Rupp, W. D., Effect of mutations in lig and pre A on UV-induced strand cutting in a uvrC strain of *Escherichia coli.* In *Molecular Mechanisms for Repair of DNA* (see ref. *17*), pp 439–442.
25. Emerit, I., Levy, A., and de Vaux Saint Cyr, C., Chromosome damaging agent of low molecular weight in the serum of New Zealand Black mice. *Cytogenet. Cell Genet.* **26**, 41–48 (1980).
26. Kondo, S., Molecular biology of 4-nitroquinoline 1-oxide in the prokaryotic system. *Carcinog. Compr. Surv.* **6**, 47–64 (1981).
27. Blakeslee, J. R., Yohn, D. S., Milo, G. E., and Hart, R. W., Interaction between chemical carcinogens, oncogenic viruses and 17β-estradiol.

In *Comparative Leukemia Research 1975*, J. Climmesen and D. S. Yohn, Eds., Karger, Basel, 1976, pp 481–483.
28. Sutherland, B. M., and Oliver, R., Culture conditions affect photoreactivating enzyme levels in human fibroblasts. *Biochim. Biophys. Acta* **442**, 358–367 (1976).
29. Sutherland, B. M., Harber, L. C., and Kochevar, I. E., Pyrimidine dimer formation and repair in human skin. *Cancer Res.* **40**, 3181–3185 (1980).
30. Harm, H., Damage and repair in mammalian cells after exposure to nonionizing radiations. III. Ultraviolet and visible light irradiation of cells of placental mammals, including humans, and determination of photorepairable damage in vitro. *Mutat. Res.* **69**, 167–176 (1980).
31. Sutherland, B. M., Photoreactivating enzyme from human leukocytes. *Nature* **248**, 109–112 (1974).
32. McCormick, J. J., and Maher, V. M., DNA repair processes can alter the frequency of mutations induced in diploid human cells. *Basic Life Sci.* **15**, 315–321 (1980).
33. Parshad, R., Sanford, K. K., Jones, G. M., Tarone, R. E., Hoffman, H. A., and Grier, A. H., Susceptibility to fluorescent light-induced chromatid breaks associated with DNA repair deficiency and malignant transformation in culture. *Cancer Res.* **40**, 4415–4419 (1980).
34. Polani, P. E., DNA repair defects and chromosome instability disorders. *Ciba Found. Symp.* **66**, 81–131 (1979).
35. Hart, R. W., Hall, K. Y., and Daniel, F. B., DNA repair and mutagenesis in mammalian cells. *Photochem. Photobiol.* **28**, 131–155 (1978).
36. Hall, K. Y., Bergman, K., and Walford, R. L., DNA repair, H-2, and aging in NZB and CBA mice. *Tissue Antigens* **17**, 104–110 (1981).
37. Orgel, L. E., The maintenance of the accuracy of protein synthesis and its relevance to aging. *Proc. Natl. Acad. Sci. USA* **49**, 517–521 (1963).
38. Hart, R. W., and Setlow, R. B., Correlation between deoxyribonucleic acid excision-repair and life-span in a number of mammalian species. *Proc. Natl. Acad. Sci. USA* **71**, 2169–2173 (1974).
39. Hall, K. Y., Hart, R. W., Benirschke, A. K., and Walford, R. L., Correlation of repair of UV-induced DNA damage in primate lymphocytes and fibroblasts with maximum life span. *International Gerontological Meetings*, Hamburg, F.R.G., 1981.
40. Smith-Sonneborn, J., DNA repair and longevity assurance in *Paramecium tetraurelia*. *Science* **203**, 1115–1117 (1979).
41. Seshadri, R. S., Morley, A. A., Trainor, K. J., and Sorrell, J., Sensitivity of human lymphocytes to bleomycin increases with age. *Experientia* **35**, 233–234 (1979).
42. Lambert, B., Ringborg, U., and Skoog, L., Age-related decrease of

ultraviolet light-induced DNA repair synthesis in human peripheral leukocytes. *Cancer Res.* **39**, Part 1, 2792–2795 (1979).
43. Smith, G. S., and Walford, R. L., Influence of the main histocompatibility complex on ageing in mice. *Nature* **270**, 727–728 (1977).
44. Novak, R., Bosze, Z., Matkovics, B., and Fachet, J., Gene affecting superoxide dismutase activity linked to histocompatibility complex in H-2 congenic mice. *Science* **207**, 86–87 (1980).
45. Lafuse, W., Meruelo, D., and Edidin, M., The genetic control of liver cAMP levels in mice. *Immunogenetics* **9**, 57–65 (1979).
46. Gatti, R. A., and Walford, R. L., Immune function and features of aging in chromosomal instability syndromes. In *Immunological Aspects of Aging*, D. Segre and L. Smith, Eds., Marcel Dekker Inc., New York, NY, 1980.
47. Cutler, R. G., Evolution of longevity in primates. *J. Hum. Evol.* **5**, 169–202 (1976).
48. Cutler, R. G., Evolution of human longevity: A critical overview. *Mech. Ageing Dev.* **9**, 337–354 (1979).

Discussion

DR. FEDERALL: With this kind of research, it is desirable to use long-lived families, let's say, as compared with the general population of the short-lived family line. Would you expect to find some possible differences between these two kinds of experimental populations?

DR. HALL: It is very hard to do because, when you are testing an individual, you have only his background—you have no idea how long the individual is going to live. Because the assay itself is not as sensitive as we would like, we are not picking up any individual differences right now within a species. For instance, in many cancer-susceptible families, which I have been looking at with Dr. Gatti to try to detect a difference in DNA-repair potentials and cancer susceptibility of a family, there is no statistical evidence of individual variances. So, I would hesitate to extend the assay to anything like that.

In the studies with mice, I do not find any kind of age-related pattern for repair in the NZB. One interesting thing I am beginning to find is that the source of lymphocytes—for instance, from the spleen or from the thymus—shows a difference in repair even when selecting for only one cell population. That is a bit puzzling and I can only speculate that it is related to variations in the state of differentiation.

Molecular Approaches to Human Immune Functions and Disorders

Randolph Wall and Andrew Saxon

Structures of Immunoglobulin Molecules and Genes

Immunoglobulin molecules consist of two identical light chains and two identical heavy chains. Each chain is composed of a series of homologous domains: the variable (V) region, beginning at the NH_3 terminus, and the remainder, forming the constant (C) region. The V regions are responsible for antigen binding and may have thousands of different sequences. The C-regions, which embody the various effector functions of the molecule, have only a few alternative sequences. The various classes of immunoglobulins (IgM, IgD, IgG, IgE, IgA) have different biological functions and are distinguished by different heavy chains (μ, δ, γ, ϵ, α), as defined by their C regions (C_μ, C_δ, C_γ, C_ϵ, C_α). The light chains in an immunoglobulin molecule can be either κ or λ class (containing V regions and either C_λ or C_κ regions). For most immunoglobulin classes, the four-chain molecule is secreted as a monomer. However, IgM and IgA are also secreted as pentamers and dimers, respectively. Immunoglobulin molecules in these multimeric complexes are covalently linked to a J (or joining) chain molecule (reviewed in *1*).

The genetics and diversity of immunoglobulin genes have long fascinated molecular biologists. The application of the powerful techniques of cloning recombinant DNA and sequencing nucleic acids have generated a largely complete picture of the multiplicity, organization, and dynamics of immunoglobulin genes in the mouse. Immunoglobulin genes are "split genes" (*2*). The gene segments (exons) that code for the V-region and the C-region domains are separated from each other by noncoding DNA sequences (introns). These split gene segments, or exons, are joined together by RNA-splicing events, which generate functional immunoglobulin messenger RNAs (3). These striking features are not unique to immunoglobulin genes. It is now clear that most genes in higher organisms are organized into intron-separated exons, which are joined by RNA splicing.

Both the chromosomal location and the organization of the mouse immunoglobulin κ, λ, and heavy-chain gene clusters are now known (Figure 1). In the case of the heavy-chain gene cluster, a continuous stretch of DNA 200 kb (1 kb = 1 kilobase = 1000 base pairs) long on mouse chromosome 12 has been cloned, and a substantial portion of this large stretch of DNA has been sequenced (reviewed in 4). Immunoglobulin genes and the sequences flanking them may amount to as much as 1–2% of the mouse genome.

Active light- and heavy-chain genes are generated by somatic DNA rearrangements that join a germline light-chain V region to a J region or a heavy-chain V region to a D region and J region (5–7). This type of DNA rearrangement is called V-region formation because these combinatorial DNA events make complete V regions. The joining of multiple germline V- and J-region gene segments contributes significantly to the immense diversity of antibodies. Immunoglobulin heavy-chain genes undergo a second kind of DNA rearrangement ("class switching"), in which the rearranged V region is moved from the C_μ region and linked to another heavy-chain C region (5, 6, 8). This accounts for the transition from IgM to IgG, IgE, or IgA expression. These two types of DNA rearrangements in immunoglobulin genes are unique among the higher eukaryotic genes studied so far. The use of combinatorial DNA mechanisms for generating diversity is also unique among the eukaryotic genes studied.

Immunoglobulin messenger RNAs, like most mRNAs in eukaryotic cells, are generated from large nuclear RNA precursors by RNA-processing events, including RNA splicing. Generally, these RNA splicing and processing events are invariant and produce only a single RNA. However, variations in RNA splicing and processing play an important role in controlling the expression of immunoglobulin genes (3). Alternative mRNA splicing pathways produce secreted and membrane-receptor forms of immunoglobulin heavy-chain mRNAs from a single gene. More complex

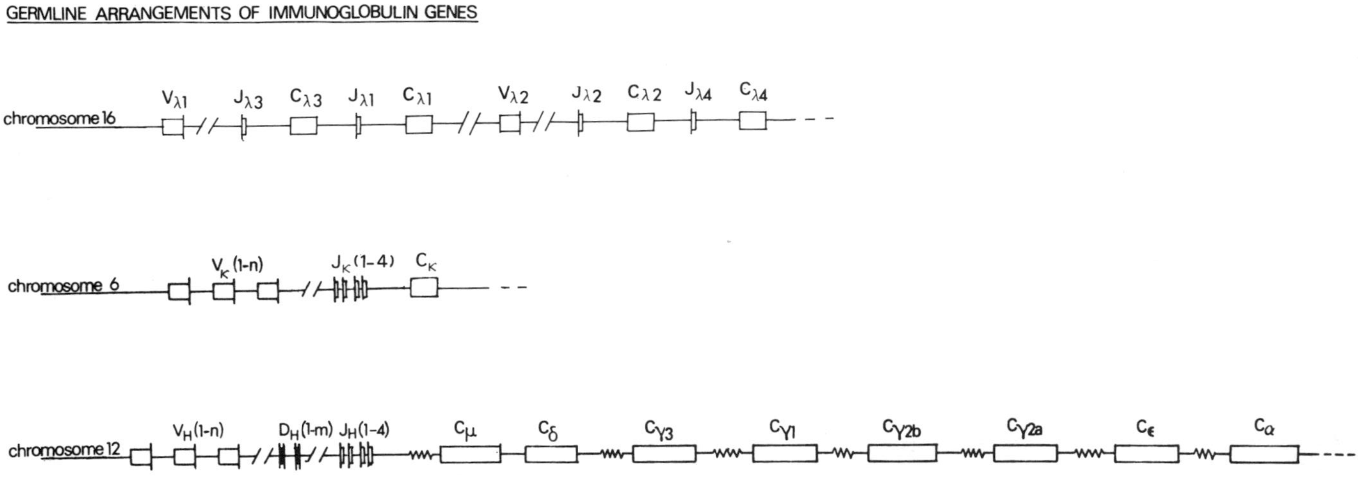

GERMLINE ARRANGEMENTS OF IMMUNOGLOBULIN GENES

Fig. 1. The germline arrangement and chromosomal location of immunoglobulin light- and heavy-chain gene segments in the mouse

pathways of RNA processing account for the co-expression of surface IgM and IgD in B lymphocytes (9). These RNA rearrangements greatly increase the versatility of immunoglobulin heavy-chain genes by generating alternative forms of mRNA. Significantly, these immunoglobulin RNA rearrangements are involved in the developmental regulation of immunoglobulin gene expression. Although such alternative patterns of RNA processing are known to exist for viral genes, immunoglobulin heavy-chain genes are the first cellular genes known to use such RNA rearrangements.

B Cell Development

Clearly, immunoglobulin genes exploit a variety of molecular mechanisms for regulating their expression. When do these DNA and RNA rearrangements occur in B cell development? Figure 2 shows a simplified scheme of B cell development, based on changes in immunoglobulin gene expression and delineated by the existence of tumor cell lines that correspond to each of these developmental steps (except the stem cell). The first cell showing immunoglobulin gene expression is the pre-B cell. These cells contain a rearranged μ gene (i.e., the C_μ-region gene segment has a rearranged V region in front of it) expressed as cytoplasmic μ heavy chains (3, 5, 6). The light-chain genes are not rearranged or detectably expressed in such pre-B cells. The next cell in this developmental scheme contains surface IgM composed of two μ chains and two identical light chains (which can be either two κ or λ light chains). Accordingly, the transition from the pre-B cell to the resting B cell occurs through rearrangement of the light-chain V region and activation of the light-chain gene.

The next developmental steps involve RNA rearrangements rather than DNA rearrangements (3, 9). Here B cells co-express μ and δ heavy chains bearing the same V region in surface IgM and IgD. When a specific antigen interacts with these surface immunoglobulin receptors, these B cells shift from the expression of membrane IgM and IgD to secretion of IgM.

The plasma cell stages in this simplified scheme of the immune response express and secrete the other classes of immunoglobulin (IgG, IgE, IgA). The transition of IgM secretion to the production of other immunoglobulin classes involves a "class switching" DNA rearrangement, in which the rearranged V region (first expressed with C_μ) is joined to another heavy-chain constant region

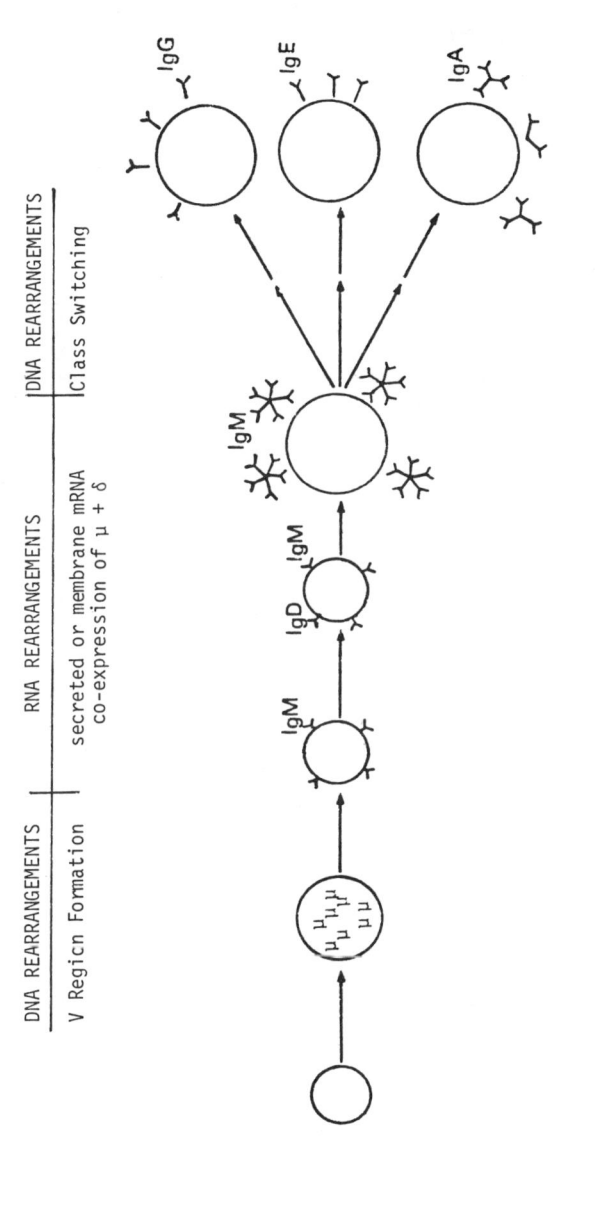

Fig. 2. A simplified scheme relating changes in immunoglobulin gene expression with B cell development stages in the mouse

(either C_γ, C_ϵ, or C_α). The mechanism for DNA rearrangements in class switchings appears to differ from that used in V-region formation (5, 6, 8).

Expression of Immune Deficiencies in Humans

Although knowledge of these events in immunoglobulin DNA and RNA rearrangement is derived from extensive studies in the mouse, the findings are directly extrapolatable to humans. All of the immunoglobulin gene structures described in the mouse are homologous to the human immunoglobulin genes studied. Humoral immune defects in humans offer a wide array of potential immunoglobulin gene defects that can further resolve the events in B cell development. Figure 3 shows our simple scheme for B cell differentiation, incorporating postulated blocks in gene expression that reflect structural defects in human immunoglobulin genes in selected immune deficiencies. This scheme is a highly simplified view of immune deficiencies in humans. Clearly, human immune deficiencies are complex in expression and can vary widely from one patient to the next. Many apparent defects in immunoglobulin gene expression appear not to result from structural alterations in the heavy- or light-chain genes, but rather from the inability of the B cell to respond to outside environmental factors (e.g., T cell help) or to altered external influences (e.g., enhanced T suppressor cell activity) (10).

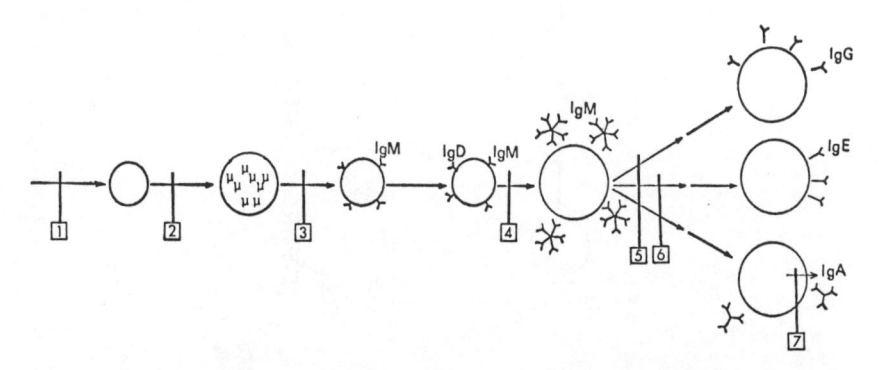

Fig. 3. A simplified scheme of some human B cell immunodeficiencies: 1, some cases of severe combined immunodeficiencies; 2, hypogammaglobulinemia with thymoma; 3, X-linked agammaglobulinemia; 4, common variable hypogammaglobulinemia; 5, immunodeficiency with increased IgM; 6, ataxia telangiectasia; and 7, IgA deficiency

Diseases of the Immune System

Certain disease states seem likely to reflect defects or changes in the immunoglobulin genes rather than regulatory defects in lymphoid cell interactions. For example, some infants with severe combined immunodeficiency apparently lack B cells, probably because of an absence of the stem cells for lymphoid development. Other children with the same syndrome may be blocked in the T cell functions that are required for B cell maturation from stem cells.

Another human immune deficiency state that may reflect a structural alteration in an immunoglobulin gene is hypogammaglobulinemia associated with thymoma. It is not clear to what extent or how the thymic tumor affects the clinical picture. These patients fail to exhibit pre-B cells with cytoplasmic μ chains and lack circulating mature B lymphocytes or plasma cells. Here there seems to be a clear failure of the B stem cells to rearrange the V region and, accordingly, failure to generate an active μ gene. These cells may never be able to start the whole process of B cell development.

The next stage of B cell development that correlates with a human B cell immunodeficiency is exemplified in X-linked agammaglobulinemia. The patients are young boys who have normal bone marrow pre-B cells characterized by the presence of large amounts of cytoplasmic μ chains without any light chains; yet B cells with surface IgM are conspicuously absent from their circulation (11). Here the defect in B cell differentiation appears to be a failure to rearrange light-chain genes (κ or λ) to generate complete IgM molecules—perhaps the result of either an aberrant rearrangement of the light-chain genes or even no functional rearrangement of the light-chain genes at all. In at least one case of X-linked agammaglobulinemia, the pre-B cells contain a rearranged and expressed μ gene as well as an aberrantly rearranged light-chain gene that does not make functional RNA or functional light chains (12).

We would predict that other types of hypogammaglobulinemia (dysgammaglobulinemia type I), where the patients have low concentrations of serum IgG and IgA with increased IgM, may result from a block in "class switching" of DNA. These immunodeficiencies are often associated with increased quantities of secreted IgM, possibly as a compensatory mechanism for the small quantities of IgG and IgA secreted in these patients. These cells may have defective "switch" sequences in front of the C_μ gene, so that they can only infrequently switch to the other isotypes and produce plasma cells secreting IgE, IgG, or IgA.

On the other hand, most cases of common variable hypogammaglobulinemia possess normal numbers of circulating B cells but fail to make normal amounts of all immunoglobulin classes. These patients' B cells cannot be activated toward immunoglobulin secretion by in vivo immunization or in vitro stimulation (13). A generalized failure to undergo appropriate RNA splicing for the generation of secreted immunoglobulin mRNAs could potentially account for this problem.

Ataxia telangiectasia is an interesting immunodeficiency syndrome characterized by IgA and IgE deficiency in many patients. Preliminary gene-mapping studies indicate that DNA from ataxia lymphoid cell lines contains apparently normal C_α genes (Taylor, Saxon, and Wall, unpublished results); thus, the failure to express IgA is not due to a deletion or gross alteration of the C_α and (and presumably D_ϵ) genes. We conclude that class switching to C_α (or to certain C_γ subclass) genes does not occur normally, and thus does not activate subsequent IgE and IgA expression.

Selective IgA deficiency is the most common human B cell immunodeficiency, affecting about one in 600 individuals. In vivo, it is characterized by failure of IgA secretion; in vitro, plasma-like cells containing IgA appear after mitogen stimulation but fail to secrete that IgA (14). Structural gene defects affecting IgA secretion could cause IgA deficiency. For instance, alteration of the secretory carboxyl-terminal region so that it cannot react with the J chain (which is required in the secretion of IgM and IgA) should selectively prevent the secretion of IgA. Similarly, glycosylation being required for immunoglobulin secretion, structural gene changes that alter or eliminate glycosylation sites on alpha-chains could block IgA secretion.

Closing Remarks

In this dawning era of genetic engineering, what are the prospects of introducing immunoglobulin genes into immune-deficient lymphoid cells and reconstituting immune-deficient individuals with cells carrying functional immunoglobulin genes? At present we feel that reliable, successful approaches for immunoglobulin gene replacement for correcting any of these immunodeficiencies are fairly far in the future. However, we are optimistic that the molecular approaches outlined here, in which we used gene mapping and gene cloning to define the molecular basis of certain B cell immune defects, represent an important and logical first step towards treating immune defects with gene therapy.

The authors acknowledge support from NIH grants CA12800, AI15251, AI16644, and AI12410. A.S. is the recipient of Allergic Diseases Academic Award, AI00326.

References

1. McHugh, Y., Yagi, M., and Koshland, M. E., In *B Lymphocytes in the Immune Response: Functional, Developmental, and Interpretative Properties.* N. Klinman, D. Mosier, I. Scher, and E. Vitetta, Eds., Elsevier/North Holland, New York, NY, 1981, pp 467–474.
2. Sanko, H., Rogers, J. H., Hüppi, K., Brack, C., Traunecker, A., Maki, R., Wall, R., and Tonegawa, S., Domains and the hinge region of an immunoglobulin heavy chain are encoded in separate DNA segments. *Nature* **277,** 627–633 (1979).
3. Wall, R., Choi, E., Carter, C., Kuehl, M., and Rogers, J., RNA processing in immunoglobulin gene expression. *Cold Spring Harbor Symp. Quant. Biol.* **45,** Pt. 2, 879–885 (1980).
4. Shimizu, A., Takehashi, N., Yaoita, Y., and Honjo, T., Organization of the constant-region gene family of the mouse immunoglobulin heavy chain. *Cell* **28,** 499–506 (1982).
5. Hood, L., Davis, M., Early, P., Calame, K., Kim, S., Crews, S., and Huang, H., Two types of DNA rearrangements in immunoglobulin genes. *Cold Spring Harbor Symp. Quant. Biol.* **45,** Pt. 2, 887–898 (1980).
6. Tonegawa, S., Sakano, H., Maki, R., Traunecker, A., Heinrich, G., Roeder, W., and Kurosawa, Y., Somatic reorganization of the immunoglobulin genes during lymphocyte differentiation. *Cold Spring Harbor Symp. Quant. Biol.* **45,** Pt. 2, 839–858 (1980).
7. Leder, P., Max, E. E., Seidman, J. G., Kwan, S. P., Scharff, M., Nau, M., and Norman, B., Recombination events that activate, diversify, and delete immunoglobulin genes. *Cold Spring Harbor Symp. Quant. Biol.* **45,** Pt. 2, 859–865 (1980).
8. Honjo, T., Kataoka, T., Yaoita, Y., Shimizu, A., Tukahashi, N., Yama-

waki-Kataoka, Y., Nikaido, T., Nakai, S., Obata, M., Kawakami, T., and Nishida, Y., Organization and reorganization of immunoglobulin heavy-chain genes. *Cold Spring Harbor Symp. Quant. Biol.* **45**, Pt. 2, 913–923 (1980).
9. Moore, K. W., Rogers, J., Hunkapiller, T., Early, P., Nottenburg, C., Weisman, I., Bazin, H., Wall, R., and Hood, L. E., Expression of IgD may use both DNA rearrangement and RNA splicing mechanisms. *Proc. Natl. Acad. Sci. USA* **78**, 1800–1804 (1981).
10. Waldmann, T. A., Blaese, R. M., Broder, S., and Krakauer, R. S., Disorders of suppressor immuno regulatory cells in the pathogenesis of immunodeficiency and autoimmunity. *Ann. Intern. Med.* **88**, 226–238 (1978).
11. Geha, R. S., Rosen, F. S., and Merler, E., Identification and characterization of the subpopulations of lymphocytes in human peripheral blood after fractionation on discontinuous gradients on albumin. The cellular defect in X-linked agammaglobulinemia. *J. Clin. Invest.* **52**, 1726–1734 (1973).
12. Cooper, M. D., Pre-B cells: Normal and abnormal development. *J. Clin. Immunol.* **1**, 81–89 (1981).
13. Ashman, R. F., Saxon, A., and Stevens, R. H., Profile of multiple lymphocyte functional defects in acquired hypogammaglobulinemia derived from in vitro cell recombination analysis. *J. Allergy Clin. Immunol.* **65**, 242–256 (1980).
14. Schwartz, S. A., Heavy chain-specific suppression of immunoglobulin synthesis and secretion by lymphocytes from patients with selective IgA deficiency. *J. Immunol.* **124**, 2034–2041 (1980).

Discussion

Q: Immunoglobulin (Ig) myelomas are much less frequent than the other type of myeloma. Would you comment on whether this is geared to a defect of switching of the B region, or to RNA splicing? What are the causes?

DR. WALL: We do not know why different isotypes in myelomas arise. I have no idea why Ig myelomas are found so rarely. Certainly, in the case of humans, the classical myeloma, which makes IgE, is a very good myeloma. The frequency at which various isotypes show up when you look at mice and humans is very different. What you are talking about may be something that is species related. I do not think it is related to the frequency with which the switching occurs, but that could be a possibility. I do not think RNA splicing is involved.

DR. GATTI: Regarding the congenital agammaglobulinemia abnormality, have you any idea how an X-linked disease would produce a problem on chromosomes?

DR. WALL: I do not, and in fact, all of these syndromes, such as ataxia talangiectasia, are characterized by many kinds of chromosomal aberrations, none of which seem necessarily to be involved with the chromosome on which the heavy chains are located. I do not know how that particular situation works. Certainly, in severe combined immunodeficiency, high concentrations of adenosine may, in fact, be inhibitory; in that case, you can consider that the enzyme has a secondary effect. In the case of X-linked congenital agammaglobulinemia, I have no idea. It may be a broader syndrome, which may or may not be related to the immunoglobulin gene. I do not think there are any known regulatory genes or immunoglobulins located on the X chromosomes.

DR. GATTI: It would have to be something like that, would it not? You have demonstrated an abnormality in this CH gene-reading pattern, which we know is an X-linked disorder; so are you saying there must be two genetic defects?

DR. WALL: To go back to ataxia telangiectasia, these are all syndromes with many different defects. It may well be that this could be a translocation that affects two different places. I think it has to be at least two genes, because I do not really see any way in which immune-response genes could be associated with the X chromosome.

Q: Consider again the patients with X-linked infantile agammaglobulinemia: When you culture the cells from the bone marrow, you get pre-B cells, that is, those that have Epstein–Barr virus receptors and produce no immunoglobulin genes; you get some that produce just μ molecules in the cytoplasm; some that produce uncoupled light chains and μ chains; and some that have the intact monomeric IgM molecule. Now, each of these has Epstein–Barr virus. You can culture the cells from these patients very easily. Do any of your molecular biology explanations help us understand those several kinds of cell lines that we can get from these patients? It looks to us as though there are steps in development of the pre-B cell.

DR. WALL: Absolutely. In fact, I simplified this, even when I talked about the mouse system. If you look at certain pre-B cells or, if, in fact, you keep pre-B cells in culture in the mouse for a long time, like Ableson virus transplant cells, some will become monomeric IgM producers although they tend to secrete it and not put it in the membrane. If the cells do put it in the membrane, they have a rearranged light-chain gene. You could probably stage these types by whether you have a rearrangement of, first, a μ gene, or, occasionally, a rearrangement of a light-chain gene where you bypass a rearrangement of a μ gene. We see those occasionally in the mouse. Rather infrequently you would have a subsequent stage where you have rearranged both the light-chain gene and the μ gene and you are making light chains. In some instances, there may be rearranged or apparently rearranged light-chain and μ-chain genes, but these for some reason do not associate, and so may be defective. That would be the molecular explanation I would put on these observations. It is a very interesting cell, because you can get more stages of these presumptive pre-B cell steps than you can in mice, where you can only obtain a μ- or a μ- plus light-chain stage.

Q: When you were talking about the transmembrane hydrophobic segments that make membrane-bound immunoglobulins on the heavy chains being about 90% normal, is that species specific, or is it cross species?

DR. WALL: When you map human and mouse genes by hybridizing the genes together, so-called heteroduplex, the membrane regions in the mouse gene hybridize just as strongly as the domains with what is presumptively the membrane region in the human gene. All we know in the mouse gene is that genes that are only 50% homologous with the rest of the genes have more than 90% homology in this membrane region, leading to the model that I propose is necessary for proper insertion in the membrane. I presume that this high homology—it is not just homology; it is sequence conservation—probably would show up in human genes as well.

Q: What diagnostic applications will your research have for immune diseases?

DR. WALL: We are in the process of restriction mapping—a technique in which DNA from bone marrow or circulating cells is digested with restriction enzymes, which cut at very specific sites and hybridize with heavy-chain or light-chain specific probes. Once you know the structure of the gene in the normal configuration, you can begin to detect defects with only a few cells. It is a way of rapidly screening, which is already being talked about in the case of globin. In cases where there seems to be some history to suggest there would be allelic genes, people are screening for defective globin genes by taking cells and doing restriction digests and hybridizing with the globin probe. We are talking about doing the same thing with immunoglobulin genes, strictly by comparing the structure of the presumptive defective gene with what we know of the normal gene. This is obviously complicated in humans because they are not inbred like mice: in the same individual you have several alleles of, let us say, $alpha_1$ gene or $alpha_2$ gene, and that allelic difference can complicate restriction mapping. It will be worked out because you do not have—or so it appears, at least—you do not have 50 alleles, but only a couple. With restriction digest analysis, which is a sort of rapid molecular biology and can be done quickly, you could use a limited number of cells from bone marrow or from the circulation to screen for immune deficiencies. All of you will have to be buying restriction enzymes and cutting up DNA with them.

IV
THERAPEUTIC ASPECTS

Diagnosis and Treatment of Inborn Errors of Organic Acid Metabolism

Stephen D. Cederbaum

An inborn error of metabolism is defined as an inherited change in the structure of DNA, leading to the formation of an abnormal absolute or functional amount of protein. This change adversely affects the normal catalysis and modulation of the conversion of one or more precursors to various products. Although this broad definition may subsume the majority of all inherited diseases, it has generally been restricted to a smaller subset of these conditions, those in which abnormal amounts of precursors or products are actually measured. Disorders in which abnormalities in the protein product itself predominate, such as the hemoglobinopathies or dysfibrinogenemias, are generally excluded. In this discussion I will confine myself to a still more limited category: disorders involving abnormalities in the metabolism of amino acids, including those of the urea cycle and small-molecular-weight organic acids, but excluding those of fatty acid metabolism. In a following chapter Dr. Desnick will emphasize the second major category of these diseases, those that lead to the storage of larger and more complex mucopolysaccharides and glycolipids within the lysosomal compartment.

The basic tenets and principles of these disorders were enunciated in 1908, by Sir Archibald Garrod who coined the term "inborn error of metabolism" and recognized that these disorders represented genetically determined enzymic deficiencies (1). At the same time, he recognized the theoretical basis of and predicted the extraordinary heterogeneity that was to be found among and within the different disorders. As is often the case with such foresight and insight, his observations lay largely dormant, and not until 1948 was the first enzyme deficiency, acatalasemia, recognized (2). Subsequently, enzymic bases for literally hundreds of these disorders have been elucidated (3–5). More recently, advances in molecular genetics have given us progressively more insight into the mechanisms leading to the enzyme deficiencies.

Excellent progress in the diagnosis and treatment of inborn errors of organic acid metabolism has occurred during this same period, albeit at a less dizzying pace. For a score or more disorders, including the most common, excellent palliative therapy has become available, with considerable impact on society as well as the patient. We estimate conservatively that the early diagnosis and treatment of phenylketonuria (PKU) alone will lead to a net yearly saving of $50,000,000 in patient care costs and to a population of normal, productive citizens. Because effective therapy is so dependent on this early and effective diagnosis, no discussion of these inborn errors would be complete without a review of the diagnostic methods used.

Diagnosis of Inborn Errors of Organic Acid Metabolism

Except for a special category of inborn errors, amenable to mass newborn screening, and exemplified by PKU, the diagnosis of these disorders requires testing of a population at increased risk, determined by the presence of specific signs and symptoms and other clinical features. Examples are listed in Table 1. The clinical features may vary from neonatal collapse and death to a chemical aberration lacking recognizable clinical manifestations. In the former instance the relatively narrow and constricted physiological responses available to the neonate often cause the signs of neurological abnormalities, jitteriness, poor temperature control, and hypoglycemia, to be indistinguishable from those ordinarily associated with neonatal sepsis. This early onset of symptoms or the profound metabolic derangements of later or intermittent occurrence are true medical emergencies and require immediate specialized diagnostic and therapeutic responses.

Perusal of this list of symptoms immediately suggests that they are neither unique to or even highly likely to be related to inborn errors of metabolism. The study of patients for inborn errors should be confined to those circumstances in which: (*a*) one sign or symptom persists without adequate explanation; (*b*) several signs and symptoms appear together, for which no demonstrable

Table 1. **Clinical and Laboratory Clues to the Diagnosis of Inborn Errors of Metabolism**

Signs and symptoms

Neonatal collapse	Gastrointestinal
Developmental retardation	Hyperpnea
Failure to thrive	Neurological and behavioral
Cutaneous changes	abnormalities
Ocular abnormalities	Peculiar odor
Organomegaly	None apparent

Laboratory clues
Urine: odor, ketones, reducing substances
Blood: anemia, leukopenia, thrombocytopenia, acidosis, hypoglycemia, ketonemia

Course
Developmental arrest or regression
Periodicity of disease related to diet or intercurrent illness

Family history
Consanguinity
Family history of mental retardation or similar illness
Known inborn error in family member

---

cause exists; or (c) a clinical crisis makes wholly rational and stepwise evaluation dangerous and impractical.

The elements of a complete evaluation of a patient suspected of having an inborn error of metabolism are shown in Table 2. Several of these (e.g., blood glucose, plasma electrolytes, and urinary ketones) are part of the assessment of any acutely ill individual and will be available as a matter of course, although they may not always be timed appropriately for the assessment of an inborn error of metabolism. Plasma ammonia is now more frequently reported, now that it can be measured extremely reliably with commercial kits and automated analyzers. Of the other studies, the most frequently used is urinary amino acid analysis, screening tests for specific disorders, and, increasingly, chromatog-

---

Table 2. **Complete Laboratory Evaluation of Patients Suspected of Having an Inborn Error of Metabolism**

Blood sugar	Urine metabolic screening tests
Plasma and urine ketones	Urine amino acids
Blood electrolytes (or pH and bicarbonate)	Plasma amino acids
Blood lactate and pyruvate	Urine organic acids
Plasma ammonia	Plasma organic acids (?)

raphy of urinary organic acids. In some instances of acute illness, without evidence of metabolic acidosis, it may be prudent temporarily to bypass the urinary amino acid study and proceed directly to analysis of plasma amino acids. Increasingly sophisticated analysis of urinary organic acids may eventually make analysis of organic acids in plasma obsolete.

The first of the comprehensive screening tests for inborn errors of metabolism was analysis of urinary amino acids by two-dimensional paper chromatography, with subsequent staining with ninhydrin and other reagents that reacted selectively with the amino group. From its inception in the post-World War II era to the present, the analysis of amino acids in urine has been largely qualitative, involving inspection and pattern recognition by experienced individuals; results are semiquantitatively related to the urinary creatinine content. Although imperfect, this approach is more realistic than any other method, because of the inability to obtain timed specimens from young and handicapped individuals.

There is a substantial consensus that amino acid screening in high-risk (symptomatic) individuals is properly carried out with two-dimensional chromatography, either on paper or on thin-layer plates. Of the various methods available, most involve use of two solvents, acting in perpendicular dimensions, but some use high-voltage electrophoresis in the first dimension.[1] All have the virtue of separating most normally and pathologically excreted amino acids with little overlap. None are perfect. What is important is for the interpreter to become familiar with any one of these. One-dimensional chromatography gives inadequate separation of amino acids, with excessive overlap; a significant increase in a single amino acid may be overlooked because the increase in the total amino acid content of its collective spot was not recognizable.

The amino acid studies are augmented by a series of spot tests designed to assess aromatic alpha-keto acids (such as phenylpyruvic acid in PKU), disulfide compounds (in homocystinuria), carbonyl groups (acetoacetate in ketonuria and the branched-chain

---

[1] *Ed. note:* A recent issue of *Clinical Chemistry* (**28:** 737–1092, 1982) is devoted to two-dimensional gel electrophoresis, which will probably be the method of choice in the future.

alpha-keto acids) and nonglucose reducing groups (galactose). Other tests are used at the discretion of individual laboratories.

Figure 1 demonstrates an amino acid chromatogram from a single normal individual, compared with that of a mixture of amino acids of known concentration. The major amino acids are separated from one another and are assessed in relation to the artificial mixture (standards) run simultaneously in the same chromatographic tank [the identity of individual amino acids is given by Shaw et al. (6)]. The intensity of staining is directly proportional to the amount of amino acid, and the compounds can be semiquantified by inspection. Each amino acid can be quantified by spectrophotometry after elution from the paper (or plate), if appropriate standards are used. The information contained in the chromatogram is sufficiently small so that it can be accurately related to the patient's age, clinical condition, other laboratory data, and spot tests. Familiarity with the clinical literature is helpful; in experienced hands, ambiguous results are obtained in fewer than 5% of instances. Amino acids in plasma can be assessed similarly, but unless a limited and specific answer is sought, the more expensive and precise column-chromatographic approach is recommended (see, e.g., 7).

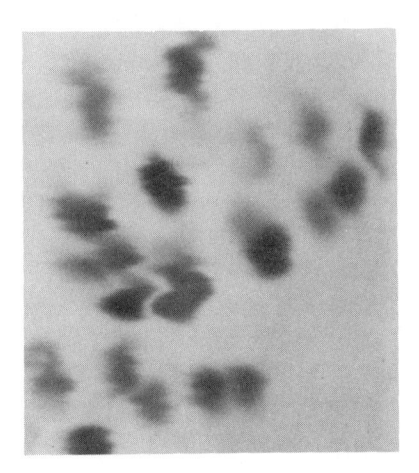

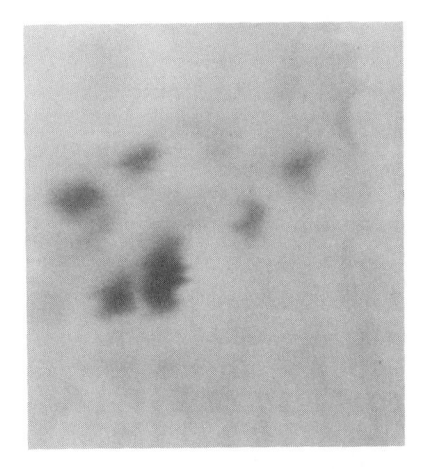

Fig. 1. Chromatogram of amino acids in urine from a normal, healthy individual

Right: An amount of urine containing 20 µg of creatinine spotted in the lower left-hand corner and subjected to two-dimensional ascending chromatography (6). *Left:* An artificial mixture of amino acids to provide a standard of migration and intensity of staining for a given chromatographic tank

Figure 2 illustrates an example of the use of this technique. The urine on the left was obtained when the PKU patient was treated and was in good metabolic balance. In this urine, the area to which phenylalanine migrates was not stained, the urine dinitrophenylhydrazine and ferric chloride tests were negative, and the plasma concentrations of phenylalanine were near normal and in the therapeutic range. Two days later, after a normal phenylalanine intake, plasma phenylalanine was up, the urinary screening tests were abnormal, and a high concentration of phenylalanine was found in the urine.

It was long intuitively clear that inborn errors involving non-ninhydrin-staining compounds must exist, but a relatively straightforward screening method had to be developed before these were diagnosed with any frequency and before the range of disorders could be defined. This technology was gas chromatography (8) and more recently, "high-performance" liquid chromatography (9). Gas chromatography is more commonly used and for the moment permits greater resolution of adjacent peaks. Most importantly, because it can be directly interfaced with a mass spectrometer, it permits unambiguous identification of a chromatographic peak.

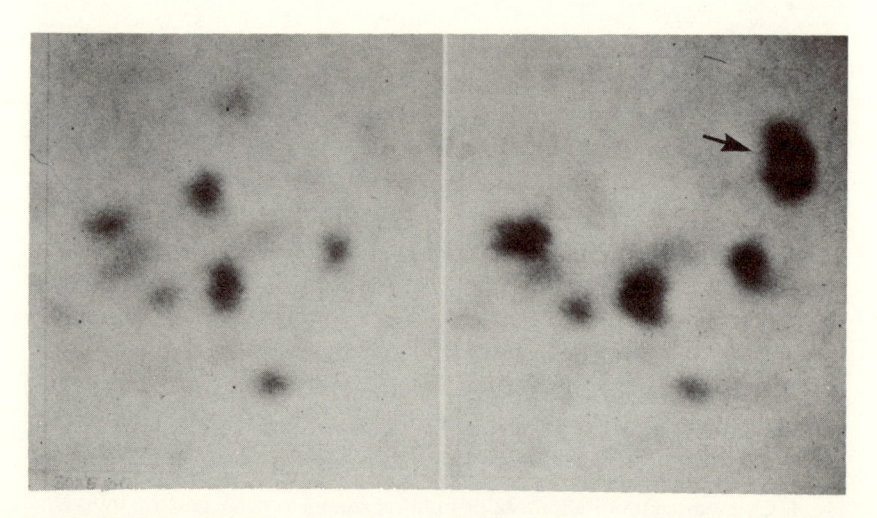

Fig. 2. Chromatograms of urinary amino acids from a patient with PKU

Left: specimen obtained when the patient was under good control. Right: specimen obtained two days after he was challenged with a normal phenylalanine intake. The arrow indicates the phenylalanine spot

The most abundant compounds that can be separated and identified by using these methods, and those most likely to be involved in inborn errors, are the organic acids. Urine is the body fluid of choice because these compounds are cleared readily. The most common methods for study involve acidification of the urine, extraction into an organic phase, and subsequent analysis by gas chromatography of the trimethylsilyl derivatives (10). Because these methods are inadequate to assess the hydrophilic compounds so important in intermediary metabolism, we recently developed a batch silica gel method for extracting all organic acids quantitatively; it is no more difficult or time consuming than the more standard methods (11). A typical urinary organic acid pattern is illustrated in Figure 3. All peaks obtained with the standard extraction are present in equal or greater abundance in our method, which we expect to become the method of choice for these studies.

Interpretation of organic acids studies is more complex and more fraught with risks than amino acids studies. Inspection of Figure 3 demonstrates the large number of peaks obtained, whose position and normal abundance cannot be retained by any ordinary intellect. The excellent reproducibility does, however, permit each peak to be defined by an invariant migration index and to be compared with the normal compounds that migrate in that area. Inspection of the chromatogram with the naked eye permits the assessment of the relative migration heights of common urinary constituents and the ascertainment of any peak of unusual magnitude. In some instances a most experienced observer may detect a more modest increase in an area of chromatogram otherwise devoid of any abundant excretory products. Statistically significant increases of excretion of a compound that do not stand out from the background are overlooked. However, current attempts to "map" these patterns with computers will facilitate comparisons between patients or between several samples from the same patient, and thus help identify abnormal results by processing the immense amount of information obtained.

In 80–90% of the cases examined, the chromatogram appears entirely normal (subject to the caveats described above) or else has a larger peak that, because of position, frequency in other patients, and clinical and laboratory criteria, can be identified and its significance inferred with a high degree of accuracy. Ten to 20% of the time, an unidentified peak of some abundance requires

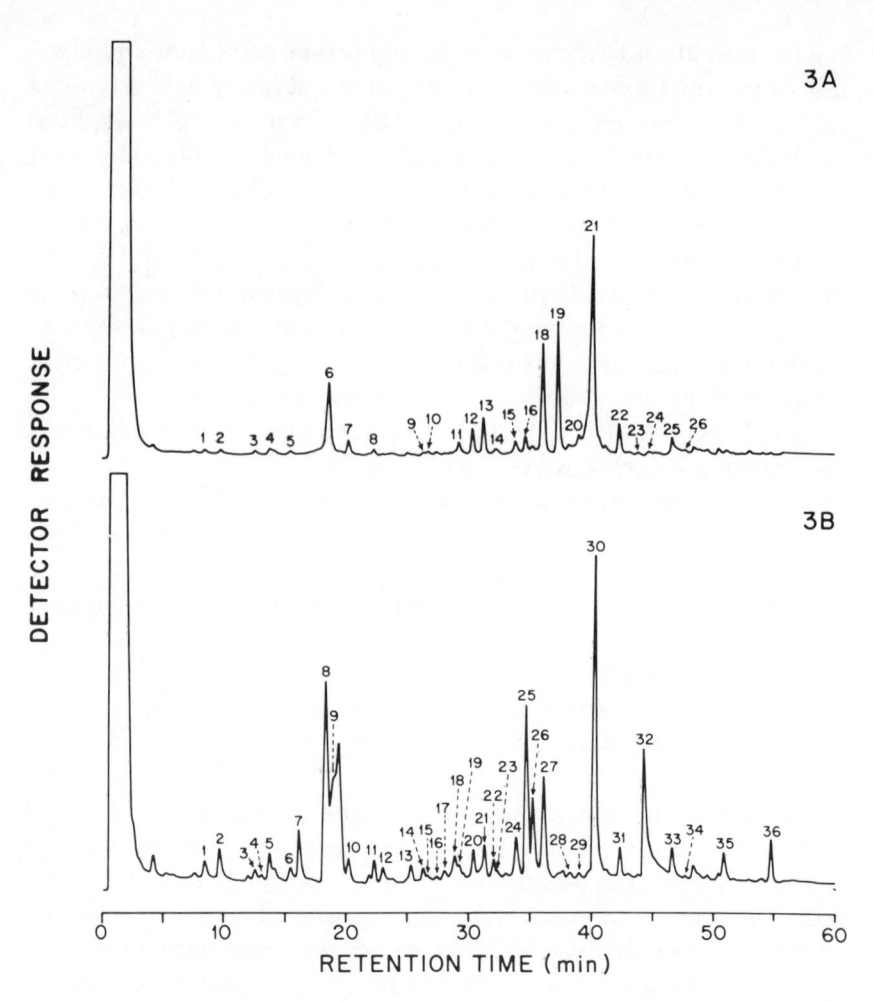

Fig. 3. Chromatogram of organic acids in urine

A, a specimen extracted with ethylacetate. *B*, the same specimen extracted by the method of Williams et al. (*11*). Note the changes in number and height of peaks

greater definition, which can be done by gas chromatography coupled with mass spectrometry (GC-MS) (*12*). We and others have sophisticated computerized GC-MS systems for automatic quantification and identification of all visible peaks in the chromatogram for which the computer is programmed. While useful in research, such a system is currently too expensive for routine clinical studies. At present, gas-chromatographic studies must be interpreted by experienced observers familiar with inborn errors and with access to mass spectrometer backup. Recently Hewlett-Packard and others have produced reliable GC-MS systems with powerful computer backup for well under $100 000. As the data-processing capability of these instruments improves, they may find a place in the general clinical laboratory for toxin studies and be available for studies of organic acids as well.

"High-performance" liquid chromatography methods are already used for the study of urinary purines and pyrimidines (*13, 14*), and procedures for glycoproteins, glycolipids, and mucopolysaccharides may soon be available; none are in widespread use now.

Recent experience with PKU and variant forms of hyperphenylalaninemia that may lead to mental retardation by other mechanisms and thus require different therapy serves as a vivid reminder of the importance of direct confirmation of the enzymic defect, especially if prenatal diagnosis or enzyme or gene therapy is to be contemplated (*15*). This principle is easily met in those disorders for which simple assays of enzymes present in cultured skin fibroblasts are available (*3*). For some of the urea-cycle defects and for phenylalanine hydroxylase (EC 1.99.1.2) deficiency, the liver is the only appropriate assay tissue, which presents formidable barriers. In disorders of the urea cycle, to be discussed extensively below, initiation of therapy based on reasonable inference rather than direct confirmation is proper, especially in view of the risks posed by the biopsy procedure itself (*16*).

Treatment of Inborn Errors of Organic Acid Metabolism

When an enzyme protein is insufficient to meet the body's metabolic needs, there are three possible consequences, illustrated in Figure 4. Given a genetic defect in the hypothetical enzyme 3, one or more substrates proximal to the block may accumulate; the product of the reaction may be deficient; a compound not normally seen in abundance in the body may accumulate as a result of the accumulation of the precursors of the missing enzyme; or a combination of all three may occur. The therapeutic strategies to be described by me, Dr. Desnick, and others have as their objective the correction of these metabolic abnormalities, focusing particularly on those that are most likely to cause symptoms.

Table 3 lists the therapeutic strategies for the treatment of inborn errors of metabolism. The ones in most common use for

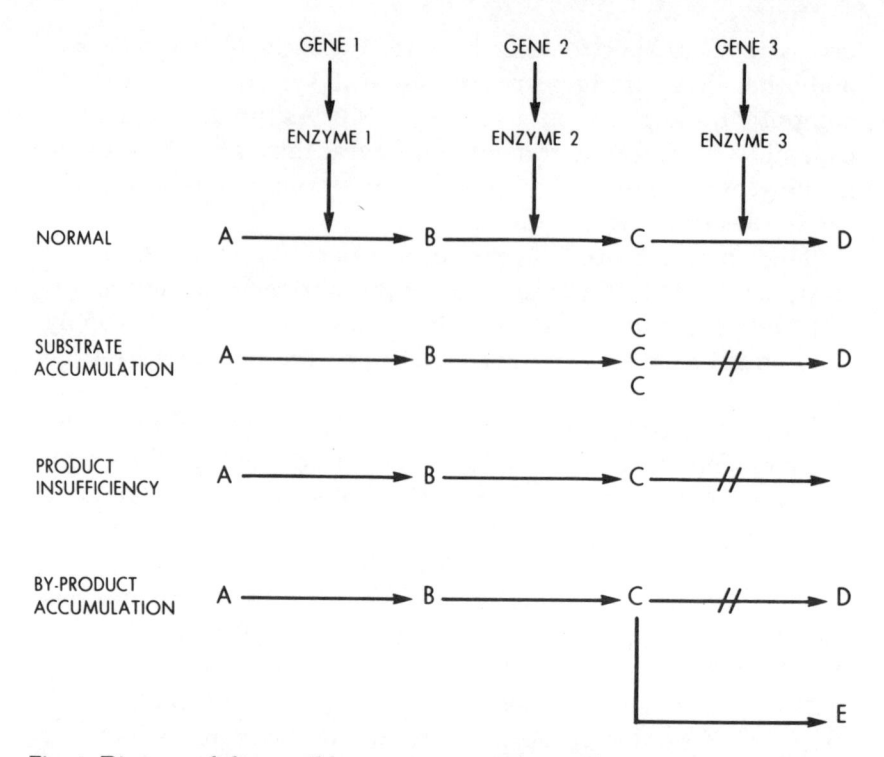

Fig. 4. Diagram of the possible consequences of an inborn error of metabolism: accumulation of substrates or precursors, deficient product formation, or the accumulation and excretion of metabolic side products

errors of organic acid metabolism are the first three: substrate limitation, product supplementation, and coenzyme supplementation. I will illustrate each of these approaches with salient examples, but will make no effort at comprehensive coverage of the many diseases in this category, which are covered in standard reference works on the subject (3, 4, 17).

The principles of the elimination diet, first developed in galactosemia (18) and PKU (19) more than a generation ago, still form the basis of most therapy for inborn errors of organic acid metabolism. In the former instance a natural diet without milk or milk products is used, whereas the latter requires a semisynthetic diet. More recently the availability of the basic building blocks of the semisynthetic diet such as Lofenalac and Phenyl-Free for PKU, MSUD diet powder for the treatment of maple syrup urine disease, and Protein-Free Base (product 80056), all from Mead-Johnson

Table 3. **Therapeutic Strategies for Inborn Errors of Metabolism**

Subtrate limitation
Substrate diversion
Product supplementation
Coenzyme (vitamin) supplementation
Enzyme induction
Enzyme replacement
   Allotransplantation
   Direct enzyme administration
   Enzyme reactor
Gene replacement

---

and Co., has made these diets more widely usable and permits them to be managed by less experienced medical personnel without extensive nutritional expertise and special dietary kitchens.

Disorders of the urea-cycle enzymes provide some of the best examples for illustrating the approaches to the treatment of inborn errors. They require both acute, short-term approaches and long-term care. They utilize the elimination diet, the diversion of substrate through an alternative pathway, and the replacement of product.

We now know that enzyme defects in each of the first four steps of the urea cycle (depicted in Figure 5)—and possibly defects in an enzyme not shown, which is responsible for activating enzyme 1—can result in neonatal hyperammonemia (*3, 4*). This chemical abnormality presents in a nonspecific manner with deteriorating neurologic status and collapse. Along with steps to deal with possible sepsis, the adverse impact of an inborn error must be moderated. Except for pyruvate dehydrogenase (EC 1.2.4.1) deficiency, which is exacerbated by glucose (*20*), the symptoms of virtually all inborn errors of organic acid metabolism are due to breakdown products of exogenous or endogenous protein or hypoglycemia. Therapeutic measures include eliminating protein from the diet, and intravenous infusion, maintaining calories and especially glucose at amounts great enough to prevent gluconeogenesis and protein breakdown. After the diagnosis, especially, but even before, if the index of suspicion is high and the situation desperate enough, peritoneal dialysis should be instituted. This is far more effective in hyperammonemia and most other disorders than exchange transfusion, which was used in earlier patients. In a series of patients undergoing between one and six double-

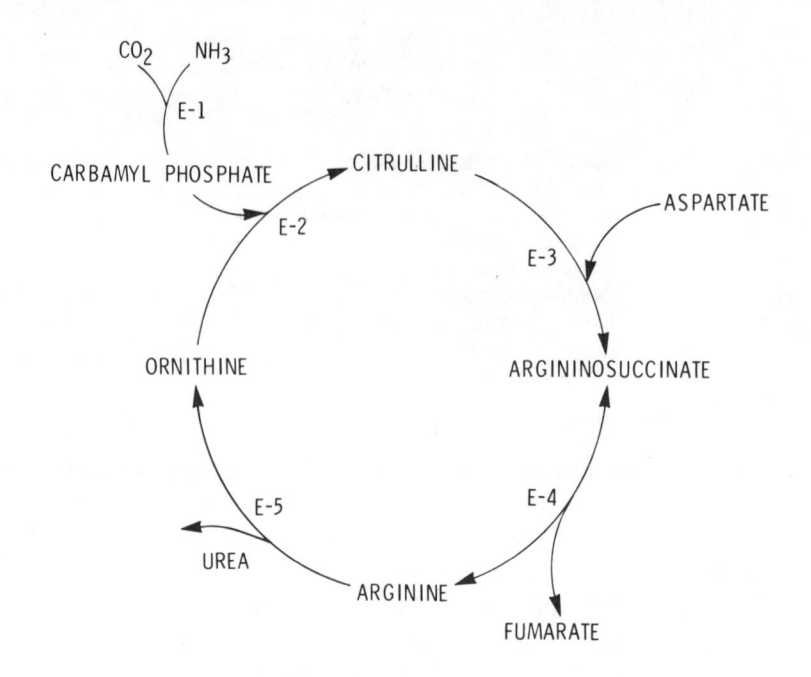

E-1 Carbamyl phosphate synthetase
E-2 Ornithine transcarbamylase
E-3 Argininosuccinic acid synthetase
E-4 Argininosuccinic acid lyase
E-5 Arginase

Fig. 5. The five steps of the urea cycle

volume exchange transfusions, the ammonia in plasma decreased by 19%; in a second group, in whom peritoneal dialysis proceeded for an average of 60 h, the ammonia decreased by 80% (*21*). Peritoneal dialysis is continued until the abnormal values are near enough normal to be maintained by ordinary means. Ammonia loss appears to occur primarily through glutamine and other amino acids and not as free ammonium ion (*21*). Of the infants reported so far with neonatal hyperammonemia due to urea-cycle defects, 50% have died, possibly because of the delay in making a specific diagnosis and instituting therapy.

Oral therapy with protein-free base, essential amino acids, and infant formula is begun as soon as possible to eliminate breakdown of endogenous protein, the amino-acid content of which cannot be regulated according to body needs. The original formulations by Snyderman et al. (*22*) and ourselves (*23*) consisted only of essential amino acids and small amounts of nonessential amino acids known to be required for growth on semisynthetic diets. More recently Batshaw, Brusilow, and their colleagues (personal communication) have used a formulation of essential amino acids, 0.75 g/kg of body weight per day, and an equal amount of protein given in the form of infant formula, the latter providing the nonessential amino acids and other nonspecific growth factors. In these patients arginine is an essential amino acid and must be given in amounts of 1.0 mmol/kg per day or more. In acute presentation, the mean plasma arginine before therapy ranged from 11 to 22 μmol/L, as compared with a normal range of 30–84 μmol/L (*16*).

The use of the nitrogen-free analogs of five essential amino acids (phenylalanine, methionine, leucine, isoleucine, and valine) proved useful, if difficult to manage (*24, 25*), but has now largely been superseded by the use of secondary pathways to promote nitrogen excretion through compounds other than urea. Credit for the work and thinking in this area must go to Batshaw and Brusilow at Johns Hopkins University, who have revolutionized the care of patients with inborn errors of urea-cycle enzymes (*16*).

The first element in this approach is the use of pharmacologic doses of arginine, especially important in argininosuccinate lyase (EC 4.3.2.1) deficiency and to a lesser extent in argininosuccinate synthetase (EC 6.3.4.5) deficiency. Argininosuccinic acid (ASA) contains both of the two ammonia nitrogens that will appear in urea and seems to be far less toxic than ammonia itself. Brusilow et al. (*26*) reasoned that ornithine might be deficient in these patients and that large doses of arginine might provide enough ornithine to permit ASA synthesis and relieve the accumulation of ammonia. The high clearance of ASA in urine made this compound ideal. Studies of arginine supplementation in argininosuccinate synthetase deficiency in fact proved this hypothesis, demonstrating dramatic decreases in concentrations of ammonia, with impressive clinical improvement despite augmented concentrations of ASA. Thus this disorder can be treated with moderate protein restriction and arginine alone (*16*). Citrulline excretion in argininosuccinate synthetase deficiency serves a similar but less effective role, because it contains only one of the two urea nitrogens and is cleared less effectively. This approach augments the accumulation of the immediate precursor of the deficient reaction, but again the precursor is less neurotoxic than ammonia.

A second approach takes advantage of a normal pathway, used to less than capacity under ordinary circumstances. The benzoate ion, found abundantly in the diet, is excreted in the urine completely after conjugation with glycine to form hippuric acid. The endogenous replacement of glycine uses one molecule of ammonia. In 1914 Lewis (27) showed that large doses of sodium benzoate caused dramatic decreases in urea excretion with waste nitrogen being excreted as hippurate, a finding recently confirmed (28). Fortunately for patients with these disorders, the capacity of the pathway is substantial and has resulted in a radically improved prognosis for these patients (16, 21). Experience with this treatment is still insufficient to state with certainty that the former fate of death within the first year of life has been substantially eliminated, but such appears to be the case (Batshaw and Brusilow, personal communication).

Followup care differs little in principle from that in the neonatal period. Purees and solids are introduced at appropriate times but are limited to low-protein foods that are exchanged for the protein in infant formula. Experience with older children with partial enzyme deficiencies suggests that the severity of acute episodes will diminish, but dietary restriction will be lifelong, and repeat hospitalizations may be required during periods of hyperammonemia induced by intercurrent illness. Distribution of protein intake throughout the day is obviously desirable.

Other inborn errors are handled in an analogous manner. Calorie intake is maximized in a balanced diet in which the precursor of the missing reaction is maintained as near the minimum daily requirement as possible, without causing malnutrition. Continual monitoring of growth, development, and concentrations of the appropriate metabolites in blood is mandatory. The use of natural foods is maximized, both to normalize the diet and to incorporate their nutrient content. Because the diets may be so unbalanced, a multivitamin supplement is usually recommended. Where appropriate, the product of a blocked reaction is given. Some disorders, such as methylmalonic acidemia that is unresponsive to vitamin B_{12}, are a constant threat to the health and life of the patient, and therapy and surveillance must be lifelong. In others, such as galactosemia past the neonatal period and PKU, the damage is insidious and directed at a developmental process. In these instances dietary therapy may be substantially relaxed in many patients in later childhood without measurable harm (15, 17); other patients react poorly to dietary relaxation and must be returned to more stringent therapy. The damage occurring in the children of untreated phenylketonuric women is a grim reminder that even in these most manageable disorders, prudence and open-mindedness are required to provide the best patient care (29).

Several enzymes deficient in inborn errors of metabolism are known to require vitamin cofactors for their function. This knowledge led to the discovery that some of these enzyme deficiencies might be corrected by the administration of pharmacologic doses of the vitamin, even when their concentrations in plasma were entirely normal (3, 4). The background and principles of this approach are illustrated by vitamin B_{12}-responsive methylmalonic acidemia, discussed later by Dr. Desnick.

Newborn Screening and Genetic Heterogeneity

Finally, I would like to comment briefly on newborn screening for metabolic disorders, an approach lying on the continuum between preemptive abortion and symptomatic therapy. The prototype for this approach is PKU. This disorder is also illustrative of some pitfalls in the screening process and the interpretation of the results (15).

PKU is caused by an inherited deficiency in phenylalanine hydroxylase, resulting in accumulation of phenylalanine in the blood and its excretion, along with some of its derivatives, in excess, in the urine. The cardinal and almost invariable clinical correlate is mental retardation. Treatment in presymptomatic or early symptomatic patients radically alters the prognosis. Virtually all those treated early and adequately have a normal IQ, although evidence for damage in cognitive function persists in a large proportion of affected individuals (15).

A reasonable and effective newborn screening program requires, among other things, that the disease when untreated cause serious handicap; that effective and accessible therapy be available; that the incidence of false positives and false negatives be low; and that the program be cost-effective. The development of the bacterial inhibition assay for phenylalanine in dried blood spots (30) allowed testing for PKU to meet these criteria, and screening for this disorder is now mandatory in virtually every jurisdiction of the developed world. Centralized and highly standardized laboratories and aggressive, specialized followup facilities are essential elements in these programs. In optimal circumstances, more than 95% of the patients are diagnosed and treated in the first two weeks of life. As a result of these programs, 1% or less of the 200 to 300 PKU patients born yearly in the United States will be seriously retarded. Before this screening technique was instituted, at least two-thirds of them would have required permanent custodial care (*31*).

The principles of PKU screening have been applied widely and successfully to neonatal hypothyroidism and galactosemia. Accurate tests for other conditions exist as well, but the rarity of these diseases impairs the cost-effectiveness of screening and has prevented their widespread adoption (*31*).

Discovery of important heterogeneity in the hyperphenylalaninemias resulted from the confluence of basic research into the reaction mechanism of phenylalanine hydroxylase and clinical observation of patients with PKU who responded poorly to biochemically effective therapy. In the late 1960s, Kaufman demonstrated that tetrahydrobiopterin was an essential cofactor in the phenylalanine hydroxylase system and that its regeneration from NADH required a second enzyme, dihydropteridine reductase (EC 1.6.99.7). He predicted that deficiency of this enzyme might also result in phenylketonuria (*32*). Because tetrahydrobiopterin is also the active cofactor in tyrosine and tryptophan hydroxylation, control of phenylalanine concentrations might therefore not be palliative in dihydropteridine reductase deficiency.

In 1975, Kaufman et al. (*33*) first described dihydropteridine reductase deficiency in a PKU patient who failed to respond to a phenylalanine-restricted diet. Subsequent examination of PKU patients has uncovered many more cases of this enzyme deficiency as well as cases of inherited deficiencies in the biosynthesis of the pteridine compounds (*34*). These so-called variants are estimated to account for about 1% of the hyperphenylalaninemic population (*34*). Because these variant patients are thought to respond favorably to replacement therapy with 5-hydroxytryptophan and L-dopa, all patients with persistent hyperphenylalaninemia are now studied for the presence of these defects (*15*).

Partial defects of phenylalanine hydroxylase, leading to various degrees of phenylalanine intolerance, have also been described. Thus, the heterogeneity predicted by molecular biology and biochemistry is rapidly being elucidated. This heterogeneity underscores the pitfalls of superficial interpretation of newborn screening studies and the importance of precise or inferential enzymic diagnosis in as many instances as possible.

Summary

The appropriate treatment for inborn errors of amino or organic acids depends on the specific site and nature of the enzymatic defect, the suspected pathogenesis of the disorder, and frequently on the age of the patient and the severity of the clinical presentation. The fundamental principle is to restore the concentrations of the perturbed metabolite toward normal by diminishing the concentrations of dietary precursor, by restoring the diminished product, or by enhancing or stabilizing the residual enzymic activity.

Current methods for the diagnosis of inborn errors of organic acid metabolism include semiquantitative analysis of urinary amino acids, plasma amino acids, and urinary organic acids by gas chromatography and mass spectrometry. Three therapeutic approaches to these disorders are substrate limitation, diversion of substrate into a normally minor pathway, and product supplementation. Special emphasis is placed on the treatment of the acute metabolic crisis by intravenous fluids and peritoneal dialysis.

This brief summary of diagnostic and therapeutic modalities illustrates the steady progress being made in the care of patients with inborn errors of organic acid metabolism. It is fair to say that the majority of diseases in this area are amenable to specific palliative if not entirely effective therapeutic approaches. Well-established diagnostic tests have been developed and a significant cadre of experts is available for their interpretation and for suggesting still other possibilities not measured by the standard approaches. For those few patients in whom therapy is impossible, correct diagnosis permits accurate genetic counselling and in many instances effective prenatal diagnosis.

Supported in part by the Mental Retardation Research Center at UCLA and USPHS grants HD-06576, HD-11298, AM-25983, HD-04612, HD-05615 and RR-00865.

References

1. Garrod, A. E., Inborn errors of metabolism (Croonian Lectures). *Lancet* **ii**, 1–7, 73–79, 142–148, 214–220 (1908).
2. Takahara, S., and Miyamoto, H., Three cases of progressive oral gangrene due to lack of catalase in the blood. *J. Otorhin. Soc. Jpn.* **51**, 163–179 (1948). Quoted in *Hereditary Disorders of Erythrocyte Metabolism*, E. Beutler, Ed., Grune & Stratton, New York, NY, 1968, p 21.
3. Stanbury, J. B., Wyngaarden, J. B., Frederickson, D. S., Goldstein, J. L., and Brown, M. S., Eds., *The Metabolic Basis of Inherited Disease*, 5th ed., McGraw Hill, New York, NY, 1983.
4. Rosenberg, L. E., and Scriver, C. R., Disorders of amino acid metabolism. In *Metabolic Control and Disease*, 8th ed., P. K. Bondy and L. E. Rosenberg, Eds., Saunders, Philadelphia, PA, 1980, pp 583–776.
5. Rosenberg, L. E., Inborn errors of metabolism. *Ibid.*, pp 73–102.
6. Shaw, K. N. F., Gutenstein, M., Jacobs, E. E., and Blascovics, J. C., Biochemical screening and monitoring of patients with phenylketonuria and variant forms of hyperphenylalaninemia. In *Phenylketonuria*, H. Bickel, F. P. Hudson, and L. I. Woolf, Eds., George Thieme Verlag, Stuttgart, 1971, pp 163–180.
7. Benson, J. V., Jr., Gordon, M. J., and Patterson, J. A., Accelerated chromatographic analyses of amino acids in physiological fluids containing glutamine and asparagine. *Anal. Biochem.* **18**, 228–240 (1967).
8. Jellum, E., Stokke, O. E., and Eldjarn, L., Screening for metabolic disorders using gas–liquid chromatography, mass spectrometry, and computer technique. *Scand. J. Clin. Lab. Invest.* **27**, 273–285 (1971).
9. Sweetman, L., Liquid partition chromatography and gas chromatography–mass spectrometry in identification of acid metabolites of amino acids. In *Heritable Disorders of Amino Acid Metabolism*, W. L. Nyhan, Ed., Wiley, New York, NY, 1974, pp 730–751.
10. Goodman, S. I., An introduction to gas chromatography–mass spectrometry and the inherited organic acidemias. *Am. J. Hum. Genet.* **32**, 781–792 (1980).
11. Williams, V. P., Ching, D. K., and Cederbaum, S. D., Adsorption of organic acids from amniotic fluid and urine onto silica gel before analysis by gas chromatography and combined gas chromatography/mass spectometry. *Clin. Chem.* **25**, 1814–1820 (1979).
12. Gates, S. C., Young, N. D., Holland, J. F., and Sweeley, C. C., Computer-aided qualitative analysis of complex biological fluids by combined gas chromatography/mass spectrometry. In *Advances in Mass Spectrometry in Biochemistry and Medicine*, **1**, A. Frigerio and N. Castagnoli, Eds., Spectrum, New York, NY, 1976, pp 483–495.

13. Evans, J. E., Tieckelmann, H., Naylor, E. W., and Guthrie, R., The measurement of urinary pyrimidine bases and nucleosides by high performance liquid chromatography. *J. Chromatogr.* **163,** 29–36 (1979).
14. Chen, S.-H., Ochs, H. D., Scott, C. R., Giblett, E. R., and Tingle, A. J., Adenosine deaminase deficiency: Disappearance of adenosine deoxynucleotides from a patient's erythrocytes after successful marrow transplantation. *J. Clin. Invest.* **62,** 1386–1389 (1978).
15. Scriver, C. R., and Clow, C. L., Phenylketonuria: Epitome of human biochemical genetics. *N. Engl. J. Med.* **303,** 1336–1342, 1394–1400 (1980).
16. Batshaw, M. L., Thomas, G. H., and Brusilow, S. W., New approaches to the diagnosis and treatment of inborn errors of urea synthesis. *Pediatrics* **68,** 290–297 (1981).
17. Raine, D. N., Ed., *The Treatment of Inherited Metabolic Disease,* American Elsevier, New York, NY, 1974.
18. Mason, H. H., and Turner, M. E., Chronic galactemia. *Am. J. Dis. Child.* **50,** 359–374 (1935).
19. Bickel, H., Gerrard, J., and Hickman, E. M., Influence of phenylalanine intake on phenylketonurics. *Lancet* **ii,** 812 (1953).
20. Cederbaum, S. D., Blass, J. P., Minkoff, N., Brown, W. J., Cotton, M. E., and Harris, S. H., Sensitivity to carbohydrate in a patient with familial intermittent lactic acidosis and pyruvate dehydrogenase deficiency. *Pediatr. Res.* **10,** 713–720 (1976).
21. Batshaw, M. L., and Brusilow, S. W., Treatment of hyperammonemic coma caused by inborn errors of urea synthesis. *J. Pediatr.* **97,** 893–900 (1980).
22. Snyderman, S. E., Sansaricq, C., Phansalkar, S. V., Schacht, R. G., and Norton, P. M., The therapy of hyperammonemia due to ornithine transcarbamylase deficiency in a male neonate. *Pediatrics* **56,** 65–73 (1975).
23. Cederbaum, S. D., Moedjono, S. J., Shaw, K. N. F., Naylor, E. W., Walzer, M., and Carter, M., Treatment of hyperargininemia due to arginase deficiency. *J. Inher. Metab. Dis.* **5,** 95–99 (1982).
24. Batshaw, M., Brusilow, S. W., and Walser, M., Treatment of carbamyl phosphate synthetase deficiency with keto-acid analogues of essential amino acids. *N. Engl. J. Med.* **292,** 1085–1090 (1975).
25. Brusilow, S. W., Batshaw, M. L., and Walser, M., Use of ketoacids in inborn errors of urea synthesis. In *Nutritional Management of Genetic Disease,* M. Winick, Ed., Wiley, New York, NY, 1979, pp 65–75.
26. Brusilow, S. W., Valle, D. L., and Batshaw, M. L., New pathways of nitrogen excretion in inborn errors of urea synthesis. *Lancet* **ii,** 452–454 (1979).

27. Lewis, H. B., Studies in the synthesis of hippuric acid in the animal organism. *J. Biol. Chem.* **18,** 225–231 (1914).
28. Brusilow, S. W., Tinker, J., and Batshaw, M. L., Amino acid acylation: A mechanism of nitrogen excretion in inborn errors of urea synthesis. *Science* **207,** 659–661 (1980).
29. Lenke, R. R., and Levy, H. L., Maternal phenylketonuria and hyperphenylalaninemia. *N. Engl. J. Med.* **303,** 1202–1208 (1980).
30. Guthrie, R., and Susi, A., A simple phenylalanine method for the detection of phenylketonuria in large populations of newborn infants. *Pediatrics* **32,** 338–343 (1963).
31. Bickel, H., Guthrie, R., and Hammersen, G., Eds., *Neonatal Screening for Inborn Errors of Metabolism.* Springer, New York, NY, 1980.
32. Kaufman, S., Unanswered questions in the primary metabolic block in phenylketonuria. In *Proceedings of the Conference on the Treatment of Phenylketonuria and Allied Disorders,* J. A. Anderson and K. F. Swaimen, Eds., U.S. Government Printing Office (HEW 68-2), Washington, DC, 1967, pp 205–209.
33. Kaufman, S., Holtzman, N. A., Milstien, S., Butler, I. J., and Krumholz, A., Phenylketonuria due to deficiency of dihydropteridine reductase. *N. Engl. J. Med.* **293,** 785–790 (1975).
34. Danks, D. M., Bartholome, K., Clayton, B. E., Curtius, H., Grobe, H., Kaufman, S., Lemming, R., Pfliederer, W., Rembold, H., and Rey, F., Malignant hyperphenylalaninemia—current status (June, 1977). *J. Inher. Metab. Dis.* **1,** 49–53 (1978).

Discussion

DR. PERRY: How many of these inborn amino acid errors are related to coenzymes rather than to the enzyme itself?

DR. CEDARBAUM: We have seen some notable examples, but probably only a small fraction of them are actually related to coenzyme defects. If you're dealing with disorders like PKU, only one in a hundred cases of hyperphenylalaninemia that are symptomatic are related to failure to regenerate this co-factor.

In case of methylmalonic acidema, about half the cases may be responsive to vitamin B_{12}. In the cases of homocystinuria, I would guess about 20 to 40% of the cases are responsive to high doses of vitamin B_6, but these are not the most common disorders. The vast majority of inborn errors are not vitamin responsive. Vitamin-responsive disorders make up a very interesting and important subgroup, but numerically they probably are not all that important.

Liver Transplantation and Portacaval Shunt in Genetic Diseases

Thomas E. Starzl

In this paper I will address two subjects: the use of portal diversion as a palliative treatment of some selected inborn errors of metabolism, and the actual provision of these patients with a missing enzyme by transplantation of a phenotypically normal new liver. Both are interesting new developments in surgery and pediatrics that, although controversial and not accepted initially, have been largely validated.

Portal Diversion

The basis for the use of portal diversion for metabolic as opposed to hemodynamic objectives was laid in the laboratory. I need not remind anyone here that the liver has a double blood supply. The hepatic artery usually provides 20–25% of the total hepatic blood flow, and the portal vein provides the remainder.

The portal blood flow is derived from blood returning from various splanchnic organs, including the pancreas, spleen, stomach, small intestine, and colon. Long before substances such as hormones were known, biologists of the 19th century concluded that this blood might contain specific and important components without which the liver could not survive. This was the accepted doctrine until an innocent little paper, one page long, upset the apple cart. In it, Nicholas Eck (1), a Russian military surgeon, described his experience with portacaval shunt in eight dogs. One of the animals died during the operation, six survived for a few days, dying of peritonitis or strangulation of the intestines and omentum, and one recovered completely and lived in the laboratory for two and one-half months. Dr. Eck blamed his associates for the fact that the dog then ran away. Revealing his thoughts about the clinical implications of this operation, he wrote, "I am conducting these experiments with the purpose of clarifying some physiologic problems, to determine whether it would be possible to treat some cases of mechanical ascites by performing such a fistula." Perhaps Dr. Eck overstated his case: he went on to say that, "the main reason to doubt that such an operation can be carried out in human beings has been removed because it was established that the blood . . . could be diverted without any danger to the body, and this by means of a perfectly safe operation." Despite the fact that he was confronted with an 88% mortality rate, he realized that the Eck fistula was technically feasible. This was more than 100 years ago.

The operation of portacaval shunt (Eck fistula), as it is usually done in the laboratory, consists of a side-to-side portacaval shunt above which the portal vein is tied off, converting the anastomosis to a completely diverting shunt (2). After such an operation, striking changes occur in the liver, the nature and rapidity of which have been completely understood in only the last 10–15 years. These changes affect the liver of all species so far studied, including humans.

The most striking morphologic change after portacaval shunt is acute atrophy of the hepatocytes to about half of their original size within less than a week. At the same time the livers accumulate fat and develop multiple and dramatic ultrastructural changes. The most specific change is depletion of the rough endoplasmic reticulum and its polyribosomes. Semiquantitative morphometric analysis shows that the rough endoplasmic reticulum is reduced to about one-fourth of its original volume. In addition, glycogen granules are depleted, and the mitochondria develop nonspecific abnormalities.

Until recently the explanation of the changes caused by Eck fistula was not known. Rather than detail the tortuous pathways we followed to determine the causes, I will skip to the final and crucial experiment (2, 3), in which we found that the changes caused by portacaval shunt in dogs could be prevented by the infusion of insulin into the tied-off central portal vein. The experiment was quite simple. We ligated the right and left portal veins in the hilum, but left the insulin-infusion catheter in one of the main portal branches. One could compare the liver lobes that were directly infused with insulin with those that were not. Thus, we looked not only at the potential protective effect in the insulin-infused lobes, but also at whether there was a carryover effect on the side not receiving insulin. There was no carryover protection. On the treated liver side, this simple procedure of infusion of insulin completely prevented the involutional changes caused by portacaval shunt. We concluded that many or most of the changes caused by portacaval shunt were due to endogenous insulin bypassing the liver. This work in experimental pathology was the product of K. A. Porter of St. Mary's Hospital and Medical School in London, with whom we have collaborated for many years (3–7).

So far, I have discussed only the striking morphologic changes caused by portacaval shunt. In addition, portal diversion causes profound changes in metabolism, the following example of which is especially relevant to clinical applications. As we have demonstrated in dogs and humans, cholesterol synthesis is greatly decreased in livers deprived of a portal blood supply (8). Bilheimer and Brown of Southwestern University, Dallas, showed the same thing in a patient upon whom I had operated.

Glycogen Storage Disease

In 1963, armed with some of the above information, we began a series of operations on patients with glycogen storage disease (6, 7) (Table 1). The patients had Types I, III, and VI disease, mostly Type I (glucose-6-phosphatase deficiency). After the operation there was a substantial amelioration of the metabolic perturbations of the patients. Those with Type I disease all had hyperlipidemia, which was alleviated immediately. Abnormalities of

Table 1. **Inborn Errors Treated with Portacaval Shunt**

Disease	No. of cases	Length of followup, years
Glycogen storage	11	2–20
Hyperlipidemia	7	2–6.5 [a]
α_1-Antitrypsin deficiency	3	1.5–5

[a] The xanthomas shrank or disappeared. The serum cholesterol decreased to 38–68% of the preportacaval shunt value. In five of the seven, the cardiovascular status stabilized.

coagulation and uric acid metabolism improved. The most striking occurrence was a growth spurt in these patients, who were all stunted. After portacaval shunt, the patients grew at the rate of 0.5–1 cm a month, during the first postoperative year. These growth spurts could be seen and documented by roentgenographic techniques of bone assessment. One child experienced such major growth that her bone age increased from 3.5 to seven years in the first 11 postoperative months. The bones lengthened and became mineralized, and new growth centers appeared in the wrists and elsewhere.

The full explanation of these striking effects is not yet clear. The blunted peripheral insulin response to a glucose meal, which is typical of Type I disease, was greatly increased after the shunt. Insulin being a powerful growth factor, perhaps the increased insulinemia was a factor in the growth. Not surprisingly, the one symptom that was not promptly relieved by portacaval shunt was the nocturnal hypoglycemia found in most patients.

One of my associates on this project, Dr. Harry Greene, later moved to Vanderbilt and introduced there the very interesting alternative form of therapy of continuous enteral alimentation (9). He provided continuous overnight feeding by nasogastric tube or by a gastrostomy and showed that many of the same benefits of portacaval shunt could be obtained thereby.[1] Consequently, I now recommend that continuous alimentation be carried out as the first option, with portacaval shunt reserved for a back-up treatment. The treatment of glycogen storage disease has been truly revolutionized in the last 20 years, first by portal diversion and then by continuous alimentation.

Familial Hypercholesterolemia

Familial hypercholesterolemia is a disease for which there is no such alternative (Table 1). Portacaval shunt often is the only effective form of treatment. The first patient treated was a nine-year-old girl with homozygous Type II hyperlipidemia, who had a massive myocardial infarction six weeks before portacaval shunt was performed (8, 10). She was taken to the operating room from

---

[1] *Ed. note:* Dr. Greene discussed this technique in the preceding volume in this series, *Human Nutrition: Clinical and Biochemical Aspects*, P. J. Garry, Ed., Am. Assoc. Clin. Chem., Washington, DC, 1981, pp 383–397.

the Intensive Care Unit at the University of Colorado, from which it was apparent that she would never emerge (*8, 10, 11*).

Homozygous familial hypercholesterolemia is characterized by deposits of xanthomatous material in the tendons, the skin, the coronary arteries, and the valves of the heart. The cardiovascular problems become so severe that these patients almost never live into or beyond the teen years. They often die of myocardial infarctions before puberty, and this, indeed, was the course this child was following (*10*). After portacaval shunt, her serum cholesterol, which had been about 8.00 g/L, decreased, and within six months it almost reached a normal concentration (*8*). We could easily see what happened to the xanthomatous lesions on her hands and other superficial areas, but comparable changes were taking place inside her body. The excrescences shrank and disappeared over a period of 16 months, leaving only faint skin stains. The child died about 18 months postoperatively, from a complication of her previous myocardial infarction. She developed a fatal arrhythmia when coming home from school.

The serum cholesterol concentrations of the other six patients we treated, five children and one adult, also decreased. A summary of the results in the first seven hyperlipidemia cases after two to 6.5 years' survival is given in Table 1. The xanthomas all shrank or completely disappeared. The serum cholesterol invariably decreased in parallel with decreases in low-density lipoproteins. The cardiovascular disease, interestingly enough, improved or stabilized in most patients as the cutaneotendinous lesions disappeared. In some of the cases, we documented by serial catheterizations a reduction in the gradient of aortic stenosis or improvement in coronary artery disease.

α-Antitrypsin Deficiency

Perhaps this third inborn error of metabolism can also be palliated with portal diversion. α_1-Antitrypsin deficiency is an inborn error that follows genetic rules, but the exact reason for the manifestations of this disorder is really not known. Although α_1-antitrypsin is synthesized by the liver, its structure is sufficiently abnormal that it cannot be transported; thus, it accumulates in the liver and probably is responsible for hepatic injury. We have treated three patients with portacaval shunt and have followed them for 1.5 to more than five years.

These patients have been remarkably stable. In two of them, we biopsied the liver at the time of the shunt and one to two years later. In one case, the amount of α_1-antitrypsin in the hepatocytes had actually decreased, as determined by morphometric analysis; and in the other, the amount remained the same. Perhaps with the depletion of rough endoplasmic reticulum the synthesis of the abnormal α_1-antitrypsin was reduced without a commensurate decrease in the excretion of this alpha-globulin through the hepatocytes. If so, a favorable metabolic equilibrium would have been established that could, in a very subtle way, allow the disease to be more compatible with long life. However, these trials are still highly experimental, and we are not recommending portal diversion to treat this liver disease.

Liver Transplantation

Liver transplantation offers a more direct approach to enzyme-deficiency disease, or inborn errors of metabolism. For any of the liver-based inborn errors I will mention here, transplantation of a phenotypically normal liver supplies or probably supplies the missing enzyme. It is a simple concept. Phenylketonuria (PKU) for example, is known to be a liver-based inborn error, and so, by definition, is curable by liver replacement. Obviously, however, less drastic approaches are preferable.

Examples also can be found in laboratory animals. Several years ago a group at the Mayo Clinic reported experiments in which Dalmatian dogs, which suffered from gout, were given livers from mongrel donors and were cured of their gout (*12*). The defect in uric acid metabolism was eliminated.

Because the concept is so childishly simple, I do not think there is any need to dwell on it. The main prerequisite to exploiting the possibilities of liver transplantation has been the need to develop better ways of preventing liver rejection.

Recent developments in immunosuppression have made possible efforts considered unrealistic only a few years ago. The key factor in these new expectations is a new drug called cyclosporin A (cyclosporine) (*13*), first used in clinical trials in kidney transplantation (*14, 15*).

Before cyclosporin A was available, the most important development in immunosuppression occurred about 20 years ago with the combined use of azathioprine (Imuran) and prednisone. With these drugs, kidney transplants became possible in other than twin recipients (*16, 17*). When, as often happened, transplanted kidneys began to be rejected after a few days or a few weeks, augmented steroid therapy allowed reversal of rejections. We also noticed that these patients subsequently developed what we called (perhaps incorrectly) partial tolerance. In many cases, the amount of immunosuppression could later be decreased. With that advantage, the patients were able to return home, have babies, go to the movies, and in general return to normal society.

This work (*16*) was done with Tom Marchioro (now at the University of Seattle in Washington) and Bill Waddell (at the University of Colorado). The technique of double-drug therapy has become the worldwide standard method of immunosuppression. Unfortunately, it was an achievement of which I personally became ashamed, because it was so limited, as illustrated by the results for nearly 5000 primary (first-time) cadaveric kidney transplantations in 105 centers from 1971 to 1976. The six-month graft survival was only 55% and the one-year survival 45% (*18*). Thus more than half of the patients given cadaveric kidneys were losing them within the first postoperative year. Moreover, the penalties, even with "success," were sometimes unacceptable and included cosmetic deformity from the steroids, infections, an increased incidence of de novo malignancies, bone disease, gastrointestinal disorders, and cataracts. Consistently good results could be obtained only with transplantation from living, related donors. Attempts to improve the outlook with antilymphocyte globulin, thoracic duct drainage, and tissue matching resulted in only small gains.

It was clear that the situation could not really change unless new drugs were developed. Such a new agent, cyclosporin A, surfaced in 1976 in a paper by Borel et al. (*13*). Cyclosporin A is an extract of two fungi. The most potent immunosuppressive agent yet described, it has no bone marrow toxicity. Until its development there had been no immunosuppressive drug, excluding steroids, that did not with chronic use depress the bone marrow.

In 1978, cyclosporin A was released for clinical trial to two groups in England—one at Cambridge, the other (for bone marrow transplantation) at the Royal Marsden Cancer Hospital near London. The first reports on whole-organ transplantation, from Calne et al. (*14, 15*) of Cambridge in 1978 and 1979, were mixed. The good news was that many cadaveric kidney recipients treated with cyclosporin A never required steroid therapy. The bad news was that three of the first 33 patients developed lymphomas. In addition, the mortality from infection was high, and one in three of the patients died. Nonetheless, the Cambridge group recommended using cyclosporin A as the sole immunosuppressive agent.

Cyclosporin A was released in the United States in late 1979, to two centers—the Peter Bent Brigham in Boston, and to us at the University of Colorado. We quickly learned that for optimal use cyclosporin A needed to be used with steroids, and not as a sole immunosuppressive agent as the English had recommended. We recommended (*19–21*) that, in addition to cyclosporin A, adults be given a five-day course of rapidly decreasing daily doses of steroids, e.g., prednisone, starting at 200 mg/day and decreasing to 20 mg daily maintenance, as the subsequent course permitted. This was a revolutionary development, because decreasing steroids to such levels, when combined with azathioprine, had required months, not days.

The control of rejection with this combination of cyclosporin A and steroids has been really quite amazing. The actual one-year survival of cadaveric kidney grafts, even during a learning phase, was 80% (*21*). That is a stunning figure, almost twice as good as the graft survival after conventional immunosuppression. At the University of Pittsburgh, where I now work, graft survival has been even higher. The combination of cyclosporin A and steroids is almost a fail-safe method of immunosuppression.

Given the background that has been developed with the kidney, there has been a powerful movement to apply the same techniques for the transplantation of other organs. For the first time, the ability to perform hepatic transplants safely and relatively reliably is in sight. The procedure usually used for liver transplantation is organ replacement. The diseased liver is removed and a cadaveric organ is put in. The new liver can be preserved for 6 to 12 h if necessary, by infusing with cold solutions. All of the structures entering and leaving the graft are installed as anatomically normal as possible. For chemists, sewing in a liver must seem naive or anti-intellectual, which it probably is, but the results can be emotionally gratifying. The longest survival after liver transplantation has been of a little girl whose operation was 12 years ago when she was four.

The problem with liver transplantation throughout the years has been that the undertaking was dangerous and unpredictable. Only 35 to 40% of the patients could be expected to survive through the first postoperative year, a situation that has changed with the use of cyclosporin A. The last year I was in Denver, we considered 14 patients for liver transplantation under the same cyclosporin–steroid therapy that we had developed for kidneys. Two patients died on the operating table. Of the other 12, 11 (92%) lived for at least a year. Even including the two operative deaths, the one-year survival rate in those liver recipients was almost 80% (20). Similar results have been obtained at the University of Pittsburgh.

Even in the early days of liver transplantation, the potential value of this technique for treating inborn errors was obvious. When liver replacement was first carried out in humans, there were changes in the recipient's alpha-protein phenotypes, haptoglobin, and group-specific components. These and subsequent observations of other phenotypes proved that the metabolic specificity of the new organ remained that of the donor for as long as the graft functioned (22).

For completely understood inborn errors, this expectation has been realized on a number of occasions (Table 2). The most experience (eight cases) has been with α_1-antitrypsin deficiency (23). After orthotopic liver transplantation, the Pi type of the recipient has become that of the donor and the abnormally low values of serum α_1-antitrypsin have increased to normal values. After liver transplantation, the accumulation of α_1-antitrypsin in a homograft has never been seen.

Another disorder that has been cured metabolically by liver replacement in spite of its unknown pathogenesis is Wilson's disease (Table 2) (24), characterized by widespread accumulation of copper in tissues. We have treated two patients with orthotopic liver transplantation. One died six years after the operation because of biliary tract complications that could not be rectified. The other is still well after more than 10 years. Both recipients underwent a protracted decoppering process, as documented by urine copper excretion. Progress could be monitored as the Kayser–Fleischer rings of the cornea receded and disappeared. Serum ceru-

Table 2. **Inborn Errors of Metabolism Corrected by Liver Transplantation**

Disease	No. of cases	Enzyme defect	Longest survival
α_1-Antitrypsin deficiency	8	Unknown	5 yr.
Wilson's disease	2	Unknown	10.5 yr.
Type IV glycogen storage disease	1	Amylo-1,4-transglucosidase (branching enzyme)	3 mo.
Tyrosinemia	2	p-Hydroxyphenylpyruvic acid oxidase	6 mo.
Niemann–Pick disease[a]	1	Sphingomyelinase	1.5 yr.
Crigler–Najjar syndrome[b]	1	Glucuronyl-transferase	1 mo.

[a] Patient treated by Dr. Pierre Daloze, Notre Dame Hospital, Montreal.
[b] Treated by auxiliary liver transplantation (see text); all other transplants were liver replacements.

loplasmin, which is almost always very low in patients with Wilson's disease, was restored to normal within a few days after transplantation and has remained so for more than 10 years in our second patient.

At least four other inborn errors with known and specific enzyme deficiencies have been treated by liver transplantation (Table 2). In a child with Niemann–Pick disease (25), a metabolic cure was obtained after orthotopic transplantation, but the pre-existing neurologic injury was not ameliorated and eventually was indirectly responsible for death. Children treated by us for Type IV glycogen storage disease and congenital tyrosinemia (26) died soon after transplantation (Table 2), but complete studies in the latter patient showed that essentially normal tyrosine metabolism had been achieved (26).

The foregoing experience was with liver replacement. Seven years ago, we attempted to treat a two-year-old child with Crigler–Najjar syndrome by transplanting an auxiliary liver. With this disease, a nearly complete absence of hepatic glucuronyl transferase makes impossible the conjugation of bilirubin by the liver. Yet, all other measures of liver function are normal, making removal of the original liver not entirely desirable. We transplanted an auxiliary liver to the right paravertebral gutter, taking its hepatic arterial supply from the aorta, and anastomosing the portal vein end-to-end to the transected recipient portal vein. Outflow was established by anastomosing the end of the graft intrahepatic inferior vena cava to the side of the recipient vena cava. The graft and recipient gallbladders were also anastomosed. The auxiliary graft produced bile immediately and by the following morning the deeply jaundiced sclera (serum bilirubin 500 mg/L) had become white and the bilirubin was normal. Unfortunately, the portal vein and hepatic artery thrombosed several days later, and the auxiliary liver was removed. The child was returned to the previous treatment with plasmapheresis and died several months later of kernicterus.

The results shown in Table 2 were obtained in an era when conventional immunosuppression was used (27). "Metabolic engineering" in the new era of better immunosuppression with cyclosporin A and steroids will become increasingly common and successful. At the University of Pittsburgh, we have already used liver transplantation to treat patients with α_1-antitrypsin deficiency, subacute Wilson's disease, tyrosinemia, Type I glycogen storage disease, and the sea blue histiocyte syndrome. With the improved new immunosuppressive therapy, these kinds of diseases will be effectively treated with increasing frequency.

References

1. Eck, N. V., K. voprosu o perevyazkie vorotnois veni. (Ligature of the portal vein). *Voen. Med. J., St. Petersburg* **130** (2), 1–2 (1877). Translated in: C. S. Child, III, Eck's fistula. *Surg. Gynecol. Obstet.* **96**, 375–376 (1953).
2. Starzl, T. E., Watanabe, K., Porter, K. A., and Putnam, C. W., Effects of insulin, glucagon, and insulin/glucagon infusions on liver morphology and the cell division after complete portacaval shunt in dogs. *Lancet* **i**, 821–825 (1976).
3. Starzl, T. E., Porter, K. A., and Putnam, C. W., Intraportal insulin protects from the liver injury of portacaval shunt in dogs. *Lancet* **ii**, 1241–1242 (1975).
4. Putnam, C. W., Porter, K. A., and Starzl, T. E., Hepatic encephalopathy and light and electron micrographic changes in baboon liver after portal diversion. *Ann. Surg.* **184**, 155–161 (1976).
5. Starzl, T. E., Lee, I. Y., Porter, K. A., and Putnam, C. W., The influence of portal blood upon lipid metabolism in normal and diabetic dogs and baboons. *Surg. Gynecol. Obstet.* **140**, 381–396 (1975).
6. Starzl, T. E., Putnam, C. W., Porter, K. A., and Benichou, J., Portaca-

val shunt for glycogen storage disease and hyperlipidemia. In *Hepatotrophic Factors,* Ciba Foundation Symp. **55,** R. Porter and J. Whelan, Eds., Elsevier/Excerpta Medica, North-Holland, Amsterdam, 1978, pp 311–325.
7. Starzl, T. E., Putnam, C. W., Porter, K. A., Halgrimson, C. G., Corman, J., Brown, B. I., Gotlin, R. W., Rodgerson, D. O., and Greene, H. L., Portal diversion for the treatment of glycogen storage disease in humans. *Ann. Surg.* **178,** 525–539 (1973).
8. Starzl, T. E., Chase, H. P., Putnam, C. W., and Porter, K. A., Portacaval shunt in hyperlipidemia. *Lancet* **ii,** 940–944 (1973).
9. Greene, H. L., Slonim, A. E., Burr, I. M., and Moran, J. R., Type I glycogen storage disease: Five years management with nocturnal intragastric feeding. *J. Pediatr.* **96,** 590–595 (1980).
10. Starzl, T. E., Chase, H. P., Putnam, C. W., and Nora, J. J., Follow-up of patient with portacaval shunt for treatment of hyperlipidemia. *Lancet* **ii,** 714–715 (1974).
11. Ahrens, E. A., Jr., Homozygous hypercholesterolaemia and the portacaval shunt. *Lancet* **ii,** 449–451 (1974).
12. Kuster, G., Shorter, R. G., Dawson, B., and Hallenbeck, O. A., Effect of allogeneic hepatic transplantation between Dalmatian and mongrel dogs on urinary excretion of uric acid. *Surg. Forum* **18,** 360–362 (1967).
13. Borel, J. F., Feurer, C., Gubler, H. U., and Stahelin, H., Biological effect of cyclosporin A: A new antilymphocytic agent. *Agents Actions* **6,** 468 (1976).
14. Calne, R. Y., Rolles, K., White, D. J. G., Thiru, S., Evans, D. B., McMaster, P., Dunn, D. C., Craddock, G. N., Henderson, R. G., Aziz, S., and Lewis, P., Cyclosporin A initially as the only immunosuppressant in 34 recipients of cadaveric organs: 32 kidneys, 2 pancreases, and 2 livers. *Lancet* **ii,** 1033–1036 (1979).
15. Calne, R. Y., White, D. J. G., Evans, D. B., Thiru, S., Henderson, D. P., Hamilton, D. V., Rolles, K., McMaster, P., Duffy, T. J., Mac Dougall, B. R. D., and Williams, R., Cyclosporin A in cadaver organ transplantation. *Br. Med. J.* **282,** 934–936 (1981).
16. Starzl, T. E., Marchioro, T. L., and Waddell, W. R., The reversal of rejection in human renal allografts with subsequent development of homograft tolerance. *Surg. Gynecol. Obstet.* **117,** 385–395 (1963).
17. Starzl, T. E., *Experience in Renal Transplantation,* W. B. Saunders Co., Philadelphia, PA, 1964, 383 pp.
18. Terasaki, P. I., Opelz, G., Graver, B., et al., National kidney recipient pool and transplant registry. *Dial. Transplant.* **6,** 22–23 (1977).
19. Starzl, T. E., Weil, R., III, Iwatsuki, S., Klintmalm, G., Schröter, G. P. J., Koep, L. J., Iwaki, Y., Terasaki, P. I., and Porter, K. A., The

use of cyclosporin A and prednisone in cadaver kidney transplantation. *Surg. Gynecol. Obstet.* **151,** 17–26 (1980).
20. Starzl, T. E., Klintmalm, G. B. G., Weil, R., III, Porter, K. A., Iwatsuki, S., and Schröter, G. P., Liver transplantation with the use of cyclosporin A and prednisone. *N. Engl. J. Med.* **305,** 266–269 (1981).
21. Starzl, T. E., Klintmalm, G. B. G., Weil, R., III, Porter, K. A., Iwatsuki, S., Schröter, G., Fernandez-Bueno, C., and MacHugh, N., Cyclosporin A and steroid therapy in 66 cadaver kidney recipients. *Surg. Gynecol. Obstet.* **153,** 486–494 (1981).
22. Alper, C. A., Raum, D., Audeh, Z., Petersen, B. H., Taylor, P. D., and Starzl, T. E., Studies of hepatic synthesis in vivo of plasma proteins including orosmucoid, tranferrin, alpha$_1$-antitrypsin, C8, and factor B. *Clin. Immunol. Immunopathol.* **16,** 84–89 (1980).
23. Hood, J. M., Koep, L. J., Peters, R. L., Schröter G. P. J., Weil, R., III, Redeker, A. G., and Starzl, T. E., Liver transplantation for advanced liver disease with alpha$_1$-antitrypsin deficiency. *N. Engl. J. Med.* **302,** 272–275 (1980).
24. Groth, C. G., Dubois, R. S., Corman, J., Gustafsson, A., Iwatsuki, S., Rodgerson, D. O., Halgrimson, C. G., and Starzl, T. E., Metabolic effects of hepatic replacement in Wilson's disease. *Transplant. Proc.* **5,** 829–833 (1973).
25. Daloze, P., Corman, J., Bloch, P., Delvin, E. E., and Glorieux, F. H., Enzyme replacement in Niemann–Pick disease by liver transplantation. *Transplant. Proc.* **7,** Suppl. 1, 607–610 (1975).
26. Fisch, R. O., McCabe, E. R. B., Doeden, D., Koep, L. J., Silverman, A., and Starzl, T. E., Homotransplantation of the liver in a patient with hepatoma in hereditary tyrosinemia. *J. Pediatr.* **93,** 592–596 (1978).
27. Starzl, T. E. (with assistance of C. W. Putnam), *Experience in Hepatic Transplantation*, W. B. Saunders Co., Philadelphia, PA, 1969, 553 pp.

Discussion

Q: What is the mechanism of cyclosporin A?

DR. STARZL: Jean Borel thought that the drug was a relatively specific inhibitor of activated T lymphocytes. That idea seems to be holding up in various in vitro experiments. Also in experimental animals and perhaps in humans, part of the population of specific suppressor cells seems to be at least passively preserved. If these two suggestions hold up, and they can be put together, they would explain the great safety with which cyclosporin A can be used. George Santos of Johns Hopkins is convinced the suppressor cell preservation is important, and several others agree with him.

DR. GREENBLATT: When you compare cyclosporin A with some of the other immunosuppressives, do you notice any difference in the virus infections?

DR. STARZL: Infections have been less, about one-fifth of what they were with conventional therapy. In Minnesota they found less fungal and almost no bacterial infection with cyclosporin A. At a Cambridge conference in September, A. G. Bird of Birmingham, England, reported six lymphomas. The lymphomas had occurred in patients who had an Epstein–Barr virus infection. The evidence that this virus caused lymphoma is circumstantial in some cases, but direct and incontrovertible in others.

Q: Does the report of an 8–14 translocation in these cases suggest that there is another event besides the cytogenetic event?

DR. STARZL: Yes. The present hypothesis is that the Epstein–Barr infection plays a background role in the sense of creating a proliferating population, and that the cytogenetic transformation is the second necessary condition. Incidentally, this kind of pathogenesis is not unique to immunosuppression under cyclosporin A. It is probable that the same events explain many of the lymphomas under conventional therapy with azathioprine and prednisone.

Q: Are there any hematopoietic ramifications following liver transplantation? Do you see any new blood types or blood products that are related to the liver?

DR. STARZL: Yes, two of the early protein phenotypes that were demonstrated to change were haptoglobin and group-specific component. Once these alpha-globins had changed phenotypes, the change persisted for the life of the patient. Since then several other phenotypes have been studied and documented in a paper by Alper et al. (22). Basically they are not too important.

Q: With liver transplantation for Niemann–Pick disease, is it realistic to hope that the extrahepatic tissues will receive a supply of the missing enzyme? I ask because I wonder if the macromolecules can be cleared from the central nervous system?

DR. STARZL: The patient I mentioned did not recover from his pre-existing neurologic status, and that was the reason for death a year and a half later. The Montreal physicians who studied the patient with Niemann–Pick disease reported the development of demonstrable sphingomyelinase in the peripheral blood.

We do know that the neurologic disorder of Wilson's disease can be strikingly reversed with provision of a new liver, but of course that is a completely different disease.

Q: The question of whether the products of the new liver can cross the blood–brain barrier and be able to mobilize the lipid material is extremely important. The possibility that this may occur is a very exciting one, but unproven.

Dr. Starzl: I hope that this occurs. The degree of reversal that can occur in a disorder such as Wilson's disease is really quite striking.

Q: Could you comment on the susceptibility to infectious disease of patients under cyclosporin A?

Dr. Starzl: The incidence of all kinds of infections is distinctly less under cyclosporin A than with conventional immunosuppression. Our preliminary impression is that bacterial and fungal infections have become extremely uncommon, occurring at about one-fifth the rate of our past experience. Patients under cyclosporin A do have a significant incidence of virus infections, but the incidence is still only half of that observed with azathioprine–prednisone therapy. Incidentally, the same kind of data is being generated by investigators of the University of Minnesota.

Q: What are the side effects of cyclosporin A?

Dr. Starzl: The incidence of lymphoma has been no greater per month of graft survival and function than with conventional immunosuppression. The most specific side effect of cyclosporin A is nephrotoxicity. However, the guidelines for management of this have been well worked out in Colorado and in Pittsburgh (20, 21). In essence, one must determine what the dose ranges are in which cyclosporin A toxicity can be expected and reduce the dose when there is a suspicion of drug injury to the kidney. The renal impairment is quickly responsive to dose reductions. So far, there have been no specific and diagnostic lesions that can be identified by conventional pathologic studies. Probably the nephrotoxicity causes proximal tubular damage. At one time, some of the European workers thought that they were seeing abnormal giant mitochondria in the renal tubules, but this has not been confirmed.

One of the unusual opportunities which we have had in the combined Colorado–Pittsburgh experience is to be able to study renal function in liver recipients and to study hepatic function in kidney recipients. By so doing, we have been able to eliminate the confusion that is inevitable when one is looking for organ toxicity with the organ that has just been transplanted. To put it more simply, it has been exceptionally difficult in renal graft recipients to study renal toxicity, but it has been simple to study renal toxicity in patients with liver transplants. The essence of management is dose manipulation.

Treatment of Inherited Metabolic Diseases: Current Status and Prospects

Robert J. Desnick

During the past two decades, considerable attention has been focused on the development of strategies to treat patients with inherited metabolic diseases. Early therapeutic endeavors primarily involved attempts to alter the disease course by metabolic manipulations (Table 1). Investigators have attempted to decrease the concentrations of an accumulated substrate (or of precursors to a metabolic block) by dietary restriction, chelation, or administration of appropriate metabolic inhibitors; or, in disorders resulting from the lack of a crucial product, to replace the normal product. Following early recognition and appropriate intervention in certain of these disorders, chemical and clinical successes have been documented. Therapeutic trials at the level of the biochemical defect have involved direct administration of the appropriate gene product, the specific active enzyme, or deficient cofactor, or the transplantation of allografts capable of producing the normal gene product. The limitations, as well as the encouraging successes, of these strategies for the treatment of genetic diseases have been the subject of recent symposia and reviews (1–4).

Current research efforts to treat these diseases are directed toward the improvement of metabolic manipulation techniques, enzyme replacement and enzyme manipulation strategies, and the evaluation of bone marrow transplantation for the correction of selected disorders. Recent attention also has focused on the potential therapeutic application of recombinant DNA technology. Theoretically, the ideal cure for these inherited diseases would be the insertion of the normal segment of DNA coding for the synthesis of a functional gene product. Therapeutic intervention at

Table 1. **Approaches for the Treatment of Inherited Metabolic Diseases**

Metabolic manipulation
  Dietary restriction
  Substrate depletion techniques
    Chelation/enhanced excretion
    Plasmapheresis/affinity binding
    Surgical-bypass procedures
  Metabolic inhibitors
  Product replacement
Gene therapy
  Production of human biologicals
  Gene transfer

Gene product therapy
  Cofactor supplementation
  Enzyme induction
  Allotransplantation
  Enzyme replacement therapy
Preventive therapy
  Heterozygote screening
  Genetic counseling
  Prenatal diagnosis

the level of the primary genetic defect, or "gene therapy," is at present precluded by our inability to insert a gene that will be properly regulated for normal expression. However, the rapid developments in recombinant DNA technology and gene transfer methodology signal the future prospects for gene therapy.

In this review I will provide an update on current therapeutic approaches, discuss recent exploratory endeavors, and highlight future prospects for the treatment of inherited metabolic diseases.

Metabolic Manipulation

As illustrated in Figure 1, therapeutic manipulations of the metabolic alteration(s) resulting from an enzymatic defect have been designed either (*a*) to limit the intake or deplete the accumulation of the toxic substrate and (or) its precursors, or (*b*) to supply adequate concentrations of crucial metabolic products. In each amenable disorder, the metabolic manipulation strategy has been based on an understanding of the pathophysiology of the disease and the nature of the accumulated substrate or deficient product. Table 2 lists the genetic diseases that have been treated by various metabolic manipulations.

Dietary Restriction

Phenylketonuria. Dietary restriction was the first therapeutically successful manipulation for an inborn error of metabolism. In 1953, Bickel et al. (5) demonstrated the value of a diet low in phenylalanine content for limiting the accumulation of the toxic substrate in patients with phenylketonuria (phenylalanine hy-

Therapeutic Strategies

SUBSTRATE: METABOLIC MANIPULATION

1. Dietary Restriction
2. Chelation/Enhanced Excretion
3. Alternate Metabolic Pathways
4. Plasmapheresis/Affinity Binding
5. Surgical Bypass Procedures
6. Metabolic Inhibitors

PRODUCT: METABOLIC MANIPULATION

7. Supply Deficient Metabolic Product

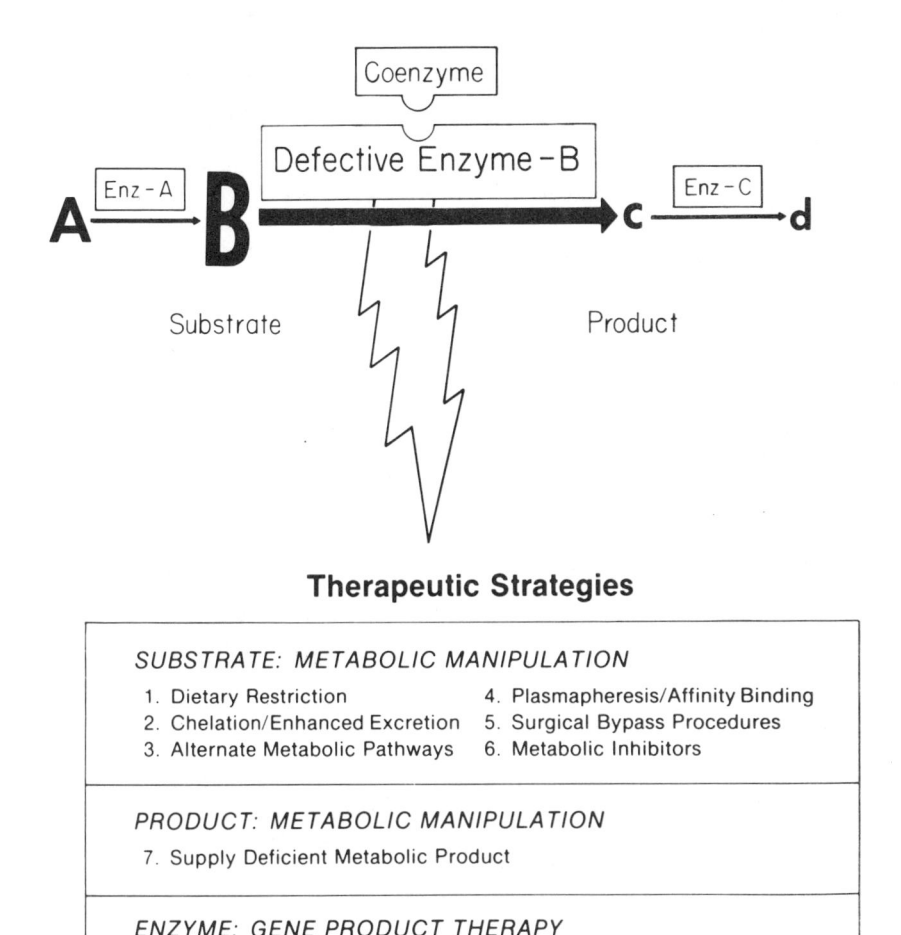

ENZYME: GENE PRODUCT THERAPY

8. Cofactor Supplementation
9. Enzyme Induction/Feedback Repression
10. Allotransplantation
11. Direct Gene Product Replacement -- Enzyme Therapy

Fig. 1. Strategies for the treatment of inherited metabolic diseases

droxylase deficiency). This disorder has served as the prototype for dietary restriction therapy, and the biochemical and clinical effectiveness of this approach has been carefully documented (6).

Three important caveats have emerged from the experience with dietary therapy in phenylketonuria. First, the question about discontinuation of the diet has been the subject of much discussion and debate. Because the disease is inborn, some investigators rec-

Table 2. Genetic Diseases Treated by Metabolic Manipulation

Dietary restriction
- Argininemia
- Argininosuccinic aciduria
- Branched-chain ketoaciduria
- Citrullinuria
- Carbamyl phosphate synthase deficiency
- Cystinosis
- Cystinuria
- Galactosemia
- Gyrate atrophy
- Hereditary fructose intolerance
- Histidinemia
- Homocystinuria
- Isovaleric acidemia
- Lactose intolerance
- Methylmalonic acidemia
- Ornithine carbamoyltransferase deficiency
- Phenylketonuria
- Propionic acidemia
- Tyrosinemia

Metabolic inhibitors
- Bartter's syndrome
- Hyperlipoproteinemia, Type III
- Infantile glycine encephalopathy
- Lesch–Nyhan syndrome
- Primary gout

Substrate depletion techniques
- Chelation/enhanced excretion
  - Argininosuccinic aciduria
  - Cystinuria
  - Familial hyperlipoproteinemia
  - Isovaleric acidemia
  - Nonketotic hyperglycinemia
  - Ornithine carbamoyltransferase deficiency
  - Primary gout
  - β-Thalassemia
  - Wilson's disease
- Plasmapheresis/affinity binding
  - Fabry's disease
  - Gaucher's disease
  - Hypercholesterolemia Type II
  - Refsum's disease
- Surgical-bypass procedures
  - Glycogenosis Type I
  - Glycogenosis Type Ib
  - Glycogenosis Type III
  - Hypercholesterolemia Type II

Product replacement
- Acrodermatitis enteropathica
- Adrenogenital syndromes
- Congenital hypothyroidism
- Hypothyroidism
- Menkes' disease
- Orotic aciduria
- Pituitary dwarfism

ommend that their patients adhere to the diet throughout life. However, most affected children cannot tolerate the taste of the special dietary preparations once they have sampled regular food. The question of long-term phenylalanine restriction has become particularly important in light of recent preliminary findings suggesting that subtle changes in cerebral function may occur in affected children after the dietary restriction is discontinued (7).

Second, the problem of maternal phenylketonuria is as yet unresolved. Because phenylketonuric women have a high risk of delivering babies with congenital malformations (8), resumption of dietary therapy during pregnancy has been recommended. However, even when dietary restriction is begun before conception, the results are variable (9,10). Clearly, the factors that predispose to fetal damage (e.g., maternal blood phenylalanine control) must be delineated and alternative forms of therapy developed if fetal toxicity is to be prevented.

Third, two new forms of hyperphenylalaninuria—one due to the deficiency of dihydropteridine reductase (*11*), the other due to a defect in tetrahydrobiopterin synthesis (*12*)—have been discovered that are not treatable by dietary restriction alone. Both of these variants involve a deficiency of tetrahydrobiopterin, the cofactor required for phenylalanine hydroxylase activity. In addition, tetrahydrobiopterin is a cofactor for both tyrosine and tryptophan hydroxylases, enzymes involved in the synthesis of the neurotransmitters, dopamine and serotonin. Thus, the amounts of DOPA and 5-hydroxytryptophan (precursors of dopamine, norepinephrine, epinephrine, and serotonin) also are decreased in these forms of phenylketonuria. Administration of DOPA, 5-hydroxytryptophan, and carbidopa, in an attempt to replace these neurotransmitter precursors, did not prove clinically effective in patients who already had neurologic damage (*11*), but appeared to be effective if initiated early in conjunction with dietary therapy (K. Tada, personal communication). More encouraging preliminary studies indicate that the direct administration of tetrahydrobiopterin may be therapeutic, particularly for patients with defective tetrahydrobiopterin biosynthesis (*13–15*).

A novel method for dietary restriction in phenylketonuria is the oral administration of gelatin capsules containing the plant enzyme, phenylalanine ammonia-lyase (*16*). This enzyme converts phenylalanine in the gut to *trans*-cinnamic acid and thereby selectively depletes the phenylalanine derived from food protein before absorption. A pilot trial of oral enzyme ingestion in an untreated patient with phenylalanine hydroxylase deficiency reduced the concentration of phenylalanine in blood by about 25%. Further experience with this enzyme will determine its usefulness in reducing the phenylalanine concentrations in blood as an adjunct to dietary therapy. In addition, this method may provide a tolerable form of substrate depletion for the management of older patients who are not on a low-phenylalanine diet, particularly previously treated patients who become pregnant.

Other dietarily treatable disorders. Subsequent experience with dietary restriction has proven effective not only for phenylketonuria, but also for other inborn errors whose pathology results from toxic substrate accumulation. These include galactosemia (*17,18*), hereditary fructose intolerance (*19*), lactose intolerance (*20*), B_6-unresponsive homocystinuria (*21,22*), B_{12}-unresponsive methylmalonic acidemia (*23,24*), branched-chain ketoaciduria (*25,26*), isovaleric acidemia (*27*), and tyrosinemia (*28*). Experimental attempts to treat cystinuria (*29,30*), cystinosis (*31*), histidinemia (*32,33*), and other aminoacidurias by appropriate dietary restriction have met with limited success. Recently, a Japanese collaborative study has shown no significant impairment of intellectual development in 77 untreated histidinemic patients, suggesting that dietary restriction was not necessary because histidinemia did not cause mental retardation (*34*). Generalized protein restriction has proven effective in urea-cycle defects, especially those with partial enzyme defects (*35*), and in certain organic acidopathies (*36*). Efforts to decrease the hyperammonemia in these disorders (caused by deficiencies of carbomyl-phosphate synthetase, ornithine carbamoyltransferase, or argininosuccinate synthetase) by the use of low-protein diets supplemented with nitrogen-free α-keto-acid analogs (ketovaline, ketoleucine, ketoisoleucine, phenyllactate, and hydroxymethionine) (*35,37,38*) require further evaluation to determine their efficacy.

Gyrate atrophy, which results from the deficient activity of ornithine-γ-aminotransferase, a pyridoxine-dependent enzyme, is a recent addition to the list of disorders in which dietary restriction has proven therapeutic. An arginine-deficient diet corrected the hyperornithinemia, ornithinuria, and lysinuria in patients with B_6-nonresponsive gyrate atrophy of the choroid and retina (*39,40*). In addition, the excretion of ornithine was increased by oral administration of α-aminoisobutyric acid, which enhances the renal clearance of dibasic amino acids. Patients receiving this diet for more than two years did not experience continued choroidoretinal degeneration and their vision improved, as measured by dark adaptation, visual field, and electroretinographic studies (*39,41*). Similar, though less dramatic, results have been obtained using a more palatable, low-protein diet instead of the semi-synthetic low-arginine diet (*42*). In addition to the visual manifestations, affected subjects also have progressive atrophy of Type II skeletal muscle fibers, presumably because of the hyperornithinemia, which leads to decreased concentrations of creatine and phosphocreatine. A trial of oral creatine supplementation produced significant enlargement of the Type II fibers after one year, without, however, improving the visual manifestations (43). These results suggest that combined dietary therapy and creatine supplementation may be optimal therapy for the B_6-unresponsive form of gyrate atrophy.

Substrate Depletion Techniques

Chelation. Another way to decrease the concentrations of noxious substrates and (or) precursors and metabolic derivatives is to administer chelators or other drugs to mobilize the excretion of these compounds. In Wilson's disease (44,45), the accumulated copper may be depleted by penicillamine, a chelating agent that binds to, mobilizes, and promotes the excretion of the intracellular copper ions. Triethylenetetramine dihydrochloride is a safe and effective copper chelator for patients with Wilson's disease who develop late drug tolerance or early penicillamine sensitivity (46,47). Penicillamine also has been used to treat cystinuria (48); the drug participates in a mixed disulfide reaction to solubilize cystine calculi and promote the urinary clearance of the more soluble cysteine–penicillamine mixed disulfide.

Cholestyramine and colestipol, nonabsorbable anion-exchange resins that bind bile acids in the intestinal lumen and thus prevent their absorption, have been administered orally to reduce cholesterol concentrations in familial hypercholesterolemia. These resins have been given in conjunction with a low-cholesterol diet (100 mg of cholesterol per day) containing less than 8% of calories as saturated fat. The increased fecal excretion of bile salts leads to an increased conversion of cholesterol to bile acids, resulting in decreased plasma concentrations of cholesterol (49). These bile-acid-binding resins also enhance catabolism of low-density lipoproteins (LDL)[1] (50), presumably by decreasing the synthesis of very-low-density lipoproteins. When these resins are combined with nicotinic acid supplementation, the concentrations of both cholesterol and LDL are decreased (51,52).

In β-thalassemia, the necessity for frequent therapeutic blood transfusions leads to iron overload and eventually to hemosiderosis. Desferrioxamine B has been used effectively to chelate the accumulated ferritin and prevent iron loading in transfusion-de-

---

[1] Abbreviations used: LDL, low-density lipoprotein; HSA, human serum albumin; G6PD, glucose-6-phosphate dehydrogenase.

pendent thalassemia (53). Therapy in primary gout has involved various uricosuric drugs (e.g., probenecid, sulfinpyrazone) to decrease the systemic uric acid accumulation by increasing its renal excretion and mobilizing the intracellular deposits of uric acid salts (54,55).

Enhanced excretion. Recent efforts to treat the urea-cycle defects have focused on the use of alternative metabolic pathways to enhance excretion of waste nitrogen in the form of metabolites other than urea, namely, urea-cycle intermediates and amino acid acylation products (56–58). This maneuver exploits the fact that certain non-urea nitrogen-containing metabolites have high excretion rates; promoting the synthesis of these urea-cycle intermediates enhances excretion of waste nitrogen. For example, the non-toxic urea-cycle intermediate, argininosuccinic acid, contains both nitrogen atoms for urea synthesis and is rapidly excreted. Dietary supplementation of pharmacologic amounts of arginine (or ornithine, or both) in patients with argininosuccinase deficiency increased nitrogen waste excretion (as argininosuccinic acid), decreased plasma concentrations of ammonium, and maintained other urea precursors within their normal ranges (57). A similar approach to promote orotic acid excretion has been suggested for ornithine carbamoyltransferase deficiency (59).

Amino acid acylation provides a second alternative pathway to increase waste nitrogen excretion (56,58). Oral administration of sodium benzoate enhances the urinary excretion of hippuric acid (the glycine conjugate of benzoic acid). Similarly, administration of phenylacetic acid results in the acylation of glutamine to form phenylacetylglutamine, a rapidly excreted nitrogen-containing compound. Preliminary trials with each of these compounds in patients with various urea-cycle enzymopathies have shown encouraging results and lack of toxicity (56–60). The combined use of both compounds might provide an effective means to promote waste nitrogen excretion in the inborn errors of urea genesis as well as in other disorders of nitrogen accumulation (56).

Another approach for substrate depletion by an alternative pathway has been used for the treatment of isovaleric acidemia (61–64). On the basis of studies of bovine glycine *N*-acylase (64), Krieger and Tanaka (61) reasoned that the administration of supplementary glycine to patients with isovaleric acidemia with high hepatic isovaleryl-CoA concentrations would promote the production of isovalerylglycine, enhance its excretion, and alleviate the patients' ketoacidosis. Indeed, prompt biochemical resolution of acidotic crises and increased isovalerylglycine excretion were observed in two patients when glycine was administered orally or rectally (61,63). One patient showed improved growth during a period of chronic glycine therapy (61), but the use of glycine to prevent acidotic episodes and improve development in these patients will require a controlled, collaborative study.

Plasmapheresis/affinity binding. Two mechanical approaches to deplete an accumulated circulating substrate include plasmapheresis and affinity binding. The former simply removes a large volume of plasma containing the toxic compound, whereas affinity binding selectively removes a compound or class of compounds from the circulation. Theoretically, the affinity-binding method is superior because plasmapheresis removes large amounts of plasma and nonselectively removes other molecules (e.g., trace metals, cofactors, and other essential compounds) that may be crucial for certain metabolic processes. Moreover, chronic plasmapheresis requires volume replacement with synthetic plasma products or fresh plasma, both involving the risk of hepatitis.

Plasmapheresis has been attempted in several disorders characterized by high circulating concentrations of specific lipids. In Refsum's disease, a disorder characterized by high concentrations of circulating phytanic acid, owing to defective phytanic acid oxidation, chronic plasmapheresis has therapeutic value. Previously, dietary restriction of phytanic acid and phytol were beneficial (65). More recently, chronic plasmapheresis has been used effectively to decrease markedly the plasma concentrations of phytanic acid; concomitant improvement in the patients' neurologic status, including peripheral nerve function, muscle strength, and stabilized vision, has been noted (65,66, and personal communication from J. Hollander and J. A. Nusbacher). Combined dietary restriction and chronic plasmapheresis should enhance therapy in this disease, phytanic acid being entirely of dietary origin and plasmapheresis effectively minimizing the concentrations of phytanic acid and perhaps depleting any substrate that is mobilized from tissues.

Plasmapheresis also has been attempted in two lysosomal storage diseases, Fabry's and Gaucher's diseases (66, and unpublished results, Desnick and E. H. Schuchman), in which the glycosphingolipids trihexosyl ceramide and glucosyl ceramide, respectively, accumulate. The rationale for this approach is based on the fact that these substrates accumulate in the plasma, where they are primarily associated with the low- and high-density lipoproteins. Trials in patients with Gaucher type 1 disease indicated that chronic plasmapheresis did not deplete sufficient amounts of substrate to be biochemically therapeutic (Desnick and Schuchman, unpublished results). However, pilot trials in patients with Fabry's disease (66, and unpublished results) suggested that this modality may deplete circulating substrates enough to warrant further evaluation, particularly because the manifestations of this disease result from lipid deposition in the vascular endothelium (67). Thus, further long-term evaluation is required to determine the efficacy of this strategy.

Plasmapheresis (68,69) and affinity binding (70,71) have been used to deplete circulating cholesterol in homozygous familial hypercholesterolemia. The affinity ligand, heparin–agarose, used for the extracorporeal binding of LDL from patients' blood, binds the lipoprotein by the formation of precipitating heparin–lipoprotein complexes. Blood drawn into a transfer bag containing heparin, heparin–agarose beads, and $CaCl_2$ is mixed, then transfused through a filter to remove the heparin–lipoprotein complexes. Repetitive use of this technique decreased the plasma cholesterol about 50%, but the cholesterol concentration returned to initial values in three to seven days after treatment. A recently developed system involving a heparin–agarose column coupled to a blood-cell processor (72) may improve the efficiency and effectiveness of this technique; this system has not been used in human trials, however. If this plasmaperfusion system is practical, then use of various affinity ligands may provide for efficient depletion of toxic, accumulated substrates from the circulation, particularly in selected amino acid and organic acid disorders, or in those diseases in which other approaches have not proven effective.

Surgical-bypass procedures. Intriguing surgical strategies have been used to treat various metabolic diseases (73). In glycogenoses types I (74), Ib (75), and III (76), the progressive incorporation of absorbed glucose into hepatic glycogen has been partly reversed by a surgical anastamosis between the portal vein and inferior vena cava. This portacaval shunt permits some of the circulating glucose that has been absorbed by the intestine to bypass the hepatocyte, where glucose is pathologically and irreversibly deposited as glycogen; the glucose-rich blood is shunted systemically to nourish the tissues. In addition to re-establishing normoglycemia, this technique has produced other documented clinical improvements in these patients, including a substantial growth spurt, increased bone age, reduction in liver size, reduction in serum concentrations of urate and lipids, and improved coagulation and glucose tolerance. A nonsurgical approach that has also proven therapeutic, particularly in preventing severe hypoglycemic episodes, is nocturnal continuous intragastric feeding (77–79). Such feedings may be the treatment of choice for affected infants and small children, prior to consideration of surgical procedures. Ileal-jejunal-bypass procedures also have diminished the hypercholesterolemia in patients with familial hypercholesterolemia, by decreasing the reabsorption of bile acids from the ileum and thus stimulating their synthesis from hepatic cholesterol (80). Partial ileal bypasses can lower the concentrations of both total and LDL-cholesterol, which suggests that the increased bile acid synthesis enhances the rate of hepatic uptake and degradation of LDL (81).

Metabolic Inhibitors

Metabolic inhibitors have been used to reduce the synthesis of accumulated substrates or precursors. In patients with Lesch–Nyhan syndrome (hypoxanthine–guanine phosphoribosyltransferase deficiency) and primary gout, allopurinol has been used therapeutically to inhibit the precursor enzyme, xanthine oxidase, in order to reduce the toxic uric acid concentrations (54,82). Clofibrate, which inhibits the synthesis or release of glyceride from the liver, effectively decreases blood lipids to normal concentrations in patients with Type III hyperlipoproteinemia (83). More recently, compactin, a specific inhibitor of 3-hydroxy-3-methylglutaryl-CoA reductase, has been used to decrease cholesterol synthesis in familial hypercholesterolemia (84). Inhibition of this enzyme decreases sterol synthesis and results in decreased concentrations of plasma LDL. Further studies with this and similar inhibitors of sterol biosynthesis are needed to determine if this approach can safely decrease cholesterol biosynthesis and trigger a therapeutic increase in the number of LDL receptors. Combined use of a bile acid sequestration resin and the enzyme inhibitor may provide the most effective therapy for this relatively common disease.

Although not a specific inhibitor of glycine biosynthesis, strychnine antagonizes the binding of glycine to receptors in the central nervous system and has been used successfully to improve the severe depression of respiratory and motor function that results from the high concentrations of glycine in cerebrospinal fluid (*85*) of patients with severe infantile glycine encephalopathy (nonketotic hyperglycinemia).

Bartter's syndrome, or hyperplasia of the juxtaglomerular apparatus, is characterized by hypokalemic alkalosis, hyper-reninemia, aldosteronism, high urinary excretion of prostaglandin (PGE$_2$), and normal blood pressure (*86,87*). Although the basic defect in this disorder is unknown, the recent finding of increased urinary excretion of 6-keto-PGF$_{1\alpha}$ suggested that the overproduction of prostacyclin (PGI$_2$) mediated both the hyper-reninemia and the hyporesponsiveness of blood pressure to pressor agents (*88*). Treatment with indomethacin, an inhibitor of prostaglandin endoperoxide synthetase (6,9-oxycyclase) (*89*), reportedly corrects the hyper-reninemia, the aldosteronism, and the high PGE$_2$ excretion (*87–90*), but not the defect in distal fractional chloride reabsorption (*91*). After prolonged therapy, however, plasma renin activity was no longer suppressed (*92*). Further understanding of the nature of the primary defect should result in the development of specific therapy.

Product Replacement

The most clinically effective metabolic manipulations involve direct product replacement in disorders whose pathogenesis results from the failure of the defective enzyme to produce a crucial metabolic product. The administration of appropriate steroids to patients with the congenital adrenal hyperplasia syndromes (*93*)—thyroxin for hypothyroidism (*94*), growth hormone for pituitary dwarfism (*95*), and uridine for orotic aciduria (*96*)—is therapeutically effective in overriding the respective inherited metabolic blocks.

Past efforts to treat Menkes' disease by copper replacement underscore the necessity for a fundamental understanding of the primary defect before the development and initiation of therapeutic endeavors. Early evidence that the primary defect was due to defective copper absorption (*97*) led several investigators to administer copper sulfate by oral (*98*), subcutaneous (*99*), or intravenous (*97,98,100,101*) routes in an attempt to treat the apparent copper deficiency. Although the serum concentrations of copper and ceruloplasmin increased to normal values (*97,100,102*), there was no clinical improvement. More recent studies (*103–106*) indicate that the defect in Menkes' disease produces increased concentrations of intracellular copper, presumably from abnormal regulation of the copper-binding protein, metallothionein. Thus, future attempts to treat this disease will require elucidation of the precise molecular defect in copper homeostasis and the development of strategies to deplete or limit intracellular copper accumulation in affected males with this X-linked disease.

In contrast to Menkes' disease, trace metal replacement has been clinically effective in acrodermatitis enteropathica. In this disorder, inherited as an autosomal recessive trait, the systemic zinc deficiency appears to result from a defective zinc-binding factor in the intestine (*107,108*). The inability to absorb and (or) transport zinc leads to bullous skin lesions, alopecia, and deficient activities of several zinc-dependent enzymes (*109–111*). Administration of human breast milk, which contains the zinc-binding factor, ameliorates the clinical manifestations (*108,112,113*), as does oral zinc supplementation; when serum concentrations of zinc approach normal, there is clinical improvement (*112,113*). Because several offspring of affected women have shown congenital abnormalities (*114*), it has been suggested that the plasma zinc concentrations of such women should be closely monitored during pregnancy. Preliminary trials of zinc sulfate supplementation to maintain normal plasma zinc values, particularly in the second and third trimesters, have resulted in normal babies (*115*).

Another disorder in which a binding or transport protein may be defective is X-linked hypophosphatemia. In this disease, a primary renal defect in phosphate resorption leads to poor bone mineralization (rickets) and hypocalcemia. Recent efforts directed at symptomatic improvement have involved oral administration of phosphate and 1,25-dihydroxycholecalciferol (*116,117*). This regimen resulted in bone mineralization and healing, lower alkaline phosphatase activity, and symptomatic improvement; however, the primary defect, renal wastage of phosphate, was not altered. In addition, this experimental regimen was associated with an increased risk for hypercalcemia and secondary hyperparathyroidism, thus necessitating careful monitoring of serum and urine concentrations of calcium.

Gene Product Therapy

Therapeutic endeavors at the level of the biochemical defect, e.g., a functionally defective enzyme or gene product, have become the focus of recent efforts to treat inherited metabolic diseases. Characterization of the molecular nature of a specific enzymatic defect provides the biochemical rationale for the development of effective gene-product strategies (see Table 3).

Cofactor Supplementation

Many enzymatic reactions require specific cofactors, often a vitamin or its derivative, for normal catalytic activity. In certain inborn errors, the enzymatic defect may involve either the binding site for a specific cofactor or vitamin [resulting in an altered affinity for apoenzyme–coenzyme binding (118)] or the abnormal transport or biosynthesis of the active form of the cofactor (119). The coenzyme may normally form part of the active site of the holoenzyme and thus participate directly in catalysis. The apoenzyme–coenzyme interaction may decrease the K_m of the reaction by altering the conformation of the enzyme. Alternatively, the coenzyme may render the holoenzyme less susceptible to intracellular degradation and thus enhance the number of catalytically active molecules.

In several of these disorders, vitamin-responsive and -nonresponsive subtypes involving the same deficient enzymatic activity have been identified, e.g., methylmalonic aciduria (119) and cystathioninuria (120). Based on in vivo and in vitro studies, it has been hypothesized that responsive and nonresponsive forms of a particular disease represent different mutations of the apoenzyme or a mutation in a gene responsible for the synthesis of the cofactor. In the responsive mutation, the cofactor-binding site of the apoenzyme may be altered to a form that is still capable of binding when large concentrations of the cofactor are provided; the nonresponsive mutation may alter irreversibly the enzyme's conformation so that the residual enzymatic activity is not increased with the administration of large doses of the appropriate

Table 3. Gene Product Therapy: Cofactor Supplementation[a]

Cofactor	Metabolic disorder	Biochemical defect
Cobalamin	Anemia	Deficiency of intrinsic factor
	Anemia	Inactive intrinsic factor
	Anemia	Ileal transport
	Methylmalonic aciduria	L-Methylmalonyl-CoA mutase
	[b] Methylmalonic aciduria	Adenosylcobalamin synthesis
	[b] Methylmalonic aciduria with homocystinuria	Adenosylcobalamin and methylcobalamin synthesis
	Transcobalamin II deficiency	Transport into cells
Folate	Congenital malabsorption of folate	Intestinal absorption
	Dihydrofolate reductase deficiency	Dihydrofolate reductase
	Formiminoglutamic aciduria	Formiminotransferase (and cyclodeaminase)
	Homocystinuria	Methylenetetrahydrofolate reductase
Biotin	β-Methylcrotonylglycinuria	β-Methylcrotonyl-CoA carboxylase
	[b] Mixed carboxylase deficiency	Holocarboxylase synthetase
	Propionic acidemia	Propionyl-CoA carboxylase
Thiamin	Branched-chain ketoaciduria	Branched-chain ketoacid decarboxylase
	Pyruvic acidemia	Pyruvate decarboxylase
	Subacute necrotizing encephalomyelopathy (Leigh)	Pyruvate carboxylase (?)
Ascorbate	Ehlers–Danlos (VI) syndrome	Collagen lysyl hydroxylase
Pyridoxine	Cystathioninuria	γ-Cystathionase
	Gyrate atrophy	Ornithine ketoacid aminotransferase
	Homocystinuria	Cystathionine β-synthase
	Hyperoxaluria	Glyoxylate:α-ketoglutarate carboligase
	Hyperoxaluria	D-Glyceric dehydrogenase
	Infantile convulsions	Glutamate decarboxylase
	Pyridoxine-responsive anemia	
	Xanthurenic aciduria	Kynureninase
Vitamin D	Familial hypophosphatemia	Defective phosphate transport/reabsorption(?)
Tetrahydropterin	Hyperphenylalaninemia	Dehydropteridine reductase
	Hyperphenylalaninemia	Defective biopterin synthesis
L-Carnitine	Carnitine deficiency	Defective carnitine transport
Zinc sulfate	Mannosidosis	α-Mannosidase

[a] Modified from Fleischer and Gaull (121).
[b] Prenatal cofactor supplementation successfully accomplished.

cofactor, or may result in either an unstable protein or no enzyme synthesis at all. Alternatively, if the absorption, transport, or synthesis of the required cofactor is impaired, supplementation with the proper cofactor derivative may partly reconstitute enzymatic activity. Even a small increase in enzymatic activity, resulting from supplementation with the proper cofactor, may significantly affect the metabolic defect. Indeed, experience with the vitamin-dependent enzymatic deficiency diseases has indicated that for certain mutations, cofactor supplementation may increase the residual activity of certain mutant holoenzyme complexes and provide biochemical and clinical improvement. This strategy for the "biochemical manipulation" of the abnormal, residual enzymatic activity has been applied to the treatment of over 25 cofactor or vitamin-responsive disorders (Table 3) (*121–123*). Recent additions include the use of pyridoxal phosphate in B_6-responsive gyrate atrophy (*124*), tetrahydropterins in hyperphenylalaninemia (*13–15*), zinc sulfate to enhance the residual α-mannosidase activity in human and bovine mannosidosis (*125,126*), ascorbate to increase residual collagen lysyl hydroxylase activity in Type VI Ehlers–Danlos syndrome (*127,128*), biotin in multiple carboxylase deficiency (*129*), and L-carnitine in carnitine-deficient cardiomyopathy (*130*).

Attention has focused on the in utero treatment of cofactor-responsive disorders. The first successful application of this strategy was the in utero treatment of a fetus prenatally diagnosed as having B_{12}-responsive methylmalonic acidemia (*131*). The mother received large doses of B_{12}, which crossed the placenta and entered the fetal circulation. This child, now eight years old, has maintained normal psychomotor development with daily oral cofactor supplementation (M. J. Mahoney, personal communication). More recently, this approach has been taken for the treatment of a fetus prenatally found to have biotin-responsive multiple carboxylase deficiency. Notably, the neonatal period was uncomplicated and the child continues to grow and develop normally at one year of age (*132*).

A form of periconceptional cofactor therapy has been advanced for the possible prevention of neural tube defects. A decreased rate of neural tube defects was noted in the offspring of women whose diets were supplemented with a commercially available multivitamin preparation (*133*) or with folate (*134*). Although the therapeutic efficacy of this approach has not been determined, the limited evidence to date suggests that administration of folate or multivitamins provides essential cofactors that decrease or prevent the occurrence of neural tube defects. The periconceptional administration of vitamins also has been proposed for the possible prevention of orofacial clefts (*135*).

Overall, the clinical effectiveness of cofactor supplementation therapy, often accompanied by other dietary manipulations, has been variable. However, even slight enhancement of enzyme activity may prove beneficial, and follow-up studies to assess clinical effectiveness are still required for some disorders. Experience with cofactor supplementation in this group of diseases has been the subject of recent reviews (*121,123*).

Enzyme Induction/Feedback Repression

Another approach at the level of the enzymatic defect involves the use of drugs that increase residual enzymatic activity. Phenobarbital and related drugs apparently stimulate the production of smooth endoplasmic reticulum as well as the synthesis of specific enzymes of the endoplasmic reticulum, including hepatic UDP-glucuronosyltransferase. These findings provide the basis for administering phenobarbital to patients with Gilbert's syndrome or Crigler–Najjar syndrome (*136*). Although enzyme modification or stabilization has not been ruled out, the drug presumably induces smooth endoplasmic reticulum synthesis and concomitantly increases the amount of UDP-glucuronosyltransferase, resulting in increased conjugation of unconjugated bilirubin and a decrease in plasma bilirubin. This approach may be of value in selected enzymatic defects that result from a decreased synthetic rate of a specific enzyme located in the smooth endoplasmic reticulum.

Enzyme induction has been used as a therapeutic modality in hereditary angioneurotic edema (*137*) and α_1-antitrypsin deficiency (*138*). Both disorders result from the defective synthesis of glycoproteins produced and secreted by the liver. Angioneurotic edema, an autosomal dominant disorder, is characterized by one-half the normal concentrations of functionally active serum C1 esterase inhibitor. In this disorder, administration of the androgen-related compound danazol (a derivative of ethisterone) increased serum concentrations of C1 inhibitor three- to fivefold in most patients; C4 was also increased. Although the mechanism of induction has not been characterized, the androgen may induce synthesis of C1 inhibitor mRNA (137). Prophylactic administration of oral danazol is effective in decreasing or preventing acute attacks of angioneurotic edema, with minimal virilization and hepatotoxicity. Recently, intravenous administration of a plasma concentrate containing C1 inhibitor has been used effectively to abate acute abdominal or laryngeal attacks and increase serum C4 activity (139).

Danazol also has been used to increase the activity of the serum antiprotease, α_1-antitrypsin, in individuals with this recessively inherited deficiency (139). After 30 days of androgen therapy, functional α_1-antitrypsin in PiZZ, PiM$_{Duarte}$Z, and PiSZ individuals increased 37%, 85%, and 87%, respectively. Electrophoretic analysis of the increased glycoprotein revealed the same patterns as those observed pre-treatment. Because PiZZ, PiM$_{Duarte}$Z, and PiSZ individuals are at risk for development of severe emphysema, danazol has been suggested as a preventive approach to improve the protease–antiprotease imbalance and impede the progression of their lung disease (139).

Enzyme repression has been used as a strategy for the treatment of the acute porphyrias. For example, acute intermittent porphyria, a dominantly inherited disorder, results from the half-normal activity of the enzyme porphobilinogen deaminase and the subsequent accumulation of its substrate and its immediate precursor, porphobilinogen and δ-aminolevulinic acid, respectively. In addition, the defect in heme biosynthesis results in decreased heme production. Heme is known to repress the activity of the first and rate-limiting enzyme in the pathway, δ-aminolevulinate synthetase by an end-product feedback inhibition (140–144). During acute attacks in acute intermittent porphyria, the concentrations of porphobilinogen and δ-aminolevulinic acid are markedly increased. Presumably, hepatic δ-aminolevulinate synthetase is induced by various drugs, dietary factors, or other metabolites as well as by the decreased production of heme secondary to the deficiency of porphobilinogen deaminase (145,146). On the assumption that heme would repress the hepatic δ-aminolevulinate synthetase activity and thereby decrease the toxic concentrations of porphobilinogen and δ-aminolevulinic acid, intravenous hematin has been infused in patients with acute attacks of acute intermittent porphyria (145–147), porphyria variegata (146,147), and coproporphyria (*146,147*). "Prompt and often dramatic recovery" was observed in over 80% of the treated attacks (*146*). The high serum concentrations of δ-aminolevulinic acid and porphobilinogen were markedly decreased, often to zero, after infusions of hematin. Thus, the use of hematin to repress hepatic activity of δ-aminolevulinate synthetase appears to have therapeutic value. Further studies of this enzyme, δ-aminolevulinate dehydratase, and porphobilinogen deaminase activities, before and after hematin infusions in patients with acute intermittent porphyria, are required to document the biochemical mechanisms underlying the hematin effect. Infusions of glucose or levulose (*148,149*), as well as folate (*150*), have also been effective in the treatment of acute attacks, and the use of hematin in conjunction with these compounds should be considered for the treatment of severe attacks.

Allotransplantation

An intriguing means for transferring normal genetic information into patients with selected structural and metabolic gene defects is allotransplantation (*151–153*). This approach exploits the grafting of cells, tissues, or organs containing normal DNA to produce active enzymes or other gene products in the recipient. For structural gene defects with pathology limited to specific organs or tissues, successful transplantation of the appropriate allograft may provide effective treatment. For inherited metabolic defects, allotransplantation of appropriate tissues may provide a strategy for the continuous synthesis of active gene products. In disorders characterized by substrate accumulation in plasma, the active enzyme in the allograft may metabolize or clear any accumulated substrate that is delivered to the transplanted tissue by the circulation. As the accumulated substrate is cleared from the plasma, a concentration gradient presumably is established between the plasma and the tissue sites of substrate deposition, allowing for the continuous resaturation of the plasma and continual clearance of the systemic substrate load. In situ metabolism would probably be the major mechanism of substrate metabolism by transplanted organs such as liver, spleen, and kidney. Alternatively, the normal allograft may synthesize active enzyme, essential cofactor, hormone, or immunocompetent factor, which is either released by the turnover of allograft cells or by direct secretion into the circulation. The active enzyme or gene product would then be distributed to the tissues where it might gain access to cells for substrate metabolism. The release and distribution of normal gene products conceivably would be a therapeutic mechanism of transplanted pancreas, bone marrow, thymus, and, to a lesser degree, liver and kidney. The selection of the allograft in a particular inherited disorder must be based on the specific nature of the defective gene product, the pathophysiology of the disease, and the probable mechanism by which the allograft might provide the normal gene product.

Figure 2 summarizes the various genetic diseases in which allotransplantation has been accomplished. Several of these endeavors were specifically designed to be therapeutic—to continuously replace defective enzymes, hormones, or immunologic factors or to effectively ameliorate the functional alterations resulting from structural gene defects.

Transplantation of Bone Marrow, Thymus, and Fetal Liver

Bone marrow, thymus, and fetal liver have been successfully transplanted for the cellular, metabolic, and immunologic correc-

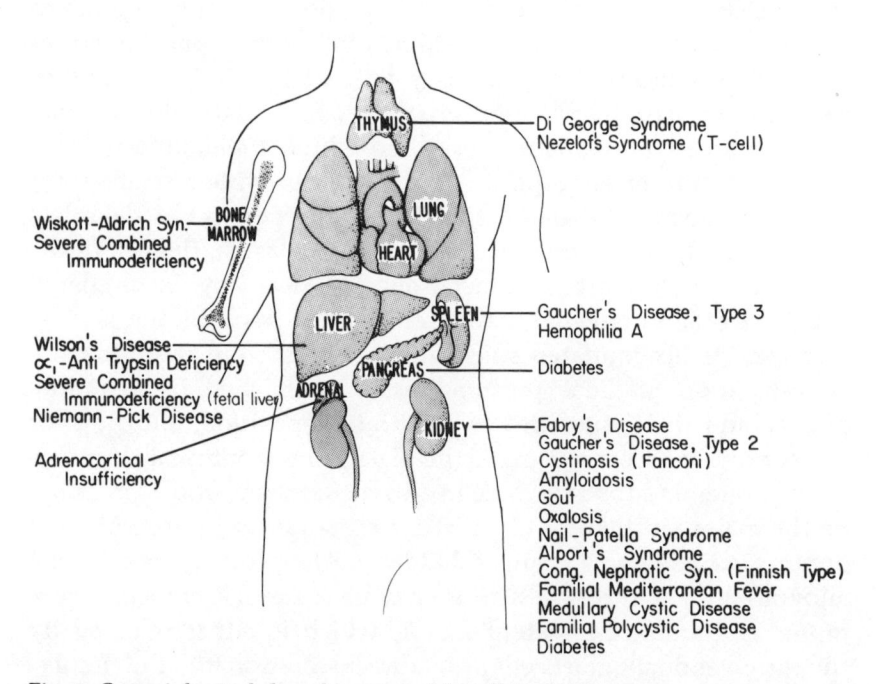

Fig. 2. Some inherited disorders treated by allotransplantation

tion of various congenital and inherited disorders (*153,154*). Bone marrow transplantation has been used to correct inherited disorders resulting from the defective function of marrow-derived cells. A major limitation of marrow transplantation has been the requirement for a histocompatible, related donor to minimize the high morbidity and mortality associated with this procedure. The first successes in bone marrow transplantation were achieved in various immunodeficiency diseases. In severe combined immunodeficiency disease, successful engraftment corrected both the humoral and cellular immune defects in affected patients (*153,155*). Marrow transplantation has also been used to reverse the cellular and immune defects in patients with various disorders including Wiscott–Aldrich syndrome (*156–158*), chronic granulomatous disease (*159*), Kostmann syndrome (*160*), Fanconi's anemia (*161*), and Chediak–Higashi syndrome (*162*). Experimental studies in mice indicate the potential of various techniques to deplete the donor marrow of lymphocytes responsible for initiating graft vs host rejection (*163*). Total lymphoid irradiation also has been used to enhance the engraftment of allogenic marrow (and minimize graft vs host rejection) to correct the β-glucuronidase deficiency in circulating cells and liver of C3H/HeJ mice (*164,165*).

Because bone marrow stem cells differentiate to form osteoclasts as well as blood cells, marrow transplantation has also been used to treat infantile severe osteopetrosis (*166*). This inherited disease results from the inability of osteoclasts to resorb bone, a process required for normal skeletal growth. Bone marrow transplantation was first achieved in the murine analog of this disease (*167*). Based on the cellular correction of the murine disorder, bone marrow transplantation was undertaken in humans. Successful engraftment restored normal osteoclastic activities, and evidence for clinical improvement has been documented (*166*).

More recently, Hobbs et al. (*168*) reported the preliminary results of bone marrow transplantation in a one-year-old child with Hurler's disease (α-L-iduronidase deficiency). They reasoned that, the majority of the clinical manifestations in this disease being the result of defective mucopolysaccharide metabolism in cells of the macrophage-monocyte system, engrafted stem cells from histocompatible donors with normal enzyme activity would provide normal cells to repopulate the reticuloendothelial system.

In addition, Hobbs (*169*) suggested that the presence of normal circulating monocytes and wandering tissue macrophages would serve as scavengers to release normal enzyme for uptake by cells in various anatomic locations (e.g., brain) for degradation of the accumulated substrates. After transplantation, the patient had decreased corneal clouding and a smaller liver and spleen. Some normalization of bone growth and a stabilized intellectual development were also reported, but these are difficult to assess because patients with Hurler's syndrome have normal or accelerated growth and mental development (rather than regression) during the first year of life (*170*). The major question remaining is whether the marrow transplant will have any effect on the progressive neurologic manifestations, which are the major debilitating features of this disease.

An "experiment of nature" argues against the ability of bone marrow transplantation to alter the course of storage diseases with neuronal pathology. In bovine mannosidosis, a chimeric calf or "freemartin" was discovered (*171*). Fusion of the placentae of the normal and mannosidosis calves resulted in the intra-uterine engraftment of normal marrow stem cells in the affected calf, in effect an "in utero bone marrow transplant." Unfortunately, the chimeric mannosidosis calf eventually died from the neurologic manifestations of this disease. This "experiment of nature" argues against the ability of engrafted normal cells to alter the course of lysosomal storage disorders (and perhaps other diseases) characterized by severe neurologic involvement.

Most recently, successful correction of β-thalassemia has been achieved by marrow transplantation in a 16-month-old affected boy (*172*). After successful engraftment of marrow from a HLA-identical normal sister, the recipient no longer has this hereditary hemoglobinopathy. This result is most encouraging and signals the use of marrow transplantation for the correction of other severe inherited hematologic disorders. The current status and problems of bone marrow transplantation have been the subject of a recent review (*173*).

Fetal liver cells also corrected the immunologic defects in severe combined immunodeficiency disease (*174*). Fetal thymus allografts have reconstituted the immunologic and thymic deficiencies in Di George's syndrome (congenital absence of the thymus) (*175*) and corrected the immunologic defect in Nezelof's syndrome, a rare T-cell immunodeficiency (176).

Orthotopic Liver Transplantation

Orthotopic liver transplantation has been characterized by limited graft survival; however, the advance of cyclosporin A has markedly prolonged graft survival, signalling the increased acceptability of the procedure (177). Even before the use of this drug, total liver allografts were accomplished in patients with Wilson's disease (178–180), α_1-antitrypsin deficiency (181–183), galactosemia (183), primary biliary atresia (183), tyrosinemia (184), and Niemann–Pick disease (185). Although the specific defect has not been identified in Wilson's disease, the concentrations of serum ceruloplasmin and copper increased from low to normal values two weeks post-transplantation. Urinary copper excretion also increased post-transplantation, and homograft biopsies have shown no copper accumulation. In one recipient, the Kaiser–Fleischer rings disappeared (180). Hepatic transplantation in α_1-antitrypsin deficiency resulted in normal concentrations of circulating α_1-antitrypsin of the donor phenotype shortly after transplantation; however, most recipients have not survived longer than one year (181,182). Liver transplantation in tyrosinemia resulted in normalization of tyrosine metabolism without dietary restriction (184); hepatic transplantation in this disease should also normalize the aminolevulinate metabolism.

A successful orthotopic liver graft was achieved in a patient with Niemann–Pick Type A disease (185). Post-transplantation, the sphingomyelinase activity in plasma, urine, and, most notably, cerebrospinal fluid appeared to be increased, suggesting that normal hepatic tissue was capable of secreting active enzyme. However, this patient died from neurologic complications. Fetal liver cells have also been transplanted into patients with Fabry's disease (186,187) and with adenosine deaminase deficient immunodeficiency disease (187); only limited data have been reported, and this approach requires further evaluation. With the advent of improved immunosuppression and graft survival (177), orthotopic liver transplantation will surely be undertaken in other genetic diseases characterized by liver failure or requiring enzymes or metabolites of hepatic origin.

Pancreatic Transplantation

Transplantation of the pancreas has been used to treat patients with juvenile diabetes mellitus (*188,189*). Almost immediately post-transplantation, the insulin concentrations became homeostatic and the glucose concentrations returned to normal. Several patients have had normal glucose and hormone values for more than one year post-transplantation. However, only about 20% of the grafts have functioned, presumably because of surgical difficulties (*190*). More encouraging results have been achieved by technical improvements that may overcome these problems (*191*).

Splenic Transplantation

Splenic allotransplantation has been used for patients with hemophilia A (*192*) and juvenile or Type 3 Gaucher's disease (*193*). Concentrations of Factor VIII were essentially unchanged; however, plasma glucocerebroside, the substrate involved in Gaucher's disease, was decreased post-transplantation. Unfortunately, these grafts were unsuccessful, owing to graft rejection.

Renal Transplantation

Extensive experience with renal transplantation has demonstrated that the kidney is one of the most successfully transplanted organs, and this treatment has been used in over a dozen genetic diseases. The majority of these disorders involve primary renal pathology, and the allograft corrects the abnormal renal function. Renal transplantation in familial polycystic disease, medullary cystic disease, familial Mediterranean fever, congenital nephrotic syndrome, Alport's syndrome, nail–patella syndrome, and amyloidosis results in excellent renal function and no apparent recurrence of the renal disease. The protein and lipid concentrations in patients with congenital nephrotic syndrome became normal after transplantation (*194*). Recipients with primary gout have normal renal function, but the hyperuricemia and gouty symptoms persist (*195*). Transplantation in a case of familial lecithin:cholesterol-acyltransferase deficiency corrected the renal insufficiency but had no effect on the metabolic disease. The abnormal lipid metabolites are slowly reaccumulating, but years of normal allograft function are expected (*196*). Results of kidney transplantation in several patients with primary oxalosis and familial Mediterranean fever with amyloidosis have been variable, owing to the rapid reaccumulation of calcium oxalate crystals and amyloid in the respective allografts (*197*).

Renal transplantation in children with cystinosis (*198*) has primarily involved allografts from their parents, who were obligate heterozygotes for the cystinotic gene. The concentrations of cystine in cornea, bone marrow, and peripheral leukocytes have not decreased post-transplantation. Although cystine has not reaccumulated in the proximal renal epithelium of the allografts, it has reaccumulated in the renal interstitial cells, presumably due to infiltration by the recipient's macrophages. However, there was no cystine reaccumulation two years after transplantation in a patient who received a cadaver allograft; perhaps the unrelated, normal allograft is more capable of handling cystine than are heterozygous kidneys.

Renal transplantation in patients with Fabry's disease (defective α-galactosidase A) was undertaken to monitor the biochemical and clinical effectiveness of enzyme transplantation. Because these patients develop renal failure, and because renal tissue contains active α-galactosidase A, a renal allograft was thought to provide active enzyme to correct the metabolic defect of Fabry's disease. Although biochemical and clinical improvement following successful renal transplantation has been reported in several recipients (*199–202*), no biochemical effect could be demonstrated in others (*203–205*).

Fibroblast Transplantation

The subcutaneous transplantation of cultured skin fibroblasts has been accomplished in patients with mucopolysaccharidoses Types I-H (*206*), II (*207–209*), III A (*209,210*), and VI (*211*). The rationale for fibroblast transplantation is based on the prior demonstration that cultured normal fibroblasts secreted enzymes that corrected the abnormal mucopolysaccharide metabolism in fibroblasts from patients with these disorders (*212–214*). Thus, the grafted normal fibroblasts presumably would continuously release enzyme for distribution and uptake by the recipient's connective-tissue cells; in addition, the grafted cells would replicate and possibly reach other tissue sites, thus providing an ever-expanding source of the normal enzyme.

Assessment of the metabolic effects of these grafts indicates mucopolysaccharide degradation (*206–210*) and the presence of low levels of enzymatic activity (*206,209,210*), although another group could not demonstrate a metabolic effect (*211*). Given the lack of clinical improvement, Gibbs concluded that fibroblast transplantation is not effective for the treatment of lysosomal storage diseases (*215*). These studies have been instructive: the initial enthusiasm for fibroblast transplantation as a therapeutic modality has been reversed by the unsuccessful outcome of these human trials. In the future, the effectiveness of various therapeutic endeavors should be assessed in animal analogues (see, e.g., *216–218*), if available, before human trials.

Erythrocyte Transfusion Therapy

Periodic erythrocyte transfusions provide a novel transplantation approach to replace the deficient adenosine deaminase in patients with severe combined immunodeficiency disease. The enzymatic defect in this disorder leads to the accumulation of adenosine, deoxyadenosine, and several of their metabolites, dATP, cAMP, and S-adenosylhomocysteine, in the plasma, erythrocytes, and lymphocytes of affected patients. Several of these metabolites inhibit normal immune function as well as interfere with normal lymphocyte differentiation and function in vitro (*219*). Matched, normal, irradiated erythrocytes containing normal adenosine deaminase activity have been infused biweekly by partial exchange transfusions (reaching heterozygous values of adenosine deaminase) into several patients with this disease (*153*). Although not as effective metabolically or clinically as bone marrow transplantation (*153,156*), erythrocyte transfusions have decreased plasma concentrations of deoxyadenosine and urinary excretion of adenosine and deoxyadenosine. The dATP concentrations became near normal in the recipients' erythrocytes and lymphocytes. Concomitantly, humoral immune function improved markedly, although cellular immune function remained somewhat impaired in the transfused patients (*153,219,220*).

Erythrocyte transfusion therapy also has proven effective for purine nucleoside phosphorylase deficiency, which is associated with severely defective T-cell immunity (*221*). Repeated erythrocyte transfusions resulted in decreased urinary concentrations of inosine, deoxyinosine, guanosine, and deoxyguanosine with concomitantly increased uric acid in urine and serum. In addition, erythrocytic 2,3-diphosphoglycerate increased, causing the oxygen dissociation curve to shift to the right. Importantly, the recipient's immunologic status was improved, but the residual dGTP concentrations may have prevented complete immunologic reconstitution (221).

Enzyme Replacement Therapy

Lacking the technology to modify or replace defective genes, investigators have turned to enzyme replacement as a potential means to treat selected inborn errors of metabolism, particularly the lysosomal storage diseases (for reviews see 1–4). The rationale for enzyme replacement therapy in selected lysosomal storage diseases evolved from two fundamental observations: the identification of lysosomes as the subcellular site of pathology, and the elucidation of the basic role of the lysosome in cellular catabolism. Thus, it was reasoned that after endocytosis and fusion of the various components of the lysosomal apparatus, exogenous enzyme would be brought into contact with the accumulated substrate for hydrolysis. The working hypothesis that exogenously supplied enzymes can be delivered to lysosomes for effective substrate catabolism has been supported by the in vitro "correction" of substrate accumulation in cultured fibroblasts. When the appropriate active enzyme was supplied in the media of cultured fibroblasts obtained from individuals with various lysosomal storage diseases, the exogenous enzyme gained access to the accumulated intracellular substrates and normalized the substrate turnover. These studies (e.g., 222–227) indicated the feasibility of enzyme replacement and, in particular, demonstrated that small quantities of exogenous enzyme could gain access to intracellular lysosomal sites and effect normal substrate metabolism.

Human Trials with Partially Purified Human Enzymes

Although the first trials of enzyme replacement were undertaken during the 1960s (2), not until the early 1970s did investigators used partially purified enzymes from humans to avoid potential immune reactions. At about the same time, animal model systems were developed for experimental evaluation and optimization of enzyme replacement strategies before trials with humans (e.g., *228*). Table 4 summarizes the results of the clinical trials of direct enzyme replacement in various lysosomal disorders. Pilot intravenous administrations of the appropriate human enzymatic activity in patients with GM_2-gangliosidosis Type 2, Sandhoff's disease [urinary β-hexosaminidase A (*229*)], Type II glycogenosis [placental α-glucosidase (*230*)], Fabry's disease [placental α-galactosidase (*231*)], and Gaucher's disease [placental β-glucosidase (*232,233*)] were in each case preceded by in vitro trials that demonstrated that the highly purified human enzyme hydrolyzed its natural substrate. The injected enzymes were rapidly cleared from the circulation and exogenous enzymatic activity was recovered in biopsied liver samples from the recipients; the approximate half-lives of activity in the circulation were between 10 and 20 min. Evidence for concomitant substrate catabolism was demonstrated by the decreased concentrations of plasma globoside [GM_2-gangliosidosis Type 2 (*229*)], hepatic glycogen [Type II glycogenosis (*230*)], plasma trihexosyl ceramide [Fabry's disease (*231*)], and plasma, erythrocytic, and hepatic glucocerebroside (*232*) or leukocyte and platelet glucocerebroside (*233*) (Gaucher's disease) found after enzyme administration.

These preliminary, but encouraging, results supported the feasibility of enzyme replacement with highly purified human enzymes. However, such treatment of disorders with primary neuronal involvement was not as promising. After the intravenous administration of enzyme to a patient with GM_2-gangliosidosis Type 2 (*229*), β-hexosaminidase A activity was rapidly cleared from the circulation, and a significant increase in β-hexosaminidase activity was detected in hepatic tissue biopsied percutaneously 45 min after injection, as compared with that in the preinjection biopsy. However, no significant increase of β-hexosaminidase A activity was observed in either lumbar or ventricular cerebrospinal fluid or in biopsied brain tissue, thus demonstrating the inability of an intravenously administered enzyme to gain access to the central nervous system (*229*). In an attempt to overcome this obstacle, von Specht et al. (*234*) intrathecally administered highly purified placental β-hexosaminidase A to two patients with GM_2-gangliosidosis Type 1 (Tay–Sachs disease). Case 1 received four intraventricular and 15 lumbar injections of pure enzyme; case 2 received weekly lumbar injections over 10 months. Although both demonstrated decreased concentrations of GM_2 ganglioside

Table 4. Human Trials with Purified Human Enzymes

Disease	Year	Enzyme administered	Source	Organ uptake	Evidence for substrate catabolism (tissue)	Ref.
Glycogenosis Type II	1973	Acid α-glucosidase	Placenta	Liver	− Liver, muscle	230
GM$_2$ gangliosidosis Type 2	1973	β-Hexosaminidase A	Urine	Liver	+ Plasma	229
Fabry	1973	α-Galactosidase A	Placenta	Liver	+ Plasma	231
Gaucher	1974	Glucocerebrosidase	Placenta	Liver	+ Liver, RBC, plasma	232
	1977	Glucocerebrosidase	Placenta		+ Lymphocytes, platelets − RBC, plasma	233
GM$_2$ gangliosidosis Type 1	1979	β-Hexosaminidase A[a]	Placenta		+ Serum	234

[a] Native and PVP-modified β-hexosaminidase administered intrathecally; all other enzymes administered intravenously. RBC, erythrocytes.

in plasma after injection, the pathologic substrate accumulation in frontal lobe biopsied pre- and post-infusion appeared unchanged by light and electron microscopy. These studies documented the constraints of the blood–brain barrier as well as the inability of intrathecally administered enzyme to gain access to neural cells. Thus, future replacement endeavors for disorders with severe neurologic involvement, such as Tay–Sachs and Niemann–Pick diseases will require the development of techniques that permit macromolecular enzymes to gain access to the neuronal sites of substrate deposition.

Animal Model Trials

To determine systematically the in vivo fate of an intravenously administered glycoprotein lysosomal hydrolase, my co-workers and I developed a murine model system in which partially purified bovine hepatic β-glucuronidase was administered intravenously to C3H/HeJ Gus^h β-glucuronidase-deficient mice (228). The heterologous enzyme was purposely chosen to assess potential immune complications. The enzyme was rapidly cleared from the circulation and preferentially taken up by the liver (70% of dose). These findings were similar to those in the human trials involving highly purified human enzymes, and identified the need to develop strategies designed to optimize the delivery of enzyme to selected target sites of pathologic substrate deposition for effective therapy.

Enzyme Delivery Strategies

Clearly, if an enzyme is to reach sites other than the liver, delivery strategies must be designed to enhance the uptake of enzyme to the crucial cell type(s) in each disease. Targeting to specific sites may require either purification of an isoenzyme from specific tissue sources or chemical modification of the enzyme; alternatively, the enzyme preparation may be immobilized in various biodegradable vesicles that can be chemically or physically modified to promote uptake by particular cells or tissues.

Two attractive strategies to enhance the target delivery of lysosomal hydrolases (and other glycoconjugates) involve (a) receptor-mediated molecular recognition processes and (b) the use of carrier vesicles such as liposomes and autologous erythrocytes. In the former, the binding of the carbohydrate moiety of the administered glycoprotein-hydrolase to a cell-specific, membrane-bound receptor signals the internalization and uptake of the molecule by components of the lysosomal apparatus. Thus, the identification of cell-specific receptor systems and the chemical modification or selection of appropriate isoenzymes may be exploited to "address-label" an enzyme to a particular cell type(s). To date, receptor-mediated uptake has been demonstrated for complex circulating glycoproteins (235–238), lysosomal hydrolases (237–242), low-density lipoproteins (243,244), and transcobalamin II (245). Because most lysosomal hydrolases are glycoproteins, the receptor-mediated glycoprotein clearance and uptake systems could be exploited for the selective delivery of an enzyme to a particular cell type or tissue. Reviews of the current status of these receptor systems are available (235,238,246,247).

Enzyme entrapment in biodegradable vesicles, such as liposomes or autologous erythrocytes, also provides a strategy for enhancing enzyme delivery to critical sites of substrate pathology as well as protecting the active enzyme from bioinactivation in the circulation and immunologic surveillance (248). Furthermore, the surface of these vesicles can be chemically modified or coated with compounds that may facilitate cell-specific uptake.

Application of receptor-mediated uptake for enzyme replacement. Receptor-mediated uptake systems offer an attractive and relatively unexploited strategy to target lysosomal enzymes to cells other than the liver. Several aspects of these recognition-marker–receptor systems may be used to enhance enzyme delivery to selected tissue or cell types, including (a) the selective removal of carbohydrate moieties from the enzyme to expose specific recognition markers or the conjugation of specific carbohydrate "address labels" onto hydrolases (249–251); (b) the use of nontoxic carbohydrates, oligosaccharides, or glycopeptides to selectively block enzyme binding for uptake by other cell types (252–256); (c) the selection and (or) modification of specific isoenzymes with "high uptake" and stability characteristics (257); or (d) some combination of the above.

The feasibility of each of these receptor-mediated strategies for enzyme replacement in selected lysosomal storage diseases already has been demonstrated in vitro and in vivo. Brady and colleagues (258) sequentially removed the sialic acid and β-galactosyl residues from purified human placental β-glucosidase. They demonstrated that the modified enzymes were taken up preferentially by isolated hepatocytes (asialio-β-glucosidase) or Kupffer cells (agalacto-β-glucosidase), presumably by the galactose and mannose/N-acetylglucosamine recognition systems, respectively. These observations indicate that specific isoenzymes may be biologically coded and (or) chemically modified to promote their differential distribution and uptake for the controlled and specific delivery of exogenous enzymes.

The coupling of specific carbohydrate residues to glycoprotein enzymes (neo-glycoproteins) offers another intriguing possibility for target delivery. Although this approach has been used to investigate carbohydrate-receptor specificities (238,242), neo-glycohydrolases have not been synthesized to date. Nonetheless, this strategy may provide an efficient means of selective cell delivery for enzymes and other therapeutic proteins and is worthy of investigation.

Rattazzi et al. (259,260) achieved some success in minimizing the hepatic uptake of β-hexosaminidase A in cats by injecting mannans before the enzyme to partially block enzyme uptake by the mannosyl/N-acetylglucosamine (and perhaps mannose 6-phosphate) recognition system. The mannan infusion did not appear to be toxic, so this approach may be useful to enhance the nonhepatic uptake of enzyme in disorders in which hepatocytes and reticuloendothelial cells are not the primary sites of pathology. Further studies are needed to assess side effects (e.g., hyperosmolality, toxicity) of the blocking compounds.

The third receptor-mediated strategy involves the selective purification of different molecular forms or tissue isoenzymes of a specific enzyme for differential uptake and survival (261,262). Selected isoenzymes may promote uptake by the pathologic target tissues via recognition of specific tissue and perhaps subcellular receptors, and may also provide additional protection from endogenous catheptic destruction.

Carrier-mediated delivery. The demonstration that enzyme can be entrapped in synthetic lipid spherules, termed liposomes (263–265), and human erythrocytes (266–270) suggested the intriguing possibility that these biodegradable vesicles may be useful as carriers of exogenous enzyme.

The effectiveness of these strategies for targeted enzyme delivery was evaluated in our murine model system and the findings have been reviewed in detail (271). Briefly, positively-charged liposomes caused a temporary labilization of the lysosomal membranes of the recipient mice, resulting in the intracellular release of endogenous, potent lysosomal hydrolases (272). In addition, cellular and humoral immune responses were elicited by negatively-charged liposomes. Moreover, the liposome vesicle itself elicited a cellular immune response by enhancing phagocytic activity in the reticuloendothelial cells of liver and spleen and activating peritoneal macrophages (272). Similar findings were reported by van Rooijen and van Nieuwmegen (273,274) after the repeated injection of free human serum albumin (HSA), free HSA and buffer-loaded negatively-charged liposomes, or liposome-entrapped HSA into rabbits. Although free HSA did not elicit an immune response, HSA entrapped in liposomes produced a marked response. An immune response was also detected after the administration of free HSA and empty liposomes, confirming the adjuvant nature of the liposome itself. These studies suggested that the adjuvant activity of macrophages was stimulated by the digestion of liposomal membranes. Other investigators have shown that positively-charged liposomes activate human complement (275) and negatively-charged liposomes interact with plasma constituents to release the entrapped markers (276). These studies also identified the potentially harmful physiologic and immunologic effects that might be associated with the use of liposomes composed of certain lipids, and emphasize the need to evaluate fully these carriers in animal models before human trials.

In contrast, studies of the in vivo fate of enzyme entrapped in autologous erythrocytes demonstrated their ability to deliver exogenous enzyme without immunologic complications (271,277). Erythrocyte-entrapped activity was primarily recovered in the liver after intravenous injection. Maximal hepatic uptake (70% of dose) occurred at 2 h and was maintained at that level for as long as 13 h post-injection; the enzyme was retained in hepatic tissues as long as 5 days, or fivefold longer than enzyme directly administered. Hepatic subcellular fractionation indicated that more than 80% of the recovered exogenous activity was detected in the lysosomally-enriched fraction at various times after administration.

Splenic uptake of erythrocyte-entrapped activity was approximately 10% of dose; however, the chemical and enzymatic modification of loaded erythrocytes significantly increased splenic uptake (271). In support of these findings, Jancik et al. (278) injected autologous neuraminidase-treated erythrocytes into rats and demonstrated that they were sequestered in the reticuloendothelial cells of the liver and spleen to a significantly greater extent than untreated control erythrocytes.

Importantly, the plasma clearance and tissue delivery of enzyme entrapped in erythrocytes appears to be dependent on the entrapment method (270), the various entrapment procedures inducing different morphologic changes that might be useful for target delivery. For example, enzyme-loaded cells that become echinocytes or stomatocytes presumably will be cleared rapidly by the reticuloendothelial system, whereas cells that tend to retain their discoid shape will be more deformable and will be retained in the circulation longer. Other modifications of the erythrocyte membrane before loading, such as treatment with sulfhydryl-active reagents (279), neuraminidase (280,281), or glutaraldehyde (282), may enhance splenic uptake. Alternatively, coating the erythrocytes with various components such as immunoglobulins may prolong the survival of the erythrocytes in the circulation. Procedures that restore deformed cells to a discoid morphology [e.g., ATP and EDTA (283)] might also be useful for treating conditions in which toxic compounds in the plasma could enter the circulating cells and be inactivated by the entrapped agent. Thus, entrapment of enzyme preparations in nonimmunogenic, biodegradable autologous erythrocytes (in contrast to liposomes) may effectively protect administered activity from the immune surveillance system, thereby avoiding untoward reactions and maximizing the amount of activity that reaches target subcellular sites of pathology.

Enzyme delivery strategies for neural uptake. The target site of many lysosomal storage diseases is the neuron. Previous replacement trials in animals and humans have demonstrated the inability of intravenously administered enzymes to cross the blood–brain barrier and gain access to neural tissue (228,229). Intrathecal administration has been attempted (234); however, no evidence of enzyme uptake in neural tissue was demonstrated. Effective replacement in these disorders requires uptake of the enzyme not only into brain tissues, but specifically into the lysosomes of the neurons in which the pathologic substrate is accumulated. This requisite presents another major obstacle because, even if a reasonable means were devised to achieve access to neural tissues, it is unlikely that the exogenous enzyme would be taken up by the lysosomes of the relatively nonphagocytic neurons. Instead, the enzyme would presumably be sequestered in the more endocytotic neuroglial cells.

Several investigators have attempted to modify the blood–brain barrier in animal systems to assess neural enzyme uptake (*284–286*). In addition, others have attempted to identify the presence of a neuron receptor for the specific uptake of exogenous enzymes (*287*). If a recognition system for specific neuronal uptake is documented, and if the mechanisms to open the blood–brain barrier prove reversible and safe, there is a potential basis to overcome the obstacles to enzyme replacement for disorders with primary neurologic involvement.

Clinical Application of Enzyme Delivery Strategies

Table 5 summarizes the application of receptor- and carrier-mediated delivery strategies in recent clinical trials of enzyme replacement. For the most part, these studies were designed to evaluate the capability of delivery strategies for the selective targeting of enzyme to the major sites of pathology in each disorder. Receptor-mediated strategies included the use of the Ashwell recognition signal for prolonged circulation of α-galactosidase A forms in Fabry's disease (*288*) and the LDL receptor-mediated uptake for α-glucosidase replacement in Type II glycogenosis (*289*).

Carrier-mediated enzyme delivery strategies also have been attempted in humans. Replacement of liposome-entrapped α-glucosidase and β-glucosidase have been attempted in Type II glycogenosis (*290*) and Type 1 Gaucher's disease (*291*), respectively. These clinical trials were conducted before the animal studies that demonstrated immune responses to liposome-entrapped antigens, and serve to underscore the need for careful evaluation in animal model systems before human use. In contrast, erythrocyte-entrapped enzyme delivery, the feasibility and safety of which were demonstrated first in animal models (*228*), was extended to the enhanced reticuloendothelial-cell uptake of β-glucosidase in patients with Type 1 Gaucher's disease (*233*).

Receptor-mediated delivery—administration of α-galactosidase A forms in Fabry's disease. In Fabry's disease, the preferential deposition of circulating substrate in the vascular endothelium is responsible

Table 5. Human Trials Exploiting Delivery Strategies

Disease	Year	Enzyme administered, source	Delivery strategy	Organ uptake	Substrate catabolism (tissue/substrate)	Ref.
Glycogenosis Type II	1976	Acid α-glucosidase, A. niger	Liposome entrapment	± liver − muscle	± liver/glycogen, muscle glycogen	290
Gaucher	1977	β-Glucocerebrosidase, placenta	Liposome entrapment		− plasma, RBC	291, 294, 295
	1977	β-Glucocerebrosidase, placenta	Erythrocyte entrapment		+ platelets, leukocytes/Glc-Cer	233, 296
Glycogenosis Type II	1979	Acid α-glucosidase, placenta	LDL-conjugated	− muscle	± muscle/glycogen	289
Fabry	1979	α-Galactosidase A, spleen(s) or plasma(p)	Receptor-mediated	+++ liver(s) + liver(p)	(s)+plasma/Gal-Gal-Glc-Cer (p)+++plasma/Gal-Gal-Glc-Cer	288, 293

RBC, erythrocytes; Gal, galactose; Glc, glucose; Cer, cerebroside.

for the major manifestations of the disease. Therefore, α-galactosidase A replacement endeavors must be directed to the depletion of the accumulated substrate in the circulation and vascular endothelium. The recent finding that α-galactosidase A forms purified from plasma and splenic tissues are differentially glycosylated (292) suggested the intriguing possibility that these enzyme forms might be biologically coded for differential distribution and retention in the plasma by exploiting the sialic acid recognition process described by Ashwell and Morell (235).

In our laboratory, highly purified α-galactosidase A from human plasma and homogeneous enzyme from human spleen (292) have been characterized. Although the two forms have similar physical and kinetic properties, they differ in their carbohydrate moieties. The plasma enzyme appears to be uniquely sialylated or markedly more sialylated than the tissue form. On the basis of these in vitro findings and the plasma-disappearance kinetics of sialylated- and asialoglycoproteins in animals (235), we hypothesized that the more sialylated plasma enzyme would have a more prolonged retention in the circulation and would mediate an increased hydrolysis of circulating substrate than would the splenic form. Two patients with Fabry's disease received multiple intravenous injections of either unentrapped splenic or plasma enzyme form (288). After injection of equivalent doses of plasma and splenic enzymes, the splenic form was rapidly cleared from the patient's circulation, with a $t_{1/2}$ of approximately 10 min; in marked contrast, the plasma form had a slower disappearance from plasma ($t_{1/2}$ about 70 min). These clearance curves were compatible with distribution of the respective enzymes in at least two compartments, the plasma form being retained longer in the injected compartment. Presumably, the differential clearance kinetics were due to the presence of sialic acid residues on the plasma form of α-galactosidase A. These findings suggest that the molecular recognition process for clearance of homologous hydrolases administered to humans was similar to the receptor-mediated uptake system described by Ashwell and Morell (235).

Although the tissue fate of these enzymes could not be determined, their differential metabolic effectiveness was underscored by their remarkably different kinetics for substrate clearance and re-accumulation. The effect of the splenic form on the circulating substrate was rapid and transient and paralleled the rapid disappearance of the enzymatic activity from the plasma. Presumably the splenic form was taken up primarily by the lysosomal apparatus of the liver, where it may have hydrolyzed accumulated substrate. In contrast, the prolonged retention of the plasma form in the circulation was associated with about a 25-fold greater substrate clearance. Repeated injections of the plasma enzyme reduced the circulating substrate to concentrations within the normal range (293).

These studies demonstrated the feasibility of enzyme replacement in Fabry's disease. The major obstacle to this goal is the need to produce adequate amounts of purified human enzyme for long-term clinical trials. Efforts to accomplish this objective will require recombinant DNA techniques to isolate the cDNA for human α-galactosidase A and express it in bacteria or yeast. The genetically engineered enzyme will then require chemical modification to attach the appropriate carbohydrate moieties that presumably are required for enzyme stability and receptor-mediated delivery.

Receptor-mediated delivery—administration of LDL-coupled α-glucosidase in Type II glycogenosis. Williams and Murray investigated the use of LDL-conjugated enzyme for the target delivery of acid α-glucosidase in a terminal patient with Type II glycogenosis (289). Because 95% of LDL is metabolized extrahepatically, replacement of the deficient enzyme with purified human α-glucosidase coupled to LDL ought to be delivered preferentially to extrahepatic sites having LDL receptors. In addition, the uptake of the LDL–enzyme complex by cultured skin fibroblasts from a patient with Type II glycogenosis was ninefold greater than the uptake of free enzyme (289). Furthermore, the half-life of the LDL-complexed activity in the fibroblasts was 2.5-fold longer than that of free enzyme.

Two doses of LDL–α-glucosidase were administered to the patient. The enzymatic activity and glycogen content were determined in muscle and hepatic biopsies and post-mortem samples. A significant increase in the α-glucosidase activity in muscle, but not in heart or liver, was detected in samples obtained at autopsy 26 days after the second infusion of 13 mg of the complex containing α-glucosidase activity of 0.5 nmol/min per milligram. Williams and Murray estimated that 77% of the administered enzyme was recovered in muscle (289). The glycogen content was decreased in liver, and to a lesser extent in muscle, but not in heart tissue as compared with data from previously autopsied patients. In addition, no adverse reactions were observed, and no antibodies to the enzyme or LDL were detected. These preliminary results indicate the feasibility of LDL–enzyme conjugates for non-neural, nonreticuloendothelial lysosomal storage diseases. Indeed, this approach may be suited to replacement endeavors in disorders with primary endothelial cell pathology, if the recipients' concentration of circulating LDL can be temporarily decreased.

Administration of liposome-entrapped α- and β-glucosidases. Negatively-charged liposomes containing *Aspergillus niger* amyloglucosidase were intravenously administered daily over seven days to an eight-month-old patient with Type II glycogenosis (290). Although her liver size decreased during the first four days of treatment, there was no other evidence of clinical effect. The patient died from heart failure on the eighth day and tissues were obtained at autopsy for analysis. Less than 1% of normal α-glucosidase activity was detected in hepatic tissue, and no activity was recovered in skeletal or cardiac muscle. The glycogen content in skeletal muscle was twice that obtained in a pre-infusion biopsy. The hepatic glycogen content (55 mg/g wt. weight) was lower than the concentrations usually seen in patients with this disease (mean 82, SD 16, mg/g), which led the investigators to suggest that hepatic catabolism had occurred. However, the design and limited nature of this trial precluded assessment of the biochemical and immunologic aspects of this therapeutic endeavor.

Belchetz and co-workers (291) attempted enzyme replacement in a patient with Type 1 Gaucher's disease by the repeated intravenous administration over a five-year period of acid β-glucosidase and ^{111}In-labeled bleomycin entrapped in negatively-charged liposomes. Neither the rate of plasma disappearance of the administered activity nor the glucosyl ceramide concentrations in plasma, erythrocytes, or other tissues were determined. Serial whole-body scans over the first nine-month period indicated a decreasing hepatic size with sequential doses and an increased rate of liposome clearance from the circulation. However, the patient experienced headaches, nausea, difficulty in concentration, sleepiness, and abdominal pain immediately after each administration of liposome-entrapped enzyme. These clinical sequelae, which presumably represent adverse physiologic and (or) immune responses to the liposome vesicle, the enzyme preparation, or both, may be similar to the adverse findings of liposome-entrapped enzyme administration in the β-glucuronidase-deficient mice (*272*).

In the following two years the patient subsequently received a course of 20 injections containing less lipid and enzyme, which markedly lessened the side effects. No adverse reactions occurred until the last injection, when the patient developed urticaria with vasculitic lesions over the knees, suggesting a Type IV delayed hypersensitivity reaction. Injections of the enzyme alone were continued; however, no evidence of clinical improvement has been documented after five years of enzyme replacement (*295*).

Administration of erythrocyte-entrapped β-glucosidase in Gaucher's disease. Beutler et al. (*233,296*) reported the first human trial of an erythrocyte-entrapped enzyme: they administered β-glucosidase in autologous erythrocytes to a patient with Type 1 Gaucher's disease. Enzyme was entrapped in erythrocytes by a dialysis technique (*269*) and administered in three doses over a five-day period. Two single doses of enzyme-entrapped resealed erythrocytes coated with anti-Rh globulin were administered six and seven months later. These enzyme-loaded erythrocytes were cleared from the circulation with a half-life of 4.8 h, compared with the slow half-life of uncoated erythrocytes (10 days) in an asplenic Gaucher recipient (*233,296*). (Gamma-globulin-coated resealed erythrocytes administered intravenously to a Gaucher's disease patient with a spleen had a half-life of 22 min. Erythrocyte half-lives were determined by labeling with ^{51}Cr.)

The erythrocyte-entrapped enzyme administrations in the asplenic patient were in series with 11 injections of unentrapped enzyme (*233*). These injections resulted in essentially no change in the substrate concentrations in the recipient's plasma or erythrocytes; however, small decreases in concentrations were observed in platelets, monocytes, and granulocytes, and the decrease in the concentration in the lymphocytes was significant.

Subsequently, Beutler et al. (*296*) infused erythrocyte-entrapped enzyme into six patients with Gaucher's disease, one of whom received 10 infusions of enzymatic activity of 56.4 nmol/min over a seven-month period. Although these studies were not associated with any significant clinical improvement, perhaps long-term endeavors utilizing greater amounts of enzymatic activity will result in clinical benefit. Because there were no significant side effects and no immune responses to the erythrocyte carrier or to the entrapped enzyme during these trials, further long-term studies of erythrocyte-entrapped active β-glucosidase should be carried out to determine the efficacy of this carrier for the treatment of Type 1 Gaucher's disease, the protection of entrapped enzymatic activity, and the target delivery of other therapeutic agents.

Prospects for Enzyme Replacement

Although the experiences to date with enzyme replacement document that purified enzymes of human origin can be safely administered, they have not proven clinically beneficial. In both the human pilot trials and the animal model studies, administration of the appropriate enzyme decreased the concentrations of its substrate in plasma and (or) biopsied tissues. However, the human trials have been only feasibility studies, undertaken when sufficient purified human enzyme was available for one or more injections. Owing to the limited availability of the enzymes and the limits of human experimentation, investigators have not determined the optimal dosage, dose frequency, distribution (tissue and subcellular), stability, or metabolic effects of the administered enzymes. Although animal model systems for several of these diseases are available (297), these pharmacologic and physiologic variables have not been adequately assessed. Moreover, investigators have recognized that the precious enzyme must be chemically modified or entrapped in carrier vehicles to direct delivery to the storage cell and tissue types. The latter problem has been emphasized by the trials of replacement therapy in Gaucher's disease by Brady et al. (298). These two obstacles, the needs to produce large amounts of purified human enzyme and to target successfully the enzyme to specific sites of pathology, must be overcome for enzyme therapy to be clinically efficacious.

It is likely that these obstacles will be surmounted. Application of recombinant DNA technology should allow us to isolate the genes directing the synthesis of these enzymes and eventually lead to the large-scale production of unlimited amounts of human enzyme (see below). Conjugation of the appropriate "address label," whether carbohydrate or protein (e.g., antibody), may provide the required delivery system. Alternatively, future advances in the development of carrier vehicles (248) may facilitate tissue-specific uptake. Needless to say, the future prospects are encouraging. Advances in recombinant DNA technology and gene expression are occurring at an unprecedented rate, and studies of receptor-mediated recognition systems continue to be an area of active and productive research. The progress made in these areas will likely find application in the treatment of selected lysosomal storage diseases in the near future.

Gene Therapy

The rapid progress in recombinant DNA technology may have important future implications for the treatment of inherited metabolic diseases. Indeed, the next decade should witness the application of these technologies to human metabolic diseases, including the production of large quantities of specific human gene products for replacement endeavors and attempts to transfer isolated normal human genes into the human genome to "cure" the primary genetic defect.

Production of Human Gene Products

Already, recombinant DNA technology has been applied to the biologic synthesis of human gene products. The first human genes isolated were those whose mRNAs were enriched in specific tissue sources (299,300) or whose polypeptide products had been previously sequenced (301,302). For example, human β-globin messages were isolated from reticulocytes and livers of patients with various thalassemias (303,304) by use of previously isolated rat and mouse cross-hybridizing DNA sequences. Because cross-hybridizing probes are not available for most human genes, various other methods have been devised to enrich for specific mRNAs. Persico et al. (305) used oligo (dT)-cellulose chromatography, sucrose gradient centrifugation, and agarose gel electrophoresis to create a pBR322 cDNA clone library enriched for sequences encoding human glucose-6-phosphate dehydrogenase (G6PD). The enrichment of G6PD mRNA was monitored by in vitro translation, and the library was subsequently screened directly by colony hybridization with a G6PD enriched ^{32}P-labeled cDNA pool isolated from HeLa cells. By a combination of these techniques seven colonies containing human G6PD sequences were isolated. Wu et al. (300) also have reported the isolation and cloning of a cDNA for another important human enzyme, argininosuccinate synthetase, by using a cell line that overproduced the enzyme and a sensitive differential filter hybridization method for screening.

The isolation of genes whose mRNAs occur in small or trace quantities has been difficult; however, Parnes et al. (306) have recently reported a modified positive selection–translation assay for the rapid screening of large numbers of clones, thereby making feasible the isolation of cDNA clones for proteins whose mRNAs represent as little as 0.03% of the total cellular mRNA. This approach was used to isolate β_2-microglobulin sequences. Another recent approach for enrichment of rare human DNA sequences of known chromosome location involves the use of human–rodent somatic cell hybrids containing a single human chromosome. The human DNA may be isolated from the rodent background by using human-specific probes, such as ^{32}P-labeled ALU sequences, under stringent hybridization conditions (307). This method has been used most extensively for the isolation of specific human X-chromosomal sequences (308,309); in principle, however, this technique should be useful for any gene whose chromosomal location has been assigned.

An alternative approach for the isolation and cloning of human DNA sequences is the use of synthetic oligonucleotides. The entire genes for several small polypeptide hormones (e.g., somatostatin, somatotropin) have been chemically synthesized, based on their amino acid sequences and the redundancy of the genetic code. In these cases, the DNA sequence was chemically synthesized from nucleotides and double-stranded DNA generated in vitro (310,311). In fact, Khorana (312) accomplished the remarkable feat of chemically synthesizing an entire, biologically functional gene, the *Escherichia coli* suppressor transfer RNA gene (207 basepairs), including the promoter and distal processing regions. Wetzel et al. (301) chemically synthesized a gene for the bovine α-thymosin polypeptide chain, inserted it into plasmid pBR322 under *lac* operon control, and achieved expression of the chimeric protein, N-α-desacetylthymosin-A, and β-galactosidase. A similar approach has been used recently to produce biologically active human insulin in *E. coli* (313).

Despite these successes, most human proteins have not been purified in large quantities, and extensive amino acid sequence data are not available. However, mixed synthetic oligonucleotide sequences complementary to as few as four amino acids (with minimal codon redundancy) have been used to screen cDNA libraries directly (*314*) or to prime reverse transcriptase and thereby generate a specific cDNA (*315*). These approaches have been used successfully for hog gastrin (*316*), human histocompatibility antigen HLA-B (*315*), rat relaxin (*317*), human β_2-microglobulin (*318*), and human fibroblast interferon (*319*).

The human double-stranded DNA segment, having been isolated or chemically synthesized, may then be inserted into bacterial plasmid or bacteriophage DNA for subsequent cloning of the recombinant molecules. Thus, the genes can be produced in large quantities for structural and other studies. Specific restriction endonuclease sites and genes conferring drug resistance are usually incorporated into the plasmid or viral vector for selection purposes. In the classic plasmid vector, pBR322, two genes for antibiotic resistance (for tetracycline and ampicillin resistance) are present. The cloned DNA is usually inserted into one of the antibiotic-resistance marker genes, rendering the plasmid sensitive to that compound. The recombinant DNA can then be used to transform *E. coli* or other bacteria. The bacteria that contain the plasmid can be detected by plating for the resistant antibiotic marker, and the plasmids that carry the recombinant DNA can be selected by their sensitivity to the other resistance marker. Bacterial clones that contain the human DNA sequence can be grown to obtain large amounts of the expressed human gene.

A major obstacle to achieving optimum expression of biologically active products from eukaryotic genes cloned in bacterial systems has been that most bacterial host systems do not perform the extensive mRNA processing and post-translational modifications (i.e., mRNA splicing, proteolysis, glycosylation) crucial to the structure and activity of these molecules. Recently, a variety of eukaryotic cloning vectors have been developed to overcome these obstacles. Most approaches involve the use of SV40-derived packaged vectors, which typically consist of two components: (*a*) defective viruses containing chimeric genomes in which the foreign DNA sequences are linked to subsets of viral DNA sequences specifying CIS-acting essential replication functions, and (*b*) adequate helper viruses capable of providing trans-replication and packaging functions needed for the propagation of the chimeric genomes. Recently, several SV40-derived dominant-selection eukaryotic expression vectors have been developed and used (*320,321*); however, the usefulness of these vectors is constrained by the size of inserts they can accommodate (about 5 kilobases) and the limited types of cells that they may infect (i.e., monkey central nervous system cells). A new eukaryotic defective-virus cloning–amplification vector has been developed involving the herpes simplex virion (*322*). This vector eliminates many of the obstacles mentioned with the SV40 systems, because it can accommodate DNA molecules up to about 150 kilobases and can infect a wide variety of host-cell species. Other investigators have used yeast to clone and express eukaryotic genes. For example, Hitzeman et al. (*323*) replaced the 5'-promoter-leader region of the human leukocyte interferon gene with that from the yeast alcohol dehydrogenase gene and subsequently inserted the fused transcriptional units into a yeast replicating-plasmid vector. Full-length, biologically active interferon molecules were produced, indicating that yeast alcohol dehydrogenase promoter was able to confer its transcriptional control on the human leukocyte interferon gene. Furthermore, these cells were able to perform the post-translational modification events necessary for the efficient expression of biologically active interferon.

These examples only highlight the remarkable technical advances occurring in this field. We can anticipate that the production of medically useful proteins will provide the human biologicals required for replacement and other therapeutic endeavors during the 1980s. In fact, commercially produced human insulin (*319*) and growth hormone (*324*) have already demonstrated their clinical benefit and safety.

Gene Transfer

The ideal treatment for inherited metabolic defects would be the permanent introduction of new genetic information into the genome of affected individuals. However, therapeutic intervention by gene transfer is currently precluded by the lack of methodology for the precise site-specific insertion of selected DNA segments with the necessary initiation, control, and intervening sequences in a manner consistent with normal transcription, translation, and regulation of gene expression.

Transfection of eukaryotic cells with exogenous nucleic acid has become an established procedure; however, the frequency and reproducibility of DNA transfer were greatly enhanced by the development of the calcium phosphate precipitation technique by Graham and van der Eb (*325*). Wigler et al. (*326*) subsequently demonstrated that nonselectable single-copy eukaryotic genes can also be transferred to mammalian cells by co-transforming these sequences into mutant recipient cells with a selectable marker, such as thymidine kinase. Other co-transformation selection systems, such as those with APRT⁻ and HGPRT⁻ recipient cells, have been used (*327*). Dominant mutant cellular genes coding for drug resistance could, in principle, also serve as selectable markers after transformation into wild-type cells. For example, Wigler et al. (*328*) transferred a mutant hamster gene coding for an altered dihydrofolate reductase (*dhfr*) to wild-type cells; transformants were subsequently selected by their increased resistance to methotrexate. These workers demonstrated that when the mutant *dhfr* was introduced into animal cells, together with the *E. coli* plasmid, pBR322, amplification of the *dhfr* sequences (after selection with methotrexate) resulted in the co-amplification of the pBR322 sequences.

Although most DNA transformation experiments have been conducted in tissue-culture systems, techniques for the insertion of specific genes plus a drug-resistance gene into bone marrow cells and the subsequent transfer of these transformed cells back into living mice have been recently reported (*329,330*). The mouse bone marrow cells were first transformed in vitro with the herpes simplex virion thymidine kinase gene (*tk*) (*329*) or *dhfr* (*330*). These genes were used because the transformed cells could be detected by their enhanced resistance to methotrexate. The treated cells were then injected into irradiated mice. In both studies, the infused cells (e.g., containing *tk* and a marker chromosome) reconstituted the blood cells of the marrow-depleted mice.

Another method for transferring genes into developing animals involves the direct microinjection of DNA sequences into the pronuclei of fertilized mouse oocytes. Subsequent analysis of the newborn progeny permits the study of transferred gene expression during normal embryonic development. This approach has proven most fruitful for studies of globin gene transfer and expression in the mouse. Stewart et al. (*331*) co-injected the human β-globin gene and the herpes simplex virion *tk* into mouse oocytes and found that two out of 62 progeny carried the DNA sequences. Notably, one of the "transformed" mice subsequently transmitted the foreign DNA to about 50% of its offspring, the frequency expected for the mendelian inheritance of a gene carried on a chromosome. This group (*331*) and others (*332,333*) have demonstrated the mendelian transmission of microinjected foreign DNA for at least two generations of mice. Although these results support the concept that microinjected DNA is, in fact, integrated into chromosomes, it is not known whether these sequences are stably integrated into unique chromosomal regions, whether these events are random, or whether the introduced foreign sequences undergo genomic mobility. The expression of microinjected viral genes has been shown in the mouse progeny, but the expression of microinjected mammalian genes has not been definitively demonstrated in these chimeric mice. Further use of this technique should provide additional insights into the integration and expression of foreign DNA in mammals.

A recent advance in the field of eukaryotic gene transfer has been achieved in a series of elegant experiments by Spradling and Rubin (*334,335*). First, they demonstrated that transposable P elements of *Drosophila* could be microinjected into *Drosophila* embryos (that lacked these elements), and that the transposable elements were integrated into chromosomal sites of the recipients. Thus, the use of this transposable element permitted the transposition of extrachromosomal DNA into the germ-line chromosomes of the *Drosophila* embryos (*334*). These findings were then extended to insert a specific *Drosophila* gene, encoding the enzyme xanthine dehydrogenase into enzyme-deficient mutant flies. The mutant flies had the rosy eye phenotype; therefore, transformed flies that expressed the normal gene would have wild-type eye color. The strategy employed was to insert the normal xanthine dehydrogenase gene into a P element (making it transposon-defective), and then co-inject normal P elements, which would code for "transposase" and permit the chromosomal integration of both the extrachromosomal P elements and those containing the xanthine dehydrogenase structural gene. In this way, they genetically transformed the mutant *Drosophila* embryos. The transformed flies had wild-type eye color, indicating that the enzymatic defect had been corrected by the transferred gene (*335*). These studies demonstrate that the use of recombinant plasmids containing endogenous transposable sequences can "target" foreign DNA to chromosomal locations for gene expression. By analogy, if such transposons can be found for human chromosomal integration, the possibility for human somatic cell transformation would be dramatically realized. Perhaps certain viruses, like the retrovirus, have such potential use for human gene transfer.

Although the developing field of eukaryotic gene transfer has only recently emerged, the novel results outlined above have already strengthened our understanding of eukaryotic gene structure, organization, and expression, and highlight the exciting future prospects of human gene therapy in selected metabolic diseases.

I thank Drs. Edward H. Schuchman and Gregory A. Grabowski for assistance with the preparation of this review, and Ms. Mary Ann Dent and Ms. Linda Lugo for their expert clerical assistance.

This review was supported in part by a grant from the March of Dimes Birth Defects Foundation (1–273), the National Institutes of Health (GM 25279), and the Clinical Research Centers Program of the Division of Research Resources, National Institutes of Health (RR 71).

References

1. Desnick, R. J., Ed., *Enzyme Therapy in Genetic Diseases,* **2,** Alan R. Liss, Inc., New York, NY, 1980.
2. Desnick, R. J., and Grabowski, G. A., Advances in the treatment of inherited metabolic diseases. *Adv. Hum. Genet.* **11,** 281–369 (1981).
3. Papadatos, C. J., and Bartsocas, C. S., Eds., *The Management of Genetic Disorders,* Alan R. Liss, Inc., New York, NY, 1979, 424 p.
4. Crawford, M. d'A., Gibbs, D. A., and Watts, R. W. E., Eds., *Advances in the Treatment of Inborn Errors of Metabolism,* John Wiley and Sons, New York, NY, 1982, 365 p.
5. Bickel, H., Gerrard, J., and Hickmans, E. M., The influence of phenylalanine intake on the chemistry and behavior of a phenylketonuric child. *Acta Pediatr.* **43,** 64–77 (1954).
6. Williamson, M. L., Koch, R., Azen, C., and Chang, G., Correlates of intelligence test results in treated phenylketonuric children. *Pediatrics* **68,** 161 (1981).
7. Koch, R., Azen, C. G., Friedman, E. G., and Williamson, M. L., Preliminary report on the effects of diet discontinuation in PKU. *J. Pediatr.* **100,** 870–875 (1982).

8. Komrower, G. M., Sardharwalla, I. B., Coutts, J. M. J., and Ingham, D., Management of maternal phenylketonuria: An emerging clinical problem. *Br. Med. J.* **i,** 1383 (1979).
9. Lenke, R. R., and Levy, H. L., Maternal phenylketonuria and hyperphenylalaninemia. An international survey of the outcome of untreated and treated pregnancies. *N. Engl. J. Med.* **303,** 1202 (1980).
10. Levy, H. L., Kaplan, G. N., and Erickson, A. M., Comparison of treated and untreated pregnancies in a mother with phenylketonuria. *J. Pediatr.* **100,** 876–880 (1982).
11. Kaufman, S., Holtzman, N. A., Milstien, S., and Krumbolz, A., Phenylketonuria due to deficiency of dihydropteridine reductase. *N. Engl. J. Med.* **293,** 785–790 (1975).
12. Kaufman, S., Berlow, S., Summer, G. K., Milstien, S., Schulman, J. D., Orloff, S., Spielberg, S., and Pueschel, S., Hyperphenylalaninemia due to a deficiency of biopterin. *N. Engl. J. Med.* **299,** 673–679 (1978).
13. Schaub, J., Daumling, S., Curtius, H.-Ch., Niederwieser, A., Bartholome, K., Viscontini, M., Schircks, B., and Bieri, J. H., Tetrahydrobiopterin therapy of atypical phenylketonuria due to defective dihydrobiopterin biosynthesis. *Arch. Dis. Child.* **53,** 674–676 (1978).
14. Niederwieser, A., Curtius, H.-Ch., Wang, M., and Leupold, D., Atypical phenylketonuria with defective biopterin metabolism. Monotherapy with tetrahydrobiopterin or sepiaptern, screening and study of biosynthesis in man. *Eur. J. Pediatr.* **138,** 110–112 (1982).
15. Kaufman, S., Kapatos, G., McInnes, R. R., Schulman, J. D., and Rizzo, W. B., Use of tetrahydropterins in the treatment of hyperphenylalaninemia due to defective synthesis of tetrahydrobiopterin: Evidence that peripherally administered tetrahydropterins enter the brain. *Pediatrics* **70,** 376–380 (1982).
16. Hoskins, J. A., Jack, G., Peiris, R. J. D., Starr, D. J. T., Wade, H. E., Wright, E. C., and Stern, J., Enzymatic control of phenylalanine intake in phenylketonuria. *Lancet* **i,** 392 (1980).
17. Nadler, H. L., Inouye, T., and Hsia, D. Y. Y., Classical galactosemia: A study of fifty cases. In *Galactosemia,* Hsia, D. Y. Y., Ed., C. C Thomas, Springfield, IL, 1969, pp 127–139.
18. Donnell, G. N., Koch, R., and Bergren, W. R., Observations on the results of management of galactosemic patients. *Ibid.,* pp 247–268.
19. Froesch, E. R., Pentosuria. In *The Metabolic Basis of Inherited Disease,* 3rd ed., Stanbury, J. G., Wyngaarden, J. B., and Fredrickson, D. S., Eds., McGraw-Hill, New York, NY, 1972, p 128.
20. Gray, G. M., The hemoglobinopathies. *Ibid.,* p 1457.
21. Komrower, G. M., Lambert, A. M., Cusworth, D. C., and Westall,

R. C., Dietary treatment of homocystinuria. *Arch. Dis. Child.* **41,** 666–671 (1966).
22. Perry, T. L., Dunn, H. G., Hansen, S., MacDougall, L., and Warrington, P. D., Early diagnosis and treatment of homocystinuria. *Pediatrics* **37,** 502–505 (1966).
23. Nyhan, W. L., Fawcett, N., Ando, T., Rennert, O. M., and Julius, R. L., Responses to dietary therapy in B_{12}-unresponsive methylmalonic acidemia. *Pediatrics* **51,** 539–548 (1973).
24. Satoh, T., Narisawa, K., Igarashi, Y., Saitoh, T., Hayasaka, K., Ichinohazama, Y., Onodera, H., Tada, K., and Oohara, K., Dietary therapy in two patients with vitamin B_{12}-unresponsive methylmalonic acidemia. *Eur. J. Pediatr.* **135,** 305–312 (1981).
25. Snyderman, E., Norton, P. M., Roitman, E., and Holt, L. E., Jr., Maple syrup urine disease, with particular reference to dietotherapy. *Pediatrics* **34,** 454–460 (1964).
26. Westall, R. G., Dietary treatment of a child with maple syrup urine disease (branched-chain ketoaciduria). *Arch. Dis. Child.* **38,** 485–491 (1963).
27. Levy, H. L., Erickson, A. M., Lott, I. T., and Kiertz, D. J., Isovaleric acidemia: Results of a family study and dietary treatment. *Pediatrics* **52,** 83–91 (1973).
28. Halverson, S., Dietary treatment of tyrosinosis. *Am. J. Dis. Child.* **113,** 38–40 (1967).
29. Kolb, F. O., Earll, J. M., and Harper, H. A., "Disappearance" of cystinuria in a patient treated with prolonged low methionine diet. *Metabolism* **16,** 378–386 (1967).
30. Zinneman, H. H., and Jones, J. E., Dietary methionine and its influence on cystine excretion in cystinuric patients. *Metabolism* **15,** 915–921 (1966).
31. Bickel, H., Lutz, P., and Schmidt, H., The treatment of cystinosis with diet or drugs. In *Cystinosis,* Schulman, J. D., Ed., DHEW publ. no. [NIH] 72–249, 1973, pp 199–223.
32. Corner, B. D., Holton, J. B., Norman, R. M., and Williams, P. M., A case of histidinemia controlled with a low histidine diet. *Pediatrics* **41,** 1074–1080 (1968).
33. Gatfield, P. D., Knights, R. M., Devereaux, M., and Pozsonye, J. P., Histidinemia: A report of four new cases in one family and effect of low histidine diet. *Can. Med. Assoc. J.* **101,** 465–469 (1969).
34. Tada, K., Tateda, H., Arashima, S., Sakai, K., Kitagawa, T., Aoki, K., Suwa, S., Kawamura, M., Oura, T., Takesada, M., Kuroda, Y., Yamashita, F., Matsuda, I., and Naruse, H., Intellectual development in patients with untreated histidinemia. *J. Pediatr.* **101,** 562–563 (1982).

35. Shih, V. H., Urea cycle disorders and other congenital hyperammonemic syndromes. In *The Metabolic Basis of Inherited Disease*, 4th ed., Stanbury, J. B., Wyngaarden, J. B., and Fredrickson, D. S., Eds., McGraw-Hill, New York, NY, 1978, pp 362–386.
36. Rosenberg, L. E., Disorders of propionate, methylmalonate, and cobalamin metabolism. *Ibid.*, p 411.
37. Batshaw, M., Brusilow, S., and Walser, M., Treatment of carbamyl phosphate synthetase deficiency with keto analogues of essential amino acids. *N. Engl. J. Med.* **292**, 1085–1090 (1975).
38. Brusilow, S. W., Batshaw, M. L., and Walser, M., Use of keto acids in inborn errors of urea synthesis. In *Nutritional Management of Genetic Disorders*, Winick, M., Ed., John Wiley and Sons, New York, NY, 1979, pp 65–75.
39. Valle, D., Walser, M., Brusilow, S. W., and Kaiser-Kupfer, M., Gyrate atrophy of the coroid and retina. *J. Clin. Invest.* **65**, 371–375 (1980).
40. Valle, D., Walser, M., Brusilow, S. W., Kaiser-Kupfer, M., and de Monastero, F., Long-term results of therapy of gyrate atrophy. *Clin. Res.* **28**, 546A (1980).
41. McInnes, R. R., Arshinoff, S. A., Bell, L., Marliss, E. B., and McCulloch, J. C., Hyperornithinaemia and gyrate atrophy of the retina: Improvement of vision during treatment with a low-arginine diet. *Lancet* **i**, 513–517 (1981).
42. Stoppoloni, G., Prisco, F., Santinelli, R., Sicuranza, G., and Rinaldi, E., Treatment of hyperornithinaemia and gyrate atrophy of choroid and retina with low-protein diet. *Lancet* **i**, 973 (1982).
43. Siplia, I., Rapola, J., Simell, O., and Vannas, A., Supplementary creatine as a treatment for gyrate atrophy of the choroid and retina. *N. Engl. J. Med.* **304**, 867–870 (1981).
44. Hsia, Y. E., Coombs, J. T., Hook, L., and Brandt, I. K., Hepatolenticular degeneration: The comparative effectiveness of D-penicillamine, potassium sulfide and diethyldithiocarbonate as decoppering agents. *J. Pediatr.* **68**, 921–926 (1966).
45. Richmond, J., Rosenoer, Y. N., Tompsett, S. L., Draper, I., and Simpson, J. A., Hepatolenticular degeneration (Wilson's disease) treated by penicillamine. *Brain* **87**, 619–638 (1964).
46. Walshe, J. M., The management of Wilson's disease with triethylenetetramine 2HCl (Trien 2HCl). In ref. *3*, pp 271–280.
47. Walshe, J. M., Treatment of Wilson's disease with trientine (triethylenetetramine) dihydrochloride. *Lancet* **i**, 643–647 (1982).
48. Crawhall, J. C., Scowen, E. F., and Watts, R. W. E., Further observations on use of D-penicillamine in cystinuria. *Br. Med. J.* **i**, 1411–1413 (1964).

49. Levy, R. I., Fredrickson, D. S., Stone, N. J., Bilheimer, D. W., Brown, W. V., Glueck, C. J., Gotto, A. M., Herbert, P. N., Kwiterovich, P. O., Langer, T., La Rosa, J., Lux, S. E., Rider, A. K., Shulman, R. S., and Sloan, H. R., Cholestyramine in type II hyperlipoproteinemia. *Ann. Intern. Med.* **79**, 51–58 (1973).
50. Shepard, J., Packard, C. J., Bicker, S., Lawrie, T. D. V., and Morgan, H. G., Cholestyramine promotes receptor-mediated low-density lipoprotein catabolism. *N. Engl. J. Med.* **302**, 1219–1222 (1980).
51. Kane, J. P., Havel, R. J., Malloy, M. J., and Tun, P., Normalization of low-density lipoproteins in familial hypercholesterolemia. *N. Engl. J. Med.* **304**, 1361–1362 (1981).
52. Illingworth, D. R., Phillipson, B. E., Rapp, J. H., and Connor, W. E., Colestipol plus nicotinic acid in treatment of heterozygous familial hypercholesterolaemia. *Lancet* **i**, 296–298 (1981).
53. Pippard, M. J., Letsky, E. A., Callender, S. T., and Weatherall, D. J., Prevention of iron loading in transfusion-dependent thalassemia. *Lancet* **i**, 1178 (1978).
54. Wyngaarden, J. B., and Kelley, W. N., Disorders of purine and pyrimidine metabolism. In *Metabolic Basis of Inherited Disease*, 4th ed. (see ref. *35*), p 989.
55. Boss, G. R., and Seegmiller, J. E., Hyperuricemia and gout. *N. Engl. J. Med.* **300**, 1459–1468 (1979).
56. Brusilow, S. W., Valle, D. L., and Batshaw, M. L., New pathways of nitrogen excretion in inborn errors of urea synthesis. *Lancet* **ii**, 452–454 (1979).
57. Brusilow, S. W., and Batshaw, M. L., Arginine therapy of argininosuccinase deficiency. *Lancet* **i**, 124–127 (1979).
58. Batshaw, M. L., Brusilow, S., Waber, L., Blom, W., Brubakk, A. M., Burton, B. K., Cann, H. M., Kerr, D., Mamunes, P., Matalon, R., Myerberg, D., and Schafer, I. A., Treatment of inborn errors of urea synthesis. Activation of alternative pathways of waste nitrogen synthesis and excretion. *N. Engl. J. Med.* **306**, 1387–1392 (1982).
59. Brubakk, A. M., Teijema, L. L., Blom, W., and Berger, R., Successful treatment of severe OTC deficiency. *J. Pediatr.* **100**, 929–931 (1982).
60. Batshaw, M., and Brusilow, S. W., Evidence of lack of toxicity of sodium phenylacetate and sodium benzoate in treating urea cycle enzymopathies. *J. Metab. Dis.* **4**, 231 (1981).
61. Krieger, I., and Tanaka, K., Therapeutic effects of glycine in isovaleric acidemia. *Pediatr. Res.* **10**, 25–29 (1976).
62. Yudkoff, M., Cohen, R. M., Puschak, R., Rothman, R., and Segal, S., Glycine therapy in isovaleric acidemia. *J. Pediatr.* **92**, 813–817 (1978).
63. Cohn, R. M., Yudkoff, M., Rothman, R., and Segal, S., Isovaleric

acidemia: Use of glycine therapy in neonates. *N. Engl. J. Med.* **299**, 996–999 (1978).
64. Bartlett, K., and Gompertz, D., The specificity of glycine N-acylase and acylglycine excretion in the organic acidemias. *Biochem. Med.* **10**, 15–21 (1974).
65. Gibberd, F. B., Page, N. G. R., Billimoria, J. D., and Retsas, S., Heredopathia atactica polyneuritiformis (Refsum's disease) treated by diet and plasma exchange. *Lancet* **i**, 575–576 (1979).
66. Moser, H. W., Braine, H., Pyeritz, R. E., Ullman, D., Murray, C., and Asbury, A., Therapeutic trial of plasmapheresis in Refsum's disease and Fabry disease. In ref. *1*, pp 491–497.
67. Johnson, D. L., and Desnick, R. J., Molecular pathology of Fabry's disease: Physical and kinetic properties of α-galactosidase in cultured endothelial cells. *Biochim. Biophys. Acta* **538**, 195–204 (1978).
68. King, M. E. E., Breslow, J. L., and Lees, R. S., Plasma-exchange therapy of homozygous familial hypercholesterolemia. *N. Engl. J. Med.* **302**, 1457–1459 (1980).
69. Witztum, J. L., Williams, J. C., Ostlund, R., Sherman, L., Siccard, G., and Schonfeld, G., Successful plasmapheresis in a 4-year-old child with homozygous familial hypercholesterolemia. *J. Pediatr.* **97**, 615–618 (1980).
70. Lupien, P.-J., Moorjani, S., and Awad, J., A new approach to the management of familial hypercholesterolemias: Removal of plasma-cholesterol based on the principle of affinity chromatography. *Lancet* **i**, 1261 (1976).
71. Lupien, P.-J., Moorjani, S., Lou, M., Brun, D., and Gagne, C., Removal of cholesterol from blood by affinity binding to heparin–agarose: Evaluation of treatment in homozygous familial hypercholesterolemia. *Pediatr. Res.* **14**, 113–117 (1980).
72. Burgstaler, E. A., Pineda, A. A., and Ellefson, R. D., Removal of plasma lipoproteins from circulating blood with a heparin–agarose column. *Mayo Clin. Proc.* **55**, 180–184 (1980).
73. Buchwald, H., and Varco, R. L., Eds., *Metabolic Surgery*, Grune and Stratton, New York, NY, 1978.
74. Riddell, A. G., Davies, R. P., and Clark, A. D., Portacaval transposition in the treatment of glycogen storage disease. *Lancet* **ii**, 1146–1148 (1966).
75. Corbeel, L., Hue, L., Lederer, B., DeBarsy, T., van Den Berghe, G., Devlieger, H., Jaeken, J., Bracke, P., and Eeckels, R., Clinical and biochemical findings before and after portacaval shunt in a girl with type Ib glycogen storage disease. *Pediatr. Res.* **15**, 58–61 (1981).
76. Starzl, T. E., Brown, B. I., Blanchard, H., and Brettschneider, L.,

Portal diversion in glycogen storage disease. *Surgery* **65,** 504–506 (1969).

77. Greene, H. L., Slonim, A. E., O'Neill, J. A., and Burr, I. M., Continuous nocturnal intragastric feeding for management of type I glycogen storage disease. *N. Engl. J. Med.* **294,** 423 (1976).

78. Fernandes, J., and Jansen, H., Glucose-6-phosphate deficient children treated by nocturnal gastric drip feeding. *Pediatr. Res.* **11,** 1016 (1977).

79. Ehrkich, R. M., Robinson, B. H., Freedman, M. H., and Howard, N. J., Nocturnal intragastric infusion of glucose in management of defective gluconeogenesis with hypoglycemia. *Am. J. Dis. Child.* **132,** 241 (1978).

80. Moore, R. B., Varco, R. L., and Buchwald, H., Metabolic surgery in the hyperlipoproteinemias. *Am. J. Cardiol.* **31,** 148–157 (1973).

81. Spengel, F. A., Jadhav, A., Duffield, R. G. M., Wood, C. B., and Thompson, G. R., Superiority of partial ileal bypass over cholestyramine in reducing cholesterol in familial hypercholesterolaemia. *Lancet* **ii,** 768–770 (1981).

82. Kelley, W. N., and Wyngaarden, J. B., The Lesch–Nyhan syndrome. In *The Metabolic Basis of Inherited Disease,* 4th ed. (see ref. *35*), p 1029.

83. Levy, R. I., Fredrickson, D. S., Schulman, R., Bilheimer, D. W., Breslow, J. L., Stone, N. J., Lux, S. E., Sloan, H. R., Krauss, R. M., and Herbert, D. N., Dietary and drug treatment of primary hyperlipoproteinemia. *Ann. Intern. Med.* **77,** 267–294 (1972).

84. Mabuchi, H., Haba, T., Tatami, R., Miyamoto, S., Sakai, Y., Wakasugi, T., Watanabe, A., Koizumi, J., and Takeda, R., Effects of an inhibitor of 3-hydroxymethylglutaryl coenzyme A reductase on serum lipoproteins and ubiquinone-10 levels in patients with familial hypercholesterolemia. *N. Engl. J. Med.* **305,** 478–517 (1981).

85. Melancon, S. B., Dallaire, L., Vincelette, P., Potier, M., and Geoffrey, G., Early treatment of severe infantile glycine encephalopathy (nonketotic hyperglycinemia) with strychnine and sodium benzoate. In ref. *3,* p 217.

86. Bartter, F. C., Pronove, P., Gill, J. R., Jr., and MacCardle, R. C., Hyperplasia of the juxtaglomerular complex with hyperaldosteronism and hypokalemic alkalosis. *Am. J. Med.* **33,** 811–828 (1962).

87. Bartter, F. C., Gill, J. R., Jr., Frolich, J. G., Bowden, R. E., Hollifield, J. W., Radfar, N., Keiser, H. R., Oates, J. A., Seyberth, H., and Taylor, A. A., Prostaglandins are overproduced by the kidneys and mediate hyperreninemia in Bartter's syndrome. *Trans. Assoc. Am. Physiol.* **89,** 77–91 (1976).

88. Gullner, G.-H., Bartter, F. C., Cerletti, C., Smith, J. B., and Gill,

J. R., Jr., Prostacyclin overproduction in Bartter's syndrome. *Lancet* **ii,** 767–770 (1979).
89. Smith, W. L., and Lands, W. E. M., Stimulation and blockade of prostaglandin biosynthesis. *J. Biol. Chem.* **246,** 6700–6704 (1971).
90. Gullner, G.-H., Gill, J. R., Jr., Bartter, F. C., and Smith, J. B., Correction of increased prostacyclin production in Bartter's syndrome by indomethacin. *Clin. Res.* **28,** 559A (1980).
91. Gill, J. R., Jr., and Bartter, F. C., Evidence for a prostaglandin defect in chloride absorption in the loop of Henle as a proximal cause of Bartter's syndrome. *Am. J. Med.* **65,** 766–772 (1978).
92. Strauss, R. G., Failure of methyldopa therapy in Bartter's syndrome. *J. Pediatr.* **85,** 101–103 (1974).
93. Brook, C. G. D., Zachmann, M., Prader, A., and Murset, G., Experience with long-term therapy in congenital adrenal hyperplasia. *J. Pediatr.* **85,** 12–19 (1974).
94. Klein, A. H., Meltzer, and S., and Kenny, F., Improved prognosis in congenital hypothyroidism treated before age three months. *J. Pediatr.* **81,** 912–915 (1972).
95. Tanner, J. M., Whitehouse, R. J., Hughes, P. C. R., and Vince, F. P., Effect of human growth hormone treatment for 1 to 7 years on growth of 100 children with growth hormone deficiency, low birth weight, inherited smallness, Turner's syndrome and other complaints. *Arch. Dis. Child.* **46,** 745–782 (1971).
96. Becroft, D. M. O., Phillips, L. I., and Simmonds, A., Hereditary orotic aciduria: Long-term therapy with uridine and a trial of uracil. *J. Pediatr.* **75,** 885–890 (1969).
97. Danks, D. M., Campbell, M. B., Stevens, B. J., Mayne, V., and Cartwright, E., Menkes hair syndrome. An inherited defect in copper absorption with widespread defects. *Pediatrics* **50,** 188–192 (1972).
98. Bucknall, W. E., Haslan, R. H., and Holtzman, N. A., Kinky hair syndrome: Response to copper therapy. *Pediatrics* **52,** 653–657 (1973).
99. Menkes, J. H., Alter, M., Steiglider, G. K., Weakly, D. R., and Sung, J. H., A sex-linked recessive disorder with retardation of growth, peculiar hair and focal cerebral and cerebellar degeneration. *Pediatrics* **29,** 764–768 (1962).
100. Dekaban, A. S., and Steusing, J. K., Menkes kinky hair disease treated with subcutaneous copper sulphate. *Lancet* **ii,** 1523 (1974). Letter.
101. Grover, W. D., and Scrutton, M. C., Copper infusion therapy in trichopoliodystrophy. *J. Pediatr.* **86,** 216–220 (1975).
102. Danks, D. M., Cartwright, E., and Stevens, B. J., Menkes steely hair (kinky hair) disease. *Lancet* **i,** 891 (1973).

103. Beratis, N. G., Price, P., LaBadie, G. U., and Hirschhorn, K., ^{64}Cu metabolism in Menkes and normal cultured skin fibroblasts. *Pediatr. Res.* **12**, 699–702 (1978).
104. Beratis, N. G., Price, P., LaBadie, G. U., and Hirschhorn, K., Copper metabolism in Menkes disease. *Pediatr. Res.* **13**, 206–210 (1979).
105. LaBadie, G. U., Hirschhorn, K., Katz, S., and Beratis, N. G., Increased copper metallothionein in Menkes cultured skin fibroblasts. *Pediatr. Res.* **15**, 257–266 (1981).
106. LaBadie, G. U., Beratis, N. G., Price, P., and Hirschhorn, K., Studies of the copper-binding proteins in Menkes' and normal cultured skin fibroblast lysates. *J. Cell. Physiol.* **106**, 369–374 (1981).
107. Evans, G. W., and Johnson, P. E., Zinc binding factor in acrodermatitis enteropathica. *Lancet* **ii**, 1310 (1976). Letter.
108. Atherton, D. J., Muller, D. P. R., Aggett, P. G., and Harries, J. T., A defect in zinc uptake by jejunal biopsies in acrodermatitis enteropathica. *Clin. Sci. Molec. Med.* **56**, 505–507 (1979).
109. Dillaha, C. J., Lorincz, A. L., and Aavik, O. R., Acrodermatitis enteropathica. Review of the literature and report of a case successfully treated with diodoquin. *J. Am. Med. Assoc.* **152**, 509–512 (1953).
110. Moynahan, E. J., Johnson, F. R., and McMinn, R. M. H., Acrodermatitis enteropathica: Demonstration of possible intestinal enzyme defect. *Proc. R. Soc. Med.* **56**, 300–301 (1963).
111. Cash, R., and Berger, C. K., Acrodermatitis enteropathica: Defective metabolism of unsaturated fatty acids. *J. Pediatr.* **74**, 717–729 (1969).
112. Moynahan, E. J., Acrodermatitis enteropathica: A lethal inherited zinc deficiency disorder. *Lancet* **ii**, 399–400 (1974).
113. Neldner, K. H., and Hambridge, K. M., Zinc therapy of acrodermatitis enteropathica. *N. Engl. J. Med.* **292**, 879–882 (1975).
114. Hambridge, K. M., Neldner, K. H., and Walravens, P. A., Zinc, acrodermatitis enteropathica and congenital malformations. *Lancet* **i**, 577–578 (1975).
115. Brenton, D. P., Jackson, M. J., and Young, A., Two pregnancies in a patient with acrodermatitis enteropathica treated with zinc sulfate. *Lancet* **ii**, 500–502 (1981).
116. Costa, T., Reade, T. M., Cole, D. E. C., Nogrady, B., Scriver, C. R., Marais, P., and Glorieux, F. H., Renal handling of phosphate (Pi) and bone mineralization in X-linked hypophosphatemia (XLH) during treatment with P_i and 1,25-$(OH)_2D_3$. *Pediatr. Res.* **14**, 521A (1980).
117. Rasmussen, H., Pechet, M., Anast, C., Mazur, A., Gertner, J., and Brodus, A. E., Long-term treatment of familial hypophosphatemic rickets with oral phosphate and 1α-hydroxyvitamin D_3. *J. Pediatr.* **99**, 16–25 (1981).

118. Lipson, M. H., Kraus, J., and Rosenberg, L. E., Affinity of cystathionine β-synthase for pyridoxal 5'-phosphate in cultured cells. A mechanism for pyridoxine-responsive homocystinuria. *J. Clin. Invest.* **66,** 188–193 (1980).
119. Fenton, W. A., and Rosenberg, L. E., Genetic and biochemical analysis of human cobalmin mutants in cell culture. *Ann. Rev. Genet.* **12,** 223–248 (1978).
120. Pascal, T. A., Gaull, G. E., Beratis, N. G., Gillam, G. M., and Tallan, H. H., Cystathionase deficiency: Evidence for genetic heterogeneity in primary cystathioninuria. *Pediatr. Res.* **12,** 125–133 (1978).
121. Fleischer, L. D., and Gaull, G. E., Enzyme manipulation by specific megavitamin therapy. In ref. *1,* pp 239–267.
122. Hsia, Y. E., Treatment in genetic diseases. In *The Prevention of Genetic Disease and Mental Retardation,* Milunsky, A., Ed., Saunders, Philadelphia, PA, 1975, pp 277–305.
123. Rosenberg, L. E., Vitamin responsive inherited metabolic disorders. *Adv. Hum. Genet.* **6,** 1–74 (1976).
124. Taka, K., Saito, T., Omura, K., Hayasaka, S., and Mizuno, K., Hyperornithinaemia associated with gyrate atrophy of the choroid and retina: *In vivo* and *in vitro* response to vitamin B$_6$. *J. Inher. Metab. Dis.* **4,** 61–62 (1981).
125. Grabowski, G. A., Walling, L., and Desnick, R. J., Human mannosidosis: *In vitro* and *in vivo* studies of cofactor supplementation. In ref. *1,* pp 319–334.
126. Jolly, R. D., Van de Water, N. S., Janmaat, A., Slack, P. M., and McKenzie, R. G., Zinc therapy in the bovine mannosidosis model. In ref. *1,* pp 305–318.
127. Elsas, L. J., Hollins, B., and Pinnell, S. R., Hydroxylysine-deficient collagen disease: Effect of ascorbic acid. *Am. J. Hum. Genet.* **26,** 28A (1974).
128. Elsas, L. J., Miller, R. L., and Pinnell, S. R., Inherited human collagen lysyl hydroxylase deficiency: Ascorbic acid response. *Clin. Res.* **24,** 294A (1976).
129. Wolf, B., Hsia, Y. E., Sweetman, L., Feldman, G., Boychuk, R. B., Bart, R. D., Crowel, D. H., DiMauro, R. M., and Nyhan, W. L., Multiple carboxylase deficiency: Clinical and biochemical improvement following neonatal biotin treatment. *Pediatrics* **68,** 113–118 (1981).
130. Waber, L. J., Valle, D., Neill, C., DiMauro, S., and Shug, A., Carnitine deficiency presenting as familial cardiomyopathy: A treatable defect in carnitine transport. *J. Pediatr.* **101,** 700–705 (1982).
131. Ampola, M. G., Mahoney, M. J., Nakamura, F., and Tanaka, K.,

Prenatal therapy of a patient with vitamin B_{12}-responsive methylmalonic acidemia. *N. Engl. J. Med.* **293,** 313–317 (1975).

132. Packman, S., Cowan, M. J., Golbus, M. S., Caswell, N. M., Sweetman, L., Burri, B. J., Nyhan, W. L., and Baker, H., Prenatal treatment of biotin-responsive multiple carboxylase deficiency. *Lancet* **i,** 1435–1440 (1982).

133. Smithells, R. W., Sheppard, S., Schorah, C. J., Seller, M. J., Nevin, N. C., Harris, R., Read, A. D., and Fielding, D. W., Apparent prevention of neural tube defects by periconceptional vitamin supplementation. *Arch. Dis. Child.* **56,** 911–918 (1981).

134. Laurence, K. M., James, N., Miller, M., Tennant, G. B., and Campbell, H., Double-blind randomized controlled trial of folate treatment before conception to prevent recurrence of neural tube defects. *Br. Med. J.* **282,** 1509–1511 (1981).

135. Tolarova, H., Periconceptional supplementation with vitamins and folic acid to prevent recurrence of cleft lip. *Lancet* **ii,** 217 (1982).

136. Thompson, R. P. H., The use and abuse of treatment in the hyperbilirubinemia syndromes. In *Treatment of Inborn Errors of Metabolism,* Seakins, J. W. T., Saunders, R. A., and Foothill, C., Eds., Livingstone, Edinburgh, 1973, pp 215–225.

137. Rosen, F. S., and Beyler, A., Hereditary angioneurotic edema and its correction with androgen therapy. In ref. *1,* pp 499–508.

138. Gadek, J. E., Fulmer, J. D., Gelfand, J. A., Frank, M. M., Petty, T. L., and Crystal, R. G., Danazol-induced augmentation of serum α_1-antitrypsin levels in individuals with marked deficiency of this antiprotease. *J. Clin. Invest.* **66,** 82–87 (1980).

139. Gadek, J. E., Hosea, S. W., Gelfand, J. A., Santaella, M., Wickerhauser, M., Triantaphyllopoulos, D. C., and Frank, M. M., Replacement therapy in hereditary angioedema with partly purified C_1 inhibitor. *N. Engl. J. Med.* **302,** 542–546 (1980).

140. Lascelles, J., The synthesis of enzymes concerned in bacteriochlorophyll formation in growing cultures of *Rhodopseudomonas spheroides. J. Gen. Microbiol.* **23,** 487–498 (1960).

141. Burnham, B., and Lascelles, J., Control of porphyrin biosynthesis through a negative-feedback mechanism. Studies with preparations of delta-aminolevulate synthetase and delta-aminolaevulate dehydratase from *Rhodopseudomonas spheroides. Biochem. J.* **87,** 462–472 (1963).

142. Granick, S., Porphyrin biosynthesis, porphyrin diseases, and induced enzyme synthesis in chemical porphyria. *Trans. N.Y. Acad. Sci.* **25,** 53–65 (1962).

143. Granick, S., The induction *in vitro* of the synthesis of δ-aminolevulinic acid synthetase in chemical porphyria. A response to certain

drugs, sex hormones and foreign chemicals. *J. Biol. Chem.* **241**, 1359–1375 (1966).
144. Waxman, A. D., Collins, A., and Tschudy, D. P., Oscillations of hepatic δ-aminolevulinic acid synthetase produced *in vivo* by heme. *Biochem. Biophys. Res. Commun.* **24**, 675–683 (1966).
145. Bonkowsky, H. L., Tschudy, D. P., Collins, A., Doherty, J., Bossenmaier, I., Cardinal, R., and Watson, C. J., Repression of the overproduction of porphyrin precursors in acute intermittent porphyria by intravenous infusions of hematin. *Proc. Natl. Acad. Sci. USA* **68**, 2725–2729 (1971).
146. Watson, C. J., Pierack, C. A., Bossenmaier, I., and Cardinal, R., Postulated deficiency of hepatic heme and repair by hematin infusions in the "inducible" hepatic porphyrias. *Proc. Natl. Acad. Sci. USA* **74**, 2118–2120 (1977).
147. Watson, C. J., Pierach, C. A., Bossenmaier, I., and Cardinal, R., Use of hematin in the acute attack of the "inducible" hepatic porphyrias. *Adv. Intern. Med.* **23**, 265–286 (1978).
148. Welland, F. H., Hellman, E. S., Gaddis, E. M., Collins, A., Hunter, G. W., Jr., and Tschudy, D. P., Factors affecting the excretion of porphyrin precursors by patients with acute intermittent porphyria. I. The effect of diet. *Metabolism* **13**, 232–250 (1964).
149. Brodie, M. J., Moore, M. R., Thompson, G. G., and Goldberg, A., The treatment of acute intermittent porphyria with levulose. *Clin. Sci. Molec. Med.* **53**, 365–371 (1977).
150. Wider de Xifra, E. A., Batlle, A. M. C., Stella, A. M., and Malamud, S., Acute intermittent porphyria—another approach to therapy. *Int. J. Biochem.* **12**, 819–822 (1980).
151. Matas, A. J., Simmons, R. L., and Desnick, R. J., Transplantation in metabolic disease. In ref. *73*, pp 177–227.
152. Matas, A. J., Desnick, R. J., Najarian, J. S., and Simmons, R. L., Clinical and experimental transplantation in enzymatic deficiency disease. *Surg. Gynecol. Obstet.* **146**, 975–986 (1978).
153. Hirschhorn, R., Treatment of genetic diseases by allotransplantation. In ref. *1*, pp 429–444.
154. Congdon, C. C., Bone marrow transplantation. *Science* **116**, 171–182 (1971).
155. Stiehm, E. R., Jr., Lawlor, G. J., Kaplan, M. S., Greenwald, H. L., Neerhout, R. C., Sengar, D. P. S., and Terasaki, P. I., Immunologic reconstitution in severe combined immunodeficiency without bone marrow chromosomal chimerism. *N. Engl. J. Med.* **286**, 797–803 (1972).
156. Bach, F. H., Albertini, R. J., and Joo, P., Bone marrow transplanta-

tion in a patient with the Wiskott–Aldrich syndrome. *Lancet* **ii**, 1364–1368 (1968).
157. Parkman, R., Rappeport, J., Geha, R., Belli, J., Cassady, R., Levey, R., Nathan, D. G., and Rosen, F. S., Complete correction of the Wiskott–Aldrich syndrome by allograft bone-marrow transplantation. *N. Engl. J. Med.* **298**, 921–927 (1978).
158. Meuwissen, H. J., Keiserman, M., Taft, E., Pollara, B., and Pickering, R. J., Marrow transplantation (MTP) in Wiskott–Aldrich Syndrome (WAS): T-cell engraftment with cyclophosphamide (CY), complete engraftment with total body irradiation. *Pediatr. Res.* **12**, 483A (1978).
159. Foroozanfar, N., Hobbs, J. R., Hugh-Jones, K., Humble, J. G., James, D. C. O., Selwyn, S., Watson, J. G., and Yamamura, M., Bone marrow transplantation from an unrelated donor for chronic granulomatous disease. *Lancet* **i**, 210–213 (1977).
160. Rappeport, J. M., Parkman, R., Newberger, PP., Camitta, B. M., and Chusid, M. J., Correction of infantile agranulocytosis (Kostmann's syndrome) by allogenic bone marrow transplantation. *Am. J. Med.* **68**, 605–609 (1980).
161. Gluckman, E., Devergie, A., Schaison, G., Bussel, A., Berger, R., Schier, J., and Bernard, J., Bone marrow transplantation in Fanconic anaemia. *Br. J. Haematol.* **45**, 557–564 (1980).
162. Elin, R. J., Reynolds, H. Y., Durbin, W. A., Wolff, S. M., and Kaznierowski, J. A., Chediak–Higashi syndrome. Reversal of increased susceptibility to infection by bone marrow transplantation. *Blood* **47**, 555–559 (1976).
163. Reisner, Y., Kapoor, N., O'Reilly, R. J., and Good, R. A., Allogenic bone marrow transplantation using stem cells fractionated by lectins: VI. *In vitro* analysis of human and monkey bone marrow cells fractionated by sheep red blood cells and soybean agglutinin. *Lancet* **ii**, 1320–1323 (1980).
164. Slavin, S., and Yatziv, S., Correction of enzyme deficiency in mice by allogenic bone marrow transplantation with total lymphoid irradiation. *Science* **210**, 1150–1152 (1980).
165. Yatziv, S., Weiss, L., Morecki, S., Fuks, Z., and Slavin, S., Long-term enzyme replacement therapy in β-glucuronidase-deficient mice by allogenic bone marrow transplantation. *J. Lab. Clin. Invest.* **99**, 792–797 (1982).
166. Coccia, P. F., Krivit, W., Cervenka, J., Clawson, C., Kersey, J. H., Kim, T. H., Nesbit, M. E., Ramsay, N. K. C., Warkentin, P. I., Teitelbaum, S. L., Kahn, A. J., and Brown, D. M., Successful bone marrow transplantation for infantile malignant osteopetrosis. *N. Engl. J. Med.* **302**, 701–708 (1980).
167. Walker, D. G., Bone resorption restored in osteopetrotic mice by

transplants of normal bone marrow and spleen cells. *Science* **190**, 784–785 (1975).
168. Hobbs, J. R., Hugh-Jones, K., Barrett, A. J., Byrom, N., Chambers, D., Henry, K., James, D. C. O., Lucas, C. F., and Rogers, T. R., Reversal of clinical features of Hurler's disease and biochemical improvement after treatment by bone-marrow transplantation. *Lancet* **ii**, 709–712 (1981).
169. Hobbs, J. R., Bone marrow transplantation for inborn errors. *Lancet* **ii**, 735–739 (1981).
170. McKusick, V. A., *Heritable Disorders of Connective Tissue*, 4th ed., C. V. Mosby Co., St. Louis, MO, 1972, pp 521–686.
171. Jolly, R. D., Thompson, K. G., Murphy, C. E., Manktelow, B. W., Bruere, A. M., and Winchester, B. G., Enzyme replacement therapy—an experiment in nature in a chimeric mannosidosis calf. *Pediatr. Res.* **10**, 219–224 (1976).
172. Thomas, E. D., Bucker, C. D., Sanders, J. E., Papayannopoulou, T., Borgna-Pignatti, C., Stefano, P. D., Sullivan, K. M., Clift, R. A., and Storb, R., Marrow transplantation for thalassemia. *Lancet* **ii**, 227–228 (1982).
173. Santos, G. W., Elfenbein, G. J., and Tutschka, P. J., Bone marrow transplantation—present status. *Transplant. Proc.* **11**, 182–190 (1979).
174. Buckley, R. H., Whisnant, J. K., Schiff, R. I., Gilbertsen, R. B., Huang, A. T., and Platt, M. S., Correction of severe combined immunodeficiency by fetal liver cells. *N. Engl. J. Med.* **294**, 1076–1081 (1976).
175. August, C. S., Rosen, F. S., Filler, R. M., Janeway, C. A., Markowski, B., and Kay, H. E. M., Implantation of a fetal thymus, restoring immunological competence in a patient with thymic aplasia (Di George's syndrome). *Lancet* **ii**, 1210–1213 (1968).
176. Tubergen, D. G., Thymus transplant in lymphopenic immunodeficiency (Nezelof's syndrome). *J. Pediatr.* **84**, 915–920 (1974).
177. Starzl, T. E., Klintmalm, G. B. G., Porter, K. A., Iwatsuki, S., and Schröter, G. P. J., Liver transplantation with use of cyclosporin A and prednisone. *N. Engl. J. Med.* **305**, 266–269 (1981).
178. Dubois, R. S., Giles, G., Rodgerson, D. O., Lilly, J., Martineau, G., Halgrimson, C. G., Schröter, G., Starzl, T. E., Sternlieb, I., and Scheinberg, I. H., Orthotopic liver transplantation for Wilson's disease. *Lancet* **i**, 505–508 (1971).
179. Groth, C. G., Dubois, R. S., Corman, J., Gustafsson, A., Iwatsuki, S., Rodgerson, D. O., Halgrimson, C. G., and Starzl, T. E., Metabolic effects of hepatic replacement in Wilson's disease. *Transplant. Proc.* **5**, 829–838 (1973).

180. Beart, R. W., Jr., Putnam, C. W., Porter, K. A., and Starzl, T. E., Liver transplantation for Wilson's disease. *Lancet* **ii**, 176 (1975).
181. Putnam, C. W., Porter, K. A., Peters, R. L., Aschcavai, M., Redeker, A. G., and Starzl, T. E., Liver replacement for alpha$_1$-antitrypsin deficiency. *Surgery* **81**, 258–292 (1977).
182. Hood, J. M., Koep, L. J., Peters, R. L., Schröter, G. P. J., Weil, R., Redeker, A. G., and Starzl, T. E., Liver transplantation for advanced liver disease with alpha-1-antitrypsin deficiency. *N. Engl. J. Med.* **302**, 272–274 (1980).
183. Macdougall, B. R. D., McMaster, P., Calne, R. Y., and Williams, R., Survival and rehabilitation after orthotopic liver transplantation. *Lancet* **i**, 1326–1328 (1980).
184. Frisch, R. O., McCabe, E. R. B., Doeden, D., Koep, L. J., Kohlhoff, J. G., Silverman, A., and Starzl, T. E., Homotransplantation of the liver in a patient with hepatoma and hereditary tyrosinemia. *J. Pediatr.* **93**, 592–596 (1978).
185. Daloze, P., Delven, E. E., Glorieux, F. H., Corman, J. L., Bettez, P., and Toussi, T., Replacement therapy for inherited enzyme deficiency: Liver orthotopic transplantation in Niemann–Pick Type A. *Am. J. Med. Genet.* **1**, 229–239 (1977).
186. Touraine, J. L., Malik, M. C., Traeger, J., Perrot, H., and Maire, I., Attempt at enzyme replacement by fetal liver transplantation in Fabry's disease. *Lancet* **i**, 1094–1095 (1979).
187. Touraine, J. L., Malik, M. C., Maire, I., Rolland, M. O., Zabot, M. T., and Mathieu, M., Fetal liver transplantation in inherited enzyme deficiencies in man. In ref. 4, p 339.
188. DiMagno, E. P., Hermon-Taylor, J., Go, V. L. W., Lillehei, R. C., and Summerskill, W. H. J., Functions of a pancreaticoduodenal allograft in man. *Gastroenterology* **61**, 363–370 (1971).
189. Jonasson, I., Transplantation of the pancreas. *Transplant. Proc.* **11**, 325–330 (1979).
190. McMaiter, P., Gibby, O. M., and Calne, R. Y., Pancreas transplantation. *Ann. R. Coll. Surg.* **68**, 47–51 (1982).
191. Groth, C. G., Lundgren, G., Klintmalm, G., Gunnarsson, R., Collste, H., Wilczek, H., Ringden, O., and Ostman, I., Successful outcome of segmental human pancreatic transplantation with enteric exocrine diversion after modifications in technique. *Lancet* **ii**, 522–524 (1982).
192. Hathaway, W. E., Mull, M. M., Githens, J. H., Groth, C. G., Marchioro, T. L., and Starzl, T. E., Attempted spleen transplant in classical hemophilia. *Transplantation* **7**, 73–80 (1969).
193. Groth, C. G., Hagenfeldt, L., Dreborg, S., Lofstrom, B., Ockerman, P. A., Samuelson, L., Svennerholm, L., Werner, B., and Westberg,

G., Splenic transplantation in a case of Gaucher disease. *Lancet* **i**, 1260–1262 (1971).
194. Hoyer, J. R., Kjellstrand, C. M., Simmons, R. L., Najarian, J. S., Mauer, S. M., Buselmeier, T. J., Michael, A. F., and Vernier, R. L., Successful renal transplantation in 3 children with congenital nephrotic syndrome. *Lancet* **i**, 1410–1412 (1973).
195. Sorensen, L. B., Suppression of the shunt pathway in primary gout by azathioprine. *Proc. Natl. Acad. Sci. USA* **55**, 571–575 (1966).
196. Flatmark, A. L., Hovig, T., Myhre, E., and Gjone, E., Renal transplantation in patients with familial lecithin:cholesterol-acyltransferase deficiency. *Transplant. Proc.* **9**, 1665–1669 (1977).
197. Deodhar, S. D., Tung, K. S. K., Zuhlke, V., and Nakamoto, S., Renal homotransplantation in a patient with primary familial oxalosis. *Arch. Pathol.* **87**, 118–124 (1969).
198. Mahoney, C. P., Striker, G. E., Fetterman, G. H., Hickman, R. O., Schneider, J., and Marchioro, T. L., Renal transplantation in childhood cystinosis: Effects of the metabolic disease and renal allografts on each other. In *Enzyme Therapy in Genetic Diseases,* Desnick, R. J., Bernlohr, R. W., and Krivit, W., Eds., Williams and Wilkins, Baltimore, MD, 1973, pp 141–148.
199. Desnick, R. J., Simmons, R. L., Allen, K. Y., Najarian, J. S., and Krivit, W., Fabry's disease: Correction of enzymatic deficiencies by renal transplantation. *Surgery* **72**, 203–210 (1972).
200. Philippart, M., Franklin, S. S., and Gordon, A., Reversal of an inborn sphingolipidosis (Fabry's disease) by kidney transplantation. *Ann. Intern. Med.* **77**, 195–200 (1972).
201. Desnick, R. J., Allen, K. Y., Simmons, R. L., Woods, J. E., Anderson, C. F., Najarian, J. S., and Krivit, W., Fabry disease: Correction of the enzymatic deficiency by renal transplantation. In *Enzyme Therapy in Genetic Disease* (see ref. *198*), pp 88–96.
202. Jacky, E., Fabrysche Erkrankung (Angiokeratoma corporis diffusum universale): Gunstiger Verlauf nach Nierentransplantation. *Schweiz. Med. Wochenschr.* **106**, 703–709 (1976).
203. Clarke, J. T. R., Guttmann, R. D., Wolfe, L. S., Beaudoin, J. G., and Morehouse, D. D., Enzyme replacement by renal allotransplantation in Fabry's disease. *N. Engl. J. Med.* **287**, 1215–1218 (1972).
204. Spense, M. W., Mackinnon, K. E., Burgess, J. K., d'Entremont, D. M., Belitsky, P., Lannon, S. G., and MacDonald, A. S., Failure to correct the metabolic defect by renal allotransplantation in Fabry's disease. *Ann. Intern. Med.* **84**, 13–20 (1976).
205. Grunfeld, J. P., LePorrier, M., Droz, D., Bensaude, I., Hinglais, N., and Crosnier, J., La transplantation renale chez les sujets atteints de maladie de Fabry. *Nouv. Presse. Med.* **4**, 2081–2086 (1975).

206. Gibbs, D. A., Spellacy, E., Roberts, A. E., and Watts, R. W. E., The treatment of lysosomal storage diseases by fibroblast transplantation: Some preliminary observations. In ref. *1,* pp 457–474.
207. Dean, M. F., Muir, H., Benson, P. F., Button, L. R., Boylston, A., and Mowbray, J., Enzyme replacement by fibroblast transplantation in a case of Hunter disease. *Nature* **261,** 323–325 (1976).
208. Dean, M. F., Stevens, R. L., Muir, H., Benson, P. F., Button, L. R., Anderson, R. L., Boylston, A., and Mowbray, J., Enzyme replacement therapy by fibroblast transplantation. *J. Clin. Invest.* **63,** 138–145 (1979).
209. Dean, M. F., Muir, H., Benson, P., and Button, L., Enzyme replacement in the mucopolysaccharidoses by fibroblast transplantation. In ref. *1,* pp 445–456.
210. Dean, M. F., Muir, H., Benson, P. F., and Button, L. R., Enzyme replacement therapy by transplantation of HLA-compatible fibroblasts in Sanfilippo A syndrome. *Pediatr. Res.* **15,** 959–963 (1981).
211. Willner, J. P., Matalon, R., Beratis, N., Ritch, R., Rose, J., Hirschhorn, K., and Desnick, R. J., Failure of fibroblast allograft for enzyme replacement in mucopolysaccharidosis Type VI. *Pediatr. Res.* **12,** 459–464 (1978).
212. Barton, R. W., and Neufeld, E. F., The Hurler corrective factor. *J. Biol. Chem.* **246,** 7773–7779 (1971).
213. Cantz, M., Chrambach, A., Bach, G., and Neufeld, E. F., The Hunter corrective factor. *J. Biol. Chem.* **247,** 5456–5462 (1972).
214. Kresse, H., and Neufeld, E. F., The Sanfilippo A corrective factor. *J. Biol. Chem.* **247,** 2164–2170 (1972).
215. Gibbs, D. A., Fibroblast transplantation in lysosomal storage diseases. In ref. *4,* pp 95–108.
216. Haskins, M. E., Jezyk, P. F., Desnick, R. J., McDonough, S. K., and Patterson, D. F., Alpha-L-iduronidase deficiency in a cat: A model of mucopolysaccharidosis I. *Pediatr. Res.* **13,** 1294–1297 (1979).
217. Jezek, P. F., Haskins, M. E., Patterson, D. F., Mellman, W. J., and Greenstein, M., Mucopolysaccharidosis in a cat with arylsulfatase B deficiency: A model of Maroteaux–Lamy syndrome. *Science* **198,** 834–840 (1977).
218. Haskins, M. E., Jezyk, P. F., Desnick, R. J., McDonough, S. K., and Patterson, D. F., Mucopolysaccharidosis in a domestic shorthaired cat—a disease distinct from that seen in the Siamese cat. *J. Am. Vet. Med. Assoc.* **175,** 384–387 (1979).
219. Hirschhorn, R., and Martin, D. W., Jr., Enzyme defects in immunodeficiency diseases. *Springer Sem. Immunopathol.* **1,** 299–320 (1978).
220. Yulish, B. S., Stern, R. C., and Polmar, S. H., Partial resolution of bone lesions. A child with severe combined immunodeficiency

disease and adenosine deaminase deficiency after enzyme-replacement therapy. *Am. J. Dis. Child.* **134,** 61–63 (1980).
221. Staal, G. E. J., Stoop, J. W., Zegers, B. J. M., Siegenbeek van Heukelom, L. H., van der Vlist, M. J. M., Wadman, S. K., and Martin, D. W., Erythrocyte metabolism in purine nucleoside phosphorylase deficiency after enzyme replacement therapy by infusion of erythrocytes. *J. Clin. Invest.* **65,** 103–108 (1980).
222. Neufeld, E. F., and Fratantoni, J. C., Inborn errors of mucopolysaccharide metabolism. *Science* **169,** 141–146 (1970).
223. Porter, M. T., Fluharty, A. L., and Kihara, H., Correction of abnormal cerebroside sulfate metabolism in cultured metachromatic leukodystrophy fibroblasts. *Science* **172,** 1263–1265 (1971).
224. O'Brien, J. S., Miller, A. L., Loverde, A. W., and Veath, M. L., Sanfilippo disease type B: Enzyme replacement and metabolic correction in cultured fibroblasts. *Science* **181,** 753–755 (1973).
225. Lagunoff, D., Nicol, D. M., and Pritzl, P., Uptake of β-glucuronidase by deficient human fibroblasts. *Lab. Invest.* **29,** 449–453 (1973).
226. Dawson, G., Matalon, R., and Li, Y. T., Correction of the enzymatic defect in cultured fibroblasts from patients with Fabry's disease: Treatment with purified α-galactosidase from ficin. *Pediatr. Res.* **7,** 684–690 (1973).
227. Cantz, M., and Kresse, H., Sandhoff's disease: Defective glycosaminoglycan catabolism in cultured fibroblasts and its correction by β-N-acetylhexosaminidase. *Eur. J. Biochem.* **47,** 581–590 (1974).
228. Thorpe, S. R., Fiddler, M. B., and Desnick, R. J., Enzyme therapy IV: A method for determining the *in vivo* fate of bovine β-glucuronidase in β-glucuronidase-deficient mice. *Biochem. Biophys. Res. Commun.* **61,** 1464–1470 (1974).
229. Johnson, W. G., Desnick, R. J., Long, D. M., Sharp, H. L., Krivit, W., Brady, B., and Brady, R. O., Intravenous injection of purified hexosaminidase A into a patient with Tay–Sachs. In *Enzyme Therapy in Genetic Diseases* (see ref. *198*), pp 120–124.
230. De Barsy, Th., Jacquemin, P., Van Hoof, F., Hers, H. G., Enzyme replacement in Pompe's disease: An attempt with purified human α-glucosidase. *Ibid.,* pp 184–190.
231. Brady, R. O., Tallman, J. F., Johnson, W. G., Gal, A. E., Leahy, W. R., Quirk, J. M., and Dekaban, A. S., Replacement therapy for inherited enzyme deficiency. *N. Engl. J. Med.* **289,** 9–14 (1973).
232. Brady, R. O., Pentchev, P. G., Gal, A. E., Hibbert, S. R., and Dekaban, A. S., Replacement therapy for inherited enzymatic deficiency. *N. Engl. J. Med.* **291,** 989–993 (1974).
233. Beutler, E., Dale, G. L., Guinto, E., and Kuhl, W., Enzyme replacement therapy in Gaucher's disease: Preliminary clinical trial of a

new enzyme preparation. *Proc. Natl. Acad. Sci. USA* **74,** 4620–4623 (1977).
234. von Specht, B. U., Geiger, G., Arnon, R., Passwell, J., Keren, G., Goldman, B., and Padeh, B., Enzyme replacement in Tay–Sachs disease. *Neurology* **29,** 858–864 (1979).
235. Ashwell, G., and Morell, A. G., The role of surface carbohydrate in the hepatic recognition of circulating glycoproteins. *Adv. Enzymol.* **41,** 99–128 (1974).
236. Brown, T. L., Henderson, L. A., Thorpe, S. R., and Baynes, J. W., The effect of α-mannose terminal oligosaccharides on the survival of glycoproteins in the circulation. *Arch. Biochem. Biophys.* **188,** 418–428 (1978).
237. Stahl, P., Six, H., Rodman, J. S., Schlesinger, P. H., Tulsiani, D. R. P., and Touster, O., Evidence for specific recognition sites of mediated clearance of lysosomal enzymes *in vivo. Proc. Natl. Acad. Sci. USA* **73,** 4045–4059 (1976).
238. Stahl, P., Rodman, J. S., Doebber, T., Miller, M. J., and Schlesinger, P., Specific recognition and uptake of lysosomal enzymes and modified glycoproteins by rat tissue. In *Protein Turnover and Lysosomal Function,* Segal, H. L., and Doyle, D. J., Eds., Academic Press, New York, NY, 1978, pp 479–496.
239. Stahl, P., Rodman, J. S., Miller, M. J., and Schlesinger, P. H., Evidence for receptor-mediated binding of glycoproteins, glycoconjugates, and lysosomal glycosidases by alveolar macrophages. *Proc. Natl. Acad. Sci. USA* **75,** 1399–1403 (1978).
240. Hudgin, R. L., Pricer, W. F., Ashwell, G. L., Stockert, F. J., and Morell, A. G., The isolation and properties of a rabbit liver binding protein specific for asialoglycoproteins. *J. Biol. Chem.* **249,** 5536–5543 (1974).
241. Morell, A. G., Gregoriadis, G., Schlenberg, F. H., Hickman, J., and Ashwell, G., The role of sialic acid in determining the survival of glycoproteins in the circulation. *J. Biol. Chem.* **246,** 1461–1467 (1971).
242. Stahl, P., Rodman, J. S., and Schlesinger, P., Clearance of lysosomal hydrolases following intravenous infusion. *Arch. Biochem. Biophys.* **177,** 594–605 (1978).
243. Brown, M. S., and Goldstein, J. L., Receptor-mediated control of cholesterol metabolism. *Science* **191,** 150–151 (1976).
244. Goldstein, J. L., and Brown, M. S., The LDL-pathway in human fibroblasts: A receptor-mediated mechanism for the regulation of cholesterol metabolism. *Curr. Topics Cell. Reg.* **11,** 147–170 (1976).
245. Youngdahl-Turner, P., Allen, R. H., and Rosenberg, L. E., Binding and uptake of transcobalamin II by human fibroblasts. *J. Clin. Invest.* **61,** 133–141 (1978).

246. Neufeld, E. F., The uptake of enzymes into lysosomes: An overview. In ref. *1*, pp 77–84.
247. Wold, R., Enzyme recognition and modification. *Ibid.*, pp 129–139.
248. Gregoriadis, B., Targeting of drugs: Implications in medicine. *Lancet* **ii**, 241–247 (1981).
249. Lee, Y. C., Stowell, C. P., and Krantz, M. J., 2-Imino-2-methoxyethyl-1-thioglycosides: New reagents for attaching sugars to proteins. *Biochemistry* **15**, 3956–3960 (1976).
250. Krantz, M. J., Holtzman, N. A., Stowell, C. P., and Lee, Y. C., Attachment of thioglycosides to proteins: Enhancement of liver membrane binding. *Biochemistry* **15**, 3963–3967 (1976).
251. Marsh, J. W., Denis, J., and Wriston, J. C., Jr., Glycosylation of *Escherichia coli* L-asparaginase. *J. Biol. Chem.* **252**, 7678–7684 (1977).
252. Sando, G. N., Synthetic inhibitors of receptor-mediated endocytosis of a lysosomal enzyme by cultured fibroblasts. *Fed. Proc.* **37**, 1502–1512 (1978).
253. Wilson, G., Effect of reductive lactose amination on the hepatic uptake of bovine pancreatic ribonuclease A dimer. *J. Biol. Chem.* **253**, 2070–2077 (1978).
254. DeWaard, A., Hickman, S., and Kornfeld, S., Isolation and properties of β-galactoside binding lectins of calf heart and lung. *J. Biol. Chem.* **251**, 7581–7590 (1976).
255. Stahl, P., Schlesinger, P. H., Rodman, J. S., and Doebber, T., Recognition of lysosomal glycosidases *in vivo* inhibited by modified glycoproteins. *Nature* **264**, 86–88 (1976).
256. Achord, D. T., Brot, F. E., and Sly, W. S., Inhibition of the rat clearance system for agalacto-orosomucoid by yeast mannans and mannose. *Biochem. Biophys. Res. Commun.* **77**, 409–415 (1977).
257. Glaser, J. H., Roozen, K. L., Brot, F. E., and Sly, W. S., Multiple isoelectric and recognition forms of human β-glucuronidase activity. *Arch. Biochem. Biophys.* **166**, 536–542 (1975).
258. Furbish, S. F., Steer, C. J., Barringer, J. A., Jones, E. A., and Brady, R. O., The uptake of native and desialylated glucocerebrosidase by rat hepatocytes and Kupffer cells. *Biochem. Biophys. Res. Commun.* **81**, 1047–1053 (1978).
259. Rattazzi, M. C., McCullough, R. A., Downing, C. J., and Kung, M.-P., Towards enzyme therapy in GM_2 gangliosidosis: β-Hexosaminidase infusion in normal cats. *Pediatr. Res.* **13**, 916–922 (1979).
260. Rattazzi, M. C., Baker, H. J., Cork, L. C., Cox, N. R., Lanse, S. B., McCullough, R. A., and Munnell, J. F., The domestic cat as a model for human GM_2 gangliosidosis: Pathogenetic and therapeutic aspects. In *Models for the Study of Inborn Errors of Metabolism*, Hommes, F. A., Ed., American Elsevier, Amsterdam, 1979, p 57.

261. Schlesinger, P., Rodman, J. S., Frey, M., Lang, S., and Stahl, P., Clearance of lysosomal hydrolases following intravenous infusion. *Arch. Biochem. Biophys.* **177,** 606–614 (1976).
262. Fiddler, M. B., and Desnick, R. J., Enzyme therapy: Differential *in vivo* retention of bovine hepatic, renal and splenic β-glucuronidases and evidence for enzyme stabilization by intermolecular exchange. *Arch. Biochem. Biophys.* **179,** 397–408 (1977).
263. Gregoriadis, G., and Ryman, B. E., Liposomes as carriers of enzymes or drugs: A new approach to the treatment of storage diseases. *Biochem. J.* **124,** 58P–63P (1971).
264. Weissman, G., Bloomgarden, D., Kaplan, R., Cohen, C., Hoffstein, S., Collins, T., Gotlieb, A., and Nagle, D., A general method for the introduction of enzymes, by means of immunoglobulin-coated liposomes into lysosomes of deficient cells. *Proc. Natl. Acad. Sci. USA* **72,** 88–92 (1975).
265. Steger, L. D., and Desnick, R. J., Enzyme therapy VI: Comparative *in vivo* fates and effects on lysosomal integrity of enzyme entrapped in negatively and positively charged liposome. *Biochim. Biophys. Acta* **464,** 530–546 (1977).
266. Thorpe, S. R., Fiddler, M. B., and Desnick, R. J., Enzyme therapy V: *In vivo* fate of erythrocyte-entrapped β-glucuronidase in β-glucuronidase-deficient mice. *Pediatr. Res.* **9,** 918–923 (1975).
267. Ihler, G. M., Glew, R. H., and Schnure, F. W., Enzyme loading of erythrocytes. *Proc. Natl. Acad. Sci. USA* **70,** 2663–2668 (1973).
268. Baker, R. F., Entry of ferritin into human red cells during hypotonic haemolysis. *Nature* **215,** 424–426 (1967).
269. Dale, G. L., Villacorte, D. F., and Beutler, E., High-yield entrapment of proteins into erythrocytes. *Biochem. Med.* **18,** 220–225 (1977).
270. Fiddler, M. B., Hudson, L. D. S., White, J. G., and Desnick, R. J., Enzyme therapy XIV: Comparison of methods for enzyme entrapment in human erythrocytes. *J. Lab. Clin. Med.* **88,** 307–318 (1980).
271. Desnick, R. J., Fiddler, M. B., Thorpe, S. R., and Steger, L. D., Enzyme entrapment in erythrocytes and liposomes for the treatment of lysosomal storage diseases. In *Biomedical Applications of Immobilized Enzymes and Proteins,* Chang, T. M. S., Ed., Academic Press, New York, NY, 1977, pp 227–244.
272. Hudson, L. D. S., Fiddler, M. B., and Desnick, R. J., Enzyme therapy X: Immune response induced by enzyme-and buffer-loaded liposomes in C3H/HeJ *Gus*[h] mice. *J. Pharmacol. Exp. Ther.* **208,** 507–514 (1979).
273. van Rooijen, N., and van Nieuwmegen, R., Liposomes in immunology: The immune response against antigen-containing liposomes. *Immunol. Commun.* **6,** 489–498 (1977).

274. van Rooijen, N., and van Nieuwmegen, R., Liposomes in immunology: Impairment of the adjuvant effects of liposomes by incorporation of the adjuvant lysolecithin and the role of macrophages. *Immunol. Commun.* **8**, 381–396 (1979).
275. Cunningham, C. M., Kingzette, M., Richards, R. L., Alving, C. R., Lint, T. F., and Gewurz, H. J., Activation of human complement by liposomes: A model for membrane activation of the alternative pathway. *Immunology* **122**, 1237–1242 (1979).
276. Finkelstein, M. C., and Weismann, G., Enzyme replacement via liposomes. Variations in lipid composition determine liposomal integrity in biological fluids. *Biochim. Biophys. Acta* **587**, 202–216 (1979).
277. Fiddler, M. B., Hudson, L. D. S., and Desnick, R. J., Enzyme therapy VIII: Immunologic evaluation of repeated administration of erythrocyte-entrapped β-glucuronidase to β-glucuronidase-deficient mice. *Biochem. J.* **168**, 141–145 (1977).
278. Jancik, J. M., Schquer, R., Andres, K. H., and von During, M., Sequestration of neuraminidase-treated erythrocytes. *Cell Tiss. Res.* **186**, 209–226 (1978).
279. Jacob, H. S., and Jandl, J. H., Effects of sulfhydryl inhibition on red blood cells II. Studies *in vivo*. *J. Clin. Invest.* **41**, 1514–1520 (1962).
280. Durocher, J. R., Payne, R. C., and Conrad, M. E., Role of sialic acid in erythrocyte survival. *Blood* **45**, 11–16 (1975).
281. Seaman, G. V. F., and Uhlenbruck, G., The surface structure of erythrocytes from some animal sources. *Arch. Biochem. Biophys.* **100**, 493–501 (1963).
282. De Loach, J., Peters, S., Pinkard, I., Glew, R., and Ihler, G., Effect of glutaraldehyde treatment on enzyme-loaded erythrocytes. *Biochim. Biophys. Acta* **496**, 136–145 (1977).
283. Weed, R. I., La Celle, P. L., and Merrill, E. W., Metabolic dependence on red cell deformability. *J. Clin. Invest.* **48**, 795–800 (1969).
284. Barringer, J. A., Rappoport, S. I., and Brady, R. O., Access of enzymes to brain following osmotic alteration of the blood–brain barrier. In ref. *1*, pp 195–205.
285. Rattazzi, M. C., Lanse, S. B., McCullough, R. A., Nester, J. A., and Jacobs, E. A., Towards enzyme replacement in GM_2 gangliosidosis: Organ deposition and induced central nervous system uptake of human β-hexosaminidase in the cat. *Ibid.,* pp 179–193.
286. Rattazzi, M. C., Appel, A. M., and Nester, J. A., Towards enzyme therapy in GM_2 gangliosidosis: Visceral organ and CNS uptake of human β-hexosaminidase in normal cats. *Am. J. Hum. Genet.* **30**, 59A (1979).
287. Kusiak, J. W., Toney, J. H., Quirk, J. M., and Brady, R. O., Specific

binding of ^{125}I-labeled β-hexosaminidase A to rat brain synaptosomes. *Proc. Natl. Acad. Sci. USA* **76,** 982–985 (1979).

288. Desnick, R. J., Dean, K. J., Grabowski, G. A., Bishop, D. F., and Sweeley, C. C., Enzyme therapy in Fabry disease: Differential *in vivo* plasma clearance and metabolic effectiveness of plasma and splenic α-galactosidase. *Proc. Natl. Acad. Sci. USA* **76,** 5326–5330 (1979).

289. Williams, J. C., and Murray, A. K., Enzyme replacement in Pompe disease with an α-glucosidase low density lipoprotein complex. In ref. *1,* pp 415–423.

290. Tyrell, D. A., Ryman, B. E., Kieton, B. R., and Dubovitz, V., Use of liposomes in treating type II glycogenosis. *Br. Med. J.* **12,** 88 (1976).

291. Belchetz, P. E., Braidman, I. P., Crawley, J. C. W., and Gregoriadis, G., Treatment of Gaucher's disease with liposome-entrapped glucocerebroside:β-glucosidase. *Lancet* **ii,** 116–117 (1977).

292. Bishop, D. F., and Desnick, R. J., Affinity purification of α-galactosidase A from human spleen, placenta and plasma with elimination of pyrogen contamination. Properties of the purified splenic enzyme and comparison to other forms. *J. Biol. Chem.* **256,** 1307–1316 (1981).

293. Desnick, R. J., Dean, K. J., Grabowski, G. A., Bishop, D. F., and Sweeley, C. C., Enzyme therapy XVII: Metabolic and immunologic evaluation of α-galactosidase A replacement in Fabry disease. In ref. *1,* pp 393–414.

294. Gregoriadis, G., Weereratne, H., Blair, H., and Bull, G. M., Liposomes in Gaucher type 1 disease: Use in enzyme therapy and the creation of an animal model. In *Gaucher Disease: A Century of Delineation and Research,* Desnick, R. J., Gatt, S., and Grabowski, G. A., Eds., Alan R. Liss, Inc., New York, NY, 1982, pp 681–701.

295. Gregoriadis, G., Neerunjun, D., Meade, T. W., Goolamali, S. K., Weereratne, H., and Bull, G., Experiences after long-term treatment of a type I Gaucher disease patient with liposome entrapped glucocerebrosidase:β-glucosidase. In ref. *1,* pp 383–392.

296. Beutler, E. L., Dale, G. L., and Kuhl, W., Replacement therapy in Gaucher disease. *Ibid.,* pp 369–381.

297. Desnick, R. J., Patterson, D. F., and Scarpelli, D. G., Eds., *Animal Models of Inherited Metabolic Diseases,* Alan R. Liss, Inc., New York, NY, 1982, 519 pp.

298. Brady, R. O., Barringer, J. A., Furbish, F. S., Stowens, D. W., and Ginns, E. I., Prospects for enzyme replacement therapy in Gaucher disease. In *Gaucher Disease: A Century of Delineation and Research* (see ref. *294*), pp 669–680.

299. Lamourous, A., Faucon Biguet, N., Samolyk, D., Privat, A., Salo-

mon, J. C., Pujol, J. F., and Mallet, J., Identification of cDNA clones coding for rat tyrosine hydroxylase antigen. *Proc. Natl. Acad. Sci. USA* **79,** 3881–3885 (1982).
300. Wu, T.-S., Bock, H.-G. O., O'Brien, W. E., and Beaudet, A. L., Cloning of cDNA for argininosuccinate synthetase mRNA and study of enzyme overproduction in a human cell line. *J. Biol. Chem.* **256,** 11826–11831 (1981).
301. Wetzel, R., Heyneker, H. L., Goeddel, D. V., Jhurani, P., Shapiro, J., Crea, R., Low, T. L. K., McClure, J. E., Thurman, G. B., and Goldstein, A. L., Production of biologically active N^α-desacetylthymosin α_1 in *Escherichia coli* through expression of a chemically synthesized gene. *Biochemistry* **19,** 6096–6104 (1980).
302. Nagata, S., Taira, H., Hall, A., Johnrud, L., Streuli, M., Escodi, J., Boll, W., Cantell, K., and Weissman, C., Synthesis in *E. coli* of a polypeptide with human leukocyte interferon activity. *Nature* **284,** 316–318 (1980).
303. Bank, A., Mears, J. G., and Ramirez, F., Disorders of human hemoglobin. *Science* **207,** 486–492 (1980).
304. Ramirez, F., Mears, J. G., Nudel, U., Bank, A., Luzzatto, L., DiPrisco, G., D'Avino, R., Pepe, G., Camardella, L., Gambino, R., Cimino, R., and Quattrin, N., Defects in DNA and globin messenger RNA in homozygotes for hemoglobin Lepore. *J. Clin. Invest.* **63,** 736–742 (1979).
305. Persico, M. G., Toniolo, D., Nobile, C., D'Urso, M., and Luzzatto, L., cDNA sequences of human glucose-6-phosphate dehydrogenase cloned in pBR322. *Nature* **294,** 778–780 (1981).
306. Parnes, J. R., Velan, B., Felsenfeld, A., Ramanathan, L., Ferrini, U., Appella, E., and Seidman, J. G., Mouse β_2-microglobulin cDNA clones: A screening procedure for cDNA clones corresponding to rare mRNAs. *Proc. Natl. Acad. Sci. USA* **78,** 2253–2257 (1981).
307. Jolly, D. J., Esty, A. C., Bernard, H. U., and Friedmann, T., Isolation of a genomic clone partially encoding human hypoxanthine phosphoribosyltransferase. *Proc. Natl. Acad. Sci. USA* **79,** 5038–5041 (1982).
308. Gusella, J. F., Keys, C., Varsanyi-Breiner, A., Kao F.-T., Jones, C., Puck, T. T., and Houseman, D., Isolation and localization of DNA segments from specific human chromosomes. *Proc. Natl. Acad. Sci. USA* **77,** 2829–2833 (1980).
309. Kao, F.-T., Hartz, J. A., Law, M. L., and Davidson, J. N., Isolation and chromosomal localization of unique DNA sequences from a human genomic library. *Proc. Natl. Acad. Sci. USA* **79,** 865–869 (1982).
310. Itakura, K., Hirose, T., Crea, R., Riggs, A. D., Heyneker, H. L., Bolivar, F., and Boyer, H. W., Expression in *Escherichia coli* of a

chemically synthesized gene for the hormone somatostatin. *Science* **198**, 1056–1063 (1977).

311. Martial, J. A., Hallewall, R. A., Baxter, J. D., and Goodman, H. M., Human growth hormone: Complementary DNA cloning and expression in bacteria. *Science* **205**, 602–606 (1979).
312. Khorana, H. G., Total synthesis of a gene. *Science* **203**, 614 (1979).
313. Goeddel, D. V., Kleid, D. G., Bolivar, F., Heyneker, H. L., Yansura, D. G., Crea, R., Hirose, T., Kraszewski, A., Itakura, K., and Riggs, A. D., Expression in *Escherichia coli* of chemically synthesized genes for human insulin. *Proc. Natl. Acad. Sci. USA* **76**, 106–110 (1979).
314. Wallace, R. B., Johnson, M. J., Hirose, T., Miyake, T., Kawashima, E. H., and Itakura, K., The use of synthetic oligonucleotides as hybridization probes. II. Hybridization of oligonucleotides of mixed sequence to rabbit β-globin DNA. *Nucleic Acids Res.* **9**, 879–894 (1981).
315. Stetler, D., Das, H., Nunberg, J. H., Saiki, R., Sheng-Dong, R., Mullis, K. B., Weissman, S. M., and Erlich, H. A., Isolation of a cDNA clone for the human HLA-DR antigen α chain by using a synthetic oligonucleotide as a hybridization probe. *Proc. Natl. Acad. Sci. USA* **79**, 5966–5970 (1982).
316 Noyes, B. E., Mevarech, M., Stein, P., and Agarhal, K. L., Detection and partial sequence analysis of gastrin mRNA by using an oligonucleotide probe. *Proc. Natl. Acad. Sci. USA* **76**, 1770–1774 (1979).
317. Hudson, P., Haley, J., Cronk, M., Shine, J., and Niall, H., Molecular cloning and characterization of cDNA sequences coding for rat relaxin. *Nature* **291**, 127–131 (1981).
318. Suggs, S., Wallace, R. B., Hirose, R., Kawashima, E. H., and Itakura, K., Use of synthetic oligonucleotides as hybridization probes: Isolation of cloned cDNA sequences for human β_2-microglobulin. *Proc. Natl. Acad. Sci. USA* **78**, 6613–6617 (1981).
319. Goedell, D. V., Heyneker, H. L., Hozumi, T., Arentzen, R., Itakura, K., Yansura, D. G., Ross, M. J., Miozzari, G., Greg, R., and Seeburg, P. H., Direct expression in *Escherichia coli* of a DNA sequence coding for human growth hormone. *Nature* **281**, 544–548 (1979).
320. Pavlakis, G. N., Hizuka, N., Gorden, P., Seeburg, P., and Hamer, D. H., Expression of two human growth hormone genes in monkey cells infected by simian virus 40 recombinants. *Proc. Natl. Acad. Sci. USA* **78**, 7398–7402 (1981).
321. Lomedico, P. T., Use of recombinant DNA technology to program eukaryotic cells to synthesize rat proinsulin: A rapid expression assay for cloned genes. *Proc. Natl. Acad. Sci. USA* **79**, 5798–5802 (1982).

322. Frenkel, N., and Spaetz, R., The herpes simplex virus amplicon: A new eukaryotic defective-virus cloning-amplifying vector. *Cell* **30**, 295–304 (1982).
323. Hitzeman, R. A., Hagie, F. E., Levine, H. L., Goeddel, D. V., Ammerer, G., and Hall, B. D., Expression of a human gene for interferon in yeast. *Nature* **293**, 717–722 (1981).
324. Hintz, R. L., Wilson, D. M., Finno, J., Rosenfeld, R. G., Bennett, A., McClellan, B., and Swift, R., Biosynthetic methionyl human growth hormone is biologically active in adult man. *Lancet* **ii**, 1276–1279 (1982).
325. Graham, F. L., and van der Eb, A. J., A new technique for the assay of infectivity of human adenovirus 5 DNA. *Virology* **52**, 456–457 (1973).
326. Wigler, M., Pellicer, A., Silverstein, S., and Axel, R., Biochemical transfer of single-copy eukaryotic genes using total cellular DNA as donor. *Cell* **14**, 725–731 (1978).
327. Wigler, M., Pellicer, A., Silverstein, S., Axel, R., Urlaub, G., and Chasin, L., DNA-mediated transfer of the adenine phosphoribosyl transferase locus into mammalian cells. *Proc. Natl. Acad. Sci. USA* **76**, 1373–1376 (1979).
328. Wigler, M., Perucho, M., Kurtz, D., Dana, S., Pellicer, A., Axel, R., and Silverstein, S., Transformation of mammalian cells with an amplifiable dominant-acting gene. *Proc. Natl. Acad. Sci. USA* **77**, 3567–3570 (1980).
329. Mercola, K. E., Stang, H. D., Browne, J., Salser, W., and Cline, M. J., Insertion of a new gene of viral origin into bone marrow cells of mice. *Science* **208**, 1033–1036 (1980).
330. Cline, M. J., Stang, H., Mercola, K., Morse, L., Ruprecht, R., Browne, J., and Salser, W., Gene transfer in intact animals. *Nature* **284**, 422–427 (1980).
331. Stewart, T. A., Wagner, E. F., and Mintz, B., Human β-globin gene sequences injected into mouse eggs, retained in adults, and transmitted to progeny. *Science* **217**, 1046–1048 (1982).
332. Gordon, J. W., and Ruddle, F. H., Integration and stable germ line transmission of genes injected into mouse pronuclei. *Science* **214**, 1244–1246 (1981).
333. Wagner, T. E., Hoppe, P. C., Jollick, J. D., Scholl, D. R., Hodinka, R. L., and Gault, J. B., Microinjection of a rabbit β-globin gene into zygotes and its subsequent expression in adult mice and their offspring. *Proc. Natl. Acad. Sci. USA* **78**, 6376–6380 (1981).
334. Spradling, A. C., and Rubin, G. M., Transposition of cloned P elements into *Drosophila* germ line chromosomes. *Science* **218**, 341–347 (1982).

335. Rubin, G. M., and Spradling, A. C., Genetic transformation of *Drosophila* with transposable element vectors. *Science* **218,** 348–353 (1982).

Discussion

Q: You said that there were dull cats and smart cats. I would be interested in knowing how you determined feline intelligence. Is there an IQ test for cats?

DR. DESNICK: First of all, these are spontaneous, naturally naturing mutations and the animals, the probands, were picked up by very astute veterinary clinicians. The University of Pennsylvania has an inborn error lab and a division of veterinary genetics interested in animal models. They have collaborated with us over the last several years and together we've worked out the defects in these two feline models. The reason we say that one is smart and one is dull is that one has Hurler's syndrome, which involves neuronal deposition of the substrate, whereas the other has mucopolysaccharidosis Type VI, which doesn't.

Whether there is such a thing as an IQ test for cats, I don't know. I rely on my veterinary colleagues to tell me about cat intelligence.

Q: When you've got a two-week-old patient suffering from isovaleric acidemia, how would some of the newer technology be helpful?

DR. DESNICK: Protein restriction and the proper kinds of metabolic manipulation are appropriate for a patient suffering from that disease. The important thing is to make the diagnosis quickly. Because that disease happens to have an unusual odor, you can pick it up pretty quickly.

Q: You seem to have abandoned efforts to send enzymes across the blood–brain barrier. Is anyone working on that sort of project?

DR. DESNICK: Yes, at least two groups are actively involved in trying to gain access to the blood–brain barrier. An investigator at Buffalo has a cat with Sandhoff's disease in which he is attempting, by air microembolism, to inject a small amount of oxygen, about 1 mL, which somehow alters the capillary junctions so that material can get across. He's had success in getting hexosaminidase across when administered through the carotid vessels. Another group at the NIH has attempted to do this in mice and in monkeys, where they administered enzyme in a similar way. Their approach is to use mannitol and other hyperosmotic solutions to alter the blood–brain barrier. The major problem with all these techniques is that, yes, you may be able to open the blood–brain barrier; you get about 1 or 2% of the enzyme you administer across into the brain; but you also put into the brain all kinds of other circulating proteins, without any idea as to their toxicity. Furthermore, to be successful, this process must be reversible; in other words, you have to be able to close the barrier securely after you open it. Finally, you have to be able to get an enzyme not only across the blood–brain barrier but also to the target site of pathology, which means you have to deliver it to the neuron. Researchers are just beginning to look at whether there are cell-specific receptors for neuronal uptake, and I think there's a lot to be studied in terms of neuron-specific uptake once you do the mechanics of opening the blood–brain barrier. Given all these problems, we concluded in our studies of Tay–Sachs that the best approaches to disorders of that sort are prevention, as Dr. Kaback discussed, and prenatal diagnosis.

Q: What are your objections to bone marrow transplantations for treatment of Hurler's disease in children in England?

Dr. Desnick: We're looking at bone marrow transplantation in the animal models because we can have one without and one with neuronal involvement. Also we can get two affected littermates and really do proper kinds of studies, where one littermate is treated, for example, with a bone marrow transplant and the other is not.

Dr. Kaback: What is your basis for believing that bone marrow transplantation will, in fact, benefit a neuron-source disease, based on all the evidence to the contrary?

Dr. Desnick: On the contrary, Michael. My hypothesis is that it won't work; but we want to be able to do the experiment. I really believe that we should do some of these crucial experiments in the animal systems first before we take an intriguing approach and go on to humans. Now, there are different thoughts on that issue, and for certain diseases I think that bone marrow transplantation might be useful. As Dr. Good will tell you, it's been done for a dozen different disorders in which they corrected the defect. As we learn how to get around the barriers of graft vs host and so forth, this is going to be a more intriguing approach. But I'm concerned about the neurologic diseases. We want to look at the animal models because there we can conclusively, rather than subjectively, show whether it is or is not an effective approach.

Q: Is this adequate therapy for Hurler's syndrome?

DR. DESNICK: I think in no way did those workers get adequate amounts of enzyme across. The best model suggesting that it won't work is probably a bovine mannosidosis, in which glycoprotein and oligosaccharides accumulate, with bony and neurologic manifestations. Bone marrow cells transfused from a twin had the effect of making the calf chimeric. Although there was depletion of the visceral substrate accumulation, there was no remarkable change in the neurological aspects of the disease.

DR. GOOD: I don't believe that bone marrow transplantation is likely to work on a disease that is basically a storage disease involving neurons themselves. But there is no question that we have been able to induce epithelial cell function by bone marrow transplantation of mesenchymally derived cells. We can do it in the thymus and we can do it in the liver; whether we can do it in the central nervous system must be addressed by experimentation. It isn't a matter of delivery of cells or delivery of enzymes. The question is, do the cells that are derived from the bone marrow have any effect on controlling enzyme function in neurons?

MEMBER OF THE AUDIENCE: Well, we've given HLA-matched leukocyte transfusions to children with storage disease of the central nervous system.

DR. GOOD: That's very different. HLA-matched cells don't have precursor cells. For example, you can't treat osteoporosis.

MEMBER OF THE AUDIENCE: Instead of getting enzymes into the gray marker molecules, perhaps you could open up the lysosomal membranes or exteriorize the lysosomes to release the marker molecules; that might be another effective therapeutic approach.

DR. DESNICK: How would you do that?

MEMBER OF THE AUDIENCE: One possibility is hyperbaric oxygen, which does seem to have a selective effect on membrane lysosomes. For example, in most burn patients who have been treated with hyperbaric oxygen, the immunologic sections of those cells seem to be depleted of lysosomes and still remain functional. This is why a few people, myself included, think that instead of trying to get enzymes into cells maybe we can get substrates out of them, but not necessarily by an enzymatic method. Do you have any thoughts?

Dr. Desnick: A group in England has been doing tissue culture studies with different lysosomal storage disease fibroblasts; they've added cytochalasin B to the culture medium and believe it may enhance excretion of the substrate. They conjecture that they are altering the cytoskeletal apparatus so as to extrude lysosomes, but the data were not clear. If you do that in vivo, you're pumping a terrific amount of this material into the circulation, which might simply be taken up elsewhere or might cause other toxic effects: indeed, you would wonder what is happening to the cytoskeletal apparatus of other cells. You may gain something in terms of substrate accumulation, but the toxicity of the therapeutic agent may be such that you do more damage than good. I understand the concept and I'm aware of this one approach, but I don't think it is a feasible one.

V

PROSPECTS

Progress in Bone Marrow Transplantation

Robert A. Good

We have begun to understand the immunological system in terms that permit some precision of manipulation and even control of its development. Although we've come a long way from the days when we knew nothing of the molecules, nothing of the cells, and even very little of the organs involved in immunity, we are really just at the beginning of the understanding that would permit us to utilize cellular engineering.

Development of the Immunological System

Both the hematopoietic system and the immunological system are in the process of constant development and renewal: this is one of the aspects that makes it possible for us to consider cellular engineering. A pluripotential stem cell can develop into lymphocyte precursors, which can develop into separate subpopulations: differentiation in these systems is going on constantly. The immunity system basically develops under the influence of microenvironments at various sites. The thymus is one site; an alternative site in birds is the thymus-like bursa of Fabricius; and, in all mammals, alternatives are probably the fetal liver and the bone marrow itself. The cells experience a kind of odyssey that takes them from the yolk sac to the fetal liver and the bone marrow; stem cells from the fetal liver or the bone marrow then emerge and come under the influence of the thymus. Stem cells are also influenced by the thymus in the pre-thymic and post-thymic stage. Similarly, the bursa of Fabricius is not the only site in birds where this development can occur, except at a certain stage in development. Thus in birds, by removing the thymus or the bursa, one can manipulate either the immunoglobulin-producing cells or the T-lymphocytes, the basis of cellular immunity. Moreover, both of these systems involve biological amplification systems to address the same fundamental effector mechanisms.

Thus far, we do not have much molecular biological understanding of what is going on in T-cell development. But we do know that there is a succession of steps and then a bifurcation of the pathway in both mice and humans, and this multiplicity and bifurcation give us a variety of different T-cells specialized for different functions.

In the scheme of B-cell development, extraordinary rearrangements of genetic material and even some added mutations take place between the pre-B-cell or the stem cell and the ultimate plasma cell and B-lymphocyte, which gives us the possibility of the miracle of immunology. As Sir Peter Medawar put it, "That miracle is that a rabbit, yet unborn, should be able to make antibody to an antigen not yet synthesized."

We now know that the immunity system is not just something for dealing with the external world, but is a highly modulated, highly controlled system that spends most of its energy talking to itself. But the immunological system also is highly modulated by external influences, especially the interaction of the three major networks of the body: the central nervous system, the endocrine network, and the immunological network, in interaction, are responsible for much of the modulation of immunity functions.

Now, in mice, our best teachers of immunology, we have learned that there is a sequence of development of the T-lymphocytes with this bifurcation and, moreover, that these lymphocytes have antigenic surface markers that define the stage of development. When the cells leave the thymus, they are more different from one another in terms of their surface markers than they were when developing in the thymus. Then subspecialization into helper cells, killer cells, or suppressor cells takes place. There is a specific phenotype, identifiable by surface antigens, for each of these functional stages. We consider these to be differentiation antigens that we can recognize and use to classify the subpopulations of the cells.

The use of monoclonal antibodies prepared by hybridoma technology against surface antigens on human thymocytes has led to the proposal of the following scheme for thymic development: early thymocytes, common thymocytes, bifurcation into subpopulations, and mature thymocytes that are specialized for helper-inductive function or cytotoxic and suppressor function.

The existence of these surface antigens as markers is great for the immunologists, but what are they doing for the cells themselves? With Dr. Robert Evans, we have developed our own series of monoclonal antibodies that can recognize all of the peripheral lymphocytes and a great majority of the thymocytes and these specialized subpopulations. With these antisera, particularly with their Fab fragments, that is, the combining end of the molecule, it's possible now to begin to analyze what these surface receptors are really doing.

The precursor T-cells and the effector T-cells with a helper inducer or suppressor function are recognizable by these highly specific monoclonal antibodies. So, we can interfere, for example, with the cytotoxicity of the T-lymphocytes—without complement and without destroying the cell—by using the anti-Leu 2a antisera, but not with the anti-Leu 1, the anti-Leu 3a, or anti-Leu 3b antisera. To a much lesser extent, we can also use anti-Leu 2b antisera to block cytotoxicity. This antiserum recognizes the same peptide recognized by anti-Leu 2a, but it reacts with an epitope on a marker peptide at the surface of the cell that is different from the epitope recognized by the anti-Leu 2a antisera. The complexity of differentiation just for the development of the B-lymphocytes and T-lymphocytes is the reason there can be many different forms of B-lymphoma and T-lymphoma. Each of these different lymphoid cancers represents a malignant deviation of one of the stages of development of the normal cells or represents one of the several subpopulations of the different lymphoid lineages that have undergone malignant transformation.

Other receptors on the B-lymphocytes include a receptor for a factor produced by T-cells, a B-cell growth factor; also, the B-cells have a receptor, the Ig molecule, that is distinct and separate for each specific antigen. In addition, there are many other surface antigens, whose function is not yet known. There is also an interesting antigenic site on the surface of B-lymphocytes such that, if you stimulate the cell by reacting an antiserum with this antigen, the cells are induced to proliferate. The stimulation of another surface receptor induces the B-cells to undergo terminal differentiation. With these new technologies, therefore, we've begun to get a handle on the controls that will permit expansion or terminal differentiation of the B-cell population; antisera against these receptors can induce either proliferation or terminal differentiation of the B-lymphocytes to plasma cells and to antibody-secreting cells. Many different receptors are on the surfaces of the lymphocytes and, although a beginning has been made, we are just beginning to understand the details of the molecular biology of the process of differentiation of B-lymphocytes and the essential chemistry involved in the interactions of the lymphoid cells.

Thymus Transplantation

The thymus, too, is being better understood. We have known for some time that the thymus is of importance around the time of birth and begins progressively to involute relatively early in life. By 15 to 20 years of age, the thymus has already begun its involution morphologically. This involution can now be quantified in terms of thymic hormone production. Both in humans and in mice the thymus is hormonally a major organ for only a short period of life.

When working with neonatally thymectomized mice, we got the idea that cellular engineering might be possible. Neonatally thymectomized mice raised in a conventional environment are very scruffy-looking little animals. They don't live very long. In the sea of microorganisms that is our world, they are very exposed, not only to bacteria but also to viruses and fungi. Raised in a germ-free environment, they may look better; transplanted with a new (syngeneic) thymus, they grow up looking entirely normal and are normal immunologically.

Further, if you inject the neonatally thymectomized mice with large numbers of differentiated lymphoid cells from an immunologically normal syngeneic animal or from donor animals matched with the thymectomized recipient according to the major histocompatibility locus, the animals develop a replicating, self-perpetuating immunological system that permits them to grow up with a relatively normal immunological system like the animals that have been treated with thymus transplants. Therefore, by cellular engineering, either with a thymus transplant, or with an adequate number of sufficiently mature T-cells, the mice can live a long life, free of autoimmunity and capable of resisting viruses, fungi, and bacteria in the environment. The trick here is to have the donor of the lymphoid cell matched with the recipient at the major histocompatibility locus.

A normal lymph node structure contains well-developed cortical areas, where the B-lymphocytes reside, and typical T-zones in the deep cortical regions or paracortical areas, which have an abundant lymphocytic population. These T-zones are almost completely lacking in lymphoid cells if neonatal thymectomy has been performed sufficiently early in life in certain strains of mice. However, they are reconstituted after a thymic transplant or after transplantation of "peripheral" spleen or lymph node cells.

But, it's not far from mice to men. One of the reasons I think mice and humans are so close immunologically and biochemically is that they are not really far apart phylogenetically. The tree shrews went our way and the ground shrews went on the way to development of mice. Thus, mice and men are close relatives, which is one thing that makes it possible for the mice to be such great and practical teachers of immunology for humans.

Consider humans with Di George's syndrome. These patients are born without a thymus. They have pretty well-developed paracortical areas in the lymph nodes. They make antibodies poorly, but they do make B-lymphocytes and plasma cells, and they do respond well by antibody production to thymus-independent antigens. They do not develop any of the T-cell-mediated immunities. But if you transplant a little wet membrane of embryonic thymus (thymus precursor), within six months they will fill up their deep cortical areas and develop a capacity for all forms of cell-mediated immunity. Often, if you have not waited too long before treating them, they will be fully reconstructed functionally simply by transplanting just a small membranous precursor of the thymus, which reconstitutes their cellular immunity and corrects the immunologic abnormality. This operation also reconstitutes them with respect to the ability to form circulating thymic hormones as well. We know this because we can now quantify several putative thymic hormones, and all increase from low to normal concentrations after transplantation of embryonic thymus in Di George's syndrome. This sustained correction of the cellular as well as the hormonal abnormalities in patients with Di George's syndrome represents the full correction of this inborn error of metabolism.

You can also make the same correction in mice that are born without a thymus or in mice that have been thymectomized. Transplanting a little membrane of epithelial tissue from the area where the thymus is about to develop—there are no lymphoid cells in such a transplant—under the renal capsule produces a well-developed thymus. The epithelium is still of donor origin, but the cells that develop in the thymus are of recipient origin. These procedures work best if the thymus donor has been matched with the recipient at the major histocompatibility locus. All of the functional and morphological aspects of the thymus develop nicely under these circumstances.

Bone Marrow Transplantation

Among patients born with six different genetically determined diseases, each of which represent inborn errors of metabolism called severe combined immunodeficiency (SCID), the thymus is entirely epithelial, without cortex and medullary development, with no Hassall's corpuscles. It's a tiny little organ and the concentrations of thymic hormone of these patients are very low. The T-cells have failed to develop in the spongy regions of the deep cortical areas of the node. There are often no cells as well in the denser stromal areas in the cortical region, where the B-cells like to be and where the germinal centers develop. The tonsils, instead of having big germinal centers and huge lymphoid and plasma cell accumulations like normal tonsils, may be completely lacking in lymphoid cells.

In 1968, after having figured out theoretically how to correct this deficiency by using stem cells from marrow and an HLA-matched sibling donor, we were able to treat a patient who was born with such a defect. This patient's family had had 12 deaths in three generations as a consequence of this disease—all males in this instance, which was an X-linked recessive form. Several autosomal recessive forms lead to a very similar disease. Because this patient had four sisters, we were able to use bone marrow from one of them that was quite well matched with the recipient at the major histocompatibility locus (it wasn't a perfect match, it was an A locus mismatch, but the C, B, D, and DR loci were matched). Drs. Richard Gatti and Dick Hong and I transplanted this patient with bone marrow from his best-matched sibling.

He was suffering from a lethal disease and we felt justified in trying this procedure even though the HLA match was not perfect. In fact, in this first instance, we completely corrected his immunological defects, but produced another disease, immunologically based aplastic anemia. We then treated this iatrogenic (caused by us) problem by another transplant from the same donor, switching the child's full hematopoietic system to that of the donor. This child, now more than 14 years after the transplant, is absolutely well in every way in which we can analyze him. He is immunologically normal. His hematopoietic system and his immunological system are both derived from his sister donor, the matched donor, because all of the cells in his bone marrow, or in his lymphoid system, or in his peripheral blood that can be induced to divide, are of female karyotype. So, he could qualify for the Olympics as a girl, but he's a strapping, vigorous, athletic male with normal immunological functions. His immunological functions were restored and his aplastic anemia cured by the first successful bone marrow transplant with a matched sibling donor.

This kind of corrective immunologic operation has now been done successfully approximately 100 times, by us as well as by others. The patients present to us perhaps at three to five months of age, often still weighing approximately birth weight. They are regularly infected with Candida or Pneumocystis or other organisms. Such children just can't live in the sea of microorganisms that occupy our ecological niche. Those infections must, if possible, be cleared up before there can be a bone marrow transplantation. Then it's like creating life: after treatment, with marrow from a matched sibling donor, these children are absolutely well, thriving, and have a sustained correction of all their immunological functions. They do not have serious graft vs host reactions, unless because of the immunologic correction they convert a persisting infection into a disease, e.g., pneumonia, when they become able to react to the infecting organism.

This approach has been used to correct not only the forms of SCID that I have indicated here may be autosomal recessive or X-linked recessive, but also adenosine deaminase deficiency as well, a disorder involving an enzymatic block. The child who represents our first successful treatment of this inborn error of metabolism is now more than 12 years old. She's a fascinating chimera because her erythrocytes and the granular leukocytes derived from her own genetic origins lack adenosine deaminase, whereas her lymphoid tissues and lymphoid cells of donor origin possess this crucial enzyme in normal amounts and are functioning normally, as a consequence of the marrow transplant from her healthy sister, which cured her.

This tells us several things. First, adenosine deaminase isn't nearly as vital for erythrocyte development and granulocyte development as it is for lymphoid cell development, where it is absolutely crucial. This is probably because the metabolites, including adenosine itself and 2-deoxyadenosine and perhaps ATP, are very toxic to the lymphoid cells. We've been able to produce this disease chemically in the laboratory by administering the tight binder of adenosine deaminase 2-deoxycoformycin, which produces a combined immunodeficiency disease that is, at first, more of a T-cell deficiency but progresses to a combined immunodeficiency with severe B-cell deficiency as well.

We've also learned that, whereas in Di George's syndrome it wasn't surprising that the thymic hormone concentrations should be so low and then come up to normal after a thymic transplantation, 18 of our 20 patients with the combined immunodeficiencies also had very low concentrations of thymic hormone. Only two had nearly normal concentrations.

If, however, instead of a thymus, we transplant bone marrow to these patients, the bone marrow cells going to the thymus appear to induce the thymic epithelium to begin to function normally, and the concentrations of thymic hormone regularly increase into the normal range. This is one of the earliest signs of a successful marrow transplant in these patients. We thus can monitor the concentrations of thymic hormones, which come up into the normal range long before the immunological system in these patients has been reconstructed. This is an important finding, because it seems to indicate that the mesenchymal cells from the bone marrow go to the bone marrow and there begin to influence functions of the epithelial cells of the thymus.

In our experience, transplanting a thymus to patients with SCID only rarely corrects the immunodeficiency—no more than one in 20 in our experience and in our evaluation of the literature. We can show in vitro that bone marrow cells cannot be induced to normal differentiation by the thymic hormone. The marrow has to be transplanted because the bone marrow origin of the immunological cells is defective; that's why you have disease of both the T- and B-cells in some of the patients, and perhaps also why the thymus function is so deficient in patients with these diseases.

Now, these are rare diseases. But six separate forms of SCID can be cured by bone marrow transplantation, and perhaps a few patients have also been treated successfully by transplantation of the thymus. What about more common diseases? We saw with our first patient, in 1968, that we could treat aplastic anemia by bone marrow transplantation when aplastic anemia complicated our first successful marrow transplant. Subsequently, we and others around the country who have bone marrow transplantation programs have been successful in treating all known forms of aplastic anemia by bone marrow transplantation. Aplastic anemias occur (*a*) following viral infection, particularly hepatitis; (*b*) following drug or chemical intoxication; (*c*) as an idiopathic disorder; and (*d*) sometimes, as a disease associated with an inborn error of metabolism—the Fanconi syndrome. The last-named patients are tricky to treat because you must suppress the immunity system with nearly lethal doses of cytotoxic drugs, although the patients are very susceptible to cytotoxins or to x-rays. Maybe the approach that Dr. Starzl showed us can make this easier. All the centers doing marrow transplantation are able to cure aplastic anemias and very much affect the mortality rate while fully correcting the cellular deficits by bone marrow transplantation.

Even the worst form of leukemia, acute myeloid leukemia, occurring in older children or young adults, is now often curable by marrow transplantation—that is, there are five- to 10-year survivors. When bone marrow transplantation was first used as a means of therapy in patients with acute myeloid leukemia, the patients were treated only at the end stage of the disease when all else had been tried and failed. Only 10% of these patients, 15% at the very best, could be transformed into long-term survivors. That, of course, was 10–15% more than would have survived without the treatment, and was sufficient to indicate that early treatment of these patients might make a real difference. Now that patients are being treated by marrow transplantation, the rate is approaching 65% long-term survivors, and these results project to perhaps 50% cures. We think graft vs host reaction plays a role in most of the deaths.

We can also treat other lethal diseases by marrow transplantation. In Wiskott–Aldrich syndrome the children are susceptible to infections by virus and fungus as well as to many bacterial diseases. Their phagocytes don't work normally. Their cells can't kill tumor cells normally—so they are also very susceptible to the development of tumors. The platelets are small and poorly functional and there is a progressive loss of both numbers and functions of T-lymphocytes. With these many abnormalities, there is little wonder that this is a highly lethal disease. All of the defects in these patients are now fully correctable by marrow transplantation. A start to change the situation occurred when Bach et al. corrected the immunologic deficiency in one such patient by giving massive doses of cyclophosphamide plus a bone marrow transplant in 1968. That patient was cured of immunodeficiency but the hematologic abnormality remained.

Then a group in Boston, led by Robertson Parkman, succeeded in marrow transplantation for complete correction of Wiskott–Aldrich syndrome. They used a combination of procarbazine and lethal radiation plus anti-lymphocyte antiserum to prepare their patients. We thought that this approach might be a little drastic and, led by Dr. Kapoor, found that these patients are adequately prepared with a modification of a busulfan regimen developed by the Baltimore group under Santos. Neither busulfan alone nor cyclophosphamide alone prepared animals for marrow transplant, but both together did: the cyclophosphamide is adequately immunosuppressive, the busulfan adequately myeloablative to succeed. When both are used in succession in humans, marrow transplants can succeed. We can now count nine patients with Wiskott–Aldrich syndrome, treated by this regimen. All nine have been corrected and apparently cured of their disease. This is a highly lethal disease with platelet abnormality, abnormality of phagocytes, and deficiency in the number and function of T-lymphocytes. The patients were given 2 mg of busulfan per kilogram of body weight per day for four days, then 50 mg of cyclophosphamide per kilogram of body weight per day for four days—a near lethal dose. With that treatment, they can undergo bone marrow transplantation and have all their hematologic and immunologic abnormalities fully corrected.

This approach has been used in our clinics for the treatment not only of Wiskott–Aldrich syndrome, but also of severe congenital neutrophil dysfunction and the most severe forms of congenital agranulocytosis (all genetically determined abnormalities of hematopoietic development). Patients have also been successfully treated for the complex immunodeficiency and hematologic abnormality that occurs in cartilage-hair hypoplasia.

As Dr. Desnick stated above, we have also shown that osteopetrosis can be cured by marrow transplantation. We learned this approach from earlier work in mice and rats. Osteopetrosis is the awful marble bone disease associated with growth failure, generalized hematopoietic failure, deafness, and blindness due to deficient function of the marrow-derived osteoclasts that function to remodel the bones.

It's clear from rodent models that, to get a sustained cure of osteopetrosis, you've got to give a bone marrow transplant in which the stem cells have achieved a sustained graft. Just transplanting normal osteoclasts can correct the abnormality for a brief period, but then the disease returns. But a proper marrow transplant, we found, with Drs. N. Kapoor, M. Sorell, and Richard O'Reilly, completely corrects this disease of the bones, and remodeling of bone and growth of the bones occur normally. In addition, the hematopoietic abnormality is corrected, and the progression to blindness and deafness in this disease is halted.

The importance of Fanconi's anemia, Wiskott–Aldrich syndrome, and SCID is that all of these patients have a very high frequency of malignancy. When we treat them by marrow transplantation and correct their aplastic anemia, their multiplicity of hematopoietic abnormalities, or their immunological defects, do we interfere with the development of malignancy? We don't know yet—it's too early to tell; but it is a crucial question to raise.

The problem is that in America, when you'd like to do a bone marrow transplant, only 25–40% of the time can you have a matched sibling donor, because only one in four sibs will match with a potential recipient at the major histocompatibility locus. Fortunately, one can use near-matching of relatives to increase the frequency of appropriate marrow donors. To treat a child with SCID, we did pioneering work in this direction when we found an uncle in the family who matched with the prospective recipient at the D and the DR locus. With our Danish co-workers, we were able safely to make the marrow transplant for this child and correct the SCID. In another case in this same family, the father was found to be a suitable donor for his little girl. Both transplants corrected the SCID, showing that one does not always need a perfectly matched sibling donor, but that sometimes an appropriately matched relative will do. One can find, by careful study of families, perhaps 5–10% additional suitable donors if the patient should need a marrow transplant.

Fetal Liver Transplants

In addition, we have been successful sometimes in treating patients with severe combined immunodeficiency by transplanting fetal liver plus thymus from the same fetal donor. Fetal liver by itself doesn't work very well. One child with severe combined immunodeficiency had also an infection with avian tuberculosis, which he couldn't resist at all. Both his SCID and the atypical acid-fast bacterial infection were treated successfully after transplantation with liver plus thymus from an aborted fetal donor.

After we had given the child an immunological system by cellular engineering, he became able to resist the avian tuberculosis. Correction of the SCID may occur slowly only after fetal liver transplantation. But fetal liver is not a suitable source of cells for hematopoietic reconstitution, although it can work sometimes. As the hematopoietic component of the fetal liver develops, it goes through a stage where it contains hematopoietic cells but does not have post-thymic immunoincompetent or post-thymic immunocompetent cells that are committed to immunologic function. Transplanting the fetal liver at this stage into experimental animals, after fatal irradiation, can correct all the abnormalities that occur consequent to the irradiation.

Current Developments in Treatment

More than 600–700 marrow transplants are now being used each year to treat a variety of genetic and acquired diseases that would be highly lethal without this treatment. These marrow transplants are indeed curing patients who otherwise can't be cured. The main problem remaining is still that of a graft vs host reaction. This reaction limits availability of donors and contributes heavily to mortality even when HLA-matched sibling donors are used. Within the last five years, however, we have succeeded with experimental animals—with mice and rats and now with monkeys and humans—to prepare the marrow so it will not initiate a graft vs host reaction. To transplant mismatched marrow successfully, we must get rid of all the "committed" cells, the post-thymic immunoincompetent as well as the post-thymic immunocompetent lymphoid cells from the marrow. We must transplant only the nondangerous marrow compartment of cells that contains the stem cells. When only the cells that have yet to go through the thymus pathway of differentiation are transplanted, the treatment is effective in mice almost 100% of the time and no graft vs host reaction is produced. We've now produced full bone marrow chimeras, which are living as long as two years after a transplant without any graft vs host reaction. With such transplants, we can thus readily and safely achieve marrow transplant across the major histocompatibility barriers.

In these experiments, the unwanted post-thymic cells are eliminated by treatment of the marrow in vitro with an antibody that is highly toxic to these cells. By treatment of marrow with such antibody with or without complement, the cells can be immunologically prepared so that the marrow can be transplanted across major histocompatibility barriers without inducing any graft vs host reaction whatever. After such marrow transplants, animals are fully functional in every way. The number of colony-forming units are normal, reflecting their vigorous hematopoietic potential. They can develop delayed allergy and reject third-party grafts normally. Their lymphoid cells are normally cytotoxic and can initiate GVHR normally. The lymphoid cells of the recipient are tolerant of donor and tolerant of recipient. They can exercise all cell-mediated lymphocytes normally; they work normally in mixed leukocyte cultures; their mitogen responses are all normal; their natural killer-cell responses are normal; and their ability to carry out antibody-dependent cell-mediated cytotoxicity functions are normal. But they can't make even a little antibody to a thymus-dependent antigen. Why not? Their T-cell numbers are normal, the B-cell numbers are normal, the accessory cell numbers are normal, the receptors on each of those cell populations are normal—to the extent that we can determine this. The animals have the capacity to make the interleukin 1, interleukin 2, and T-replacing factors normally. So why don't they work effectively in antibody synthesis to T-dependent antigens? Apparently these cells can't communicate very well with one another. There is an apparent H2 mismatch between the cells that develop through the thymus and those that develop from precursors from the same donor, the B-cell lineage, which do not need to be processed by the thymus. The cells have trouble, at first, talking to each other. But they can learn to talk to each other and they can learn to function quite normally, so we don't think the restrictions are serious. These animals appear to defend themselves well against viral infection.

Because of the major obstacle represented to bone marrow transplantation by the requirement of a matched donor, we wanted to apply this approach to monkeys and humans to make possible marrow transplantation from regularly available potential marrow donors when a matched sibling or matched relative donor is not available. We do not yet have antisera sufficiently avid or specifically directed to an appropriate antigen that will permit us to separate out or destroy all the unwanted cells. Instead, we have used the findings of investigators who were using the sugar code to get at this issue. Reisner and co-workers at the Weissman Institute had used soybean agglutinin plus peanut agglutinin to permit separation of stem cells from hazardous committed cells in mice. This treatment plus differential centrifugation eliminates all the post-thymic immunoincompetent cells as well as the immunocompetent T-cells and permits maintenance of all the stem cells. With Reisner, we have modified this method for use with humans and cynomolgus monkeys to achieve yields of 70 to 95% of the quantifiable stem cells, and to purge the marrow of unwanted T-lymphocytes and of all cells committed to develop along this lineage. We can then transplant this purged marrow in monkeys and humans and achieve hematopoietic and immunological reconstruction after lethal irradiation without inducing any graft vs host reactions.

We, and our collaborators, have now applied this approach for the treatment of 15 children with SCID, transplanting bone marrow from parents mismatched at A, B, C, D, and DR loci, but who are haplo-identical with the recipients. None of the recipients have developed any evidence of graft vs host reactions. Nine are completely reconstituted and well, and three more are partially reconstituted and well. In addition, we have used this approach to treat very high-risk leukemia patients—nearly dead in a number of instances, so that if we did induce graft vs host reaction, it wouldn't seem so disastrous. Graft vs host reaction has not been induced in this situation either with the purged marrow, and two of these patients are in long-term remission. We now are beginning to apply the method to treat patients with leukemia who are at better risk.

One thing we have learned from this new approach is that we can introduce resistance genes by marrow transplantation in experimental animals. We have also learned that we can correct the propensity of mice to develop autoimmunity and the diseases of aging by using these new techniques.

In a new approach, we have used mismatched marrow transplants to alter enzyme expression, even in organs apparently as far removed from marrow as the pancreas. Thus, with cellular engineering, especially thymus and bone marrow transplantation, we have already been able effectively to treat patients with more than 20 otherwise fatal diseases if a proper donor of hematopoietic tissue is at hand. We have been able to develop approaches that appear to be curative of inborn errors of metabolism, effective in treatment of devastating consequences of viral infections, poisonings, and even a few cancers. In our recent experimental work, we have been able greatly to broaden the potential for bone marrow transplantation by eliminating the hazard of graft vs host reaction. This is true even when donor and recipient are mismatched at the entire major histocompatibility locus. Thus far, in using these approaches for treatment of human disease, we have limited ourselves to haplo-identical donors such as parents or mismatched siblings, but in experimental animals, we have regularly been able to cross the major histocompatibility barriers entirely without inducing graft vs host disease. Using these methods in experimental studies, we have already been able to introduce resistance genes against leukemias and lymphomas by marrow transplantation in experimental animals and to treat effectively or prevent autoimmunities and to inhibit even the development of diseases of aging. We are beginning to analyze the nature of the influence that underlies the effectiveness of the introductions of these resistance genes and to anticipate that in the future, a specific chemistry of their influence can be elucidated.

We may be on the threshold of knowing enough about the immunity systems and some of the other systems of the body to consider the possibility of cellular engineering in even simpler terms. For instance, in children with an abnormality of complement function, one can give plasma from one of the family members who produces the normal complement moiety to protect the patient. This was first demonstrated in hereditary angioedema where there is a deficiency of C_1 esterase inhibitor. We now have used purified preparations to prevent and (or) abort attacks of hereditary angioneurotic edema. However, for this disease, a much more dramatic form of cellular engineering has appeared, involving induction of the missing inhibitor or induction of production.

Hereditary angioneurotic edema is a highly lethal, dominantly inherited disease, caused by the failure to produce or by production of an abnormal molecule of C_1 esterase inhibitor. These patients develop nonpainful edema, often after infections or injuries. The edema may also occur spontaneously, and it even follows menstruation in women with the disease. If this edema occurs, as it often does, in the laryngeal area, the patients may choke to death unless a physician is at hand.

Investigators at the NIH, led by Michael Frank, discovered that one could induce the production of the enzyme in this inherited disease, probably by "turning on" the recessive gene in these patients, by using danazol, a well-tolerated synthetic hormone. The activity of C_1 esterase inhibitor came up to normal values. This is engineering gene expression by hormonal manipulation to correct an otherwise highly lethal disease.

In another genetically determined disease, the affected patients have a high frequency of necrotizing skin lesions and mesenchymal disease, often resulting in end-stage kidney disease. A kidney transplant completely cured this immunodeficiency disease by supplying a complement component without which the patient could not live a satisfactory life. This component, produced by the kidney, has been maintained continuously since that transplant. As Dr. Starzl has emphasized, the possibility of treatment with transplants is now much improved because of the better means of immunosuppression available, particularly with cyclosporin A and prednisone.

A disease that occurs in A-46 mutant cattle is acrodermatitis enteropathica. Their thymus fails to develop and they have severe gastrointestinal disease and profound immunodeficiency involving the T-cell system. But the only thing really wrong with these animals is that they can't absorb zinc from the gastrointestinal tract. One can correct this disease completely just by giving the element zinc, a very simple treatment for a profound immunodeficiency.

This disease also occurs in humans, where it is characterized by central nervous system maldevelopment, an awful skin rash, SCID, and increased susceptibility to infection. Like the cattle, these patients can't absorb zinc normally from the gastrointestinal tract. The perfect and absolute cure of this human disease is simply to give the element zinc in larger amounts than is normally required, which cures all of this SCID of genetic origin. That's certainly easier than doing a bone marrow transplantation, and it is most effective. All of the abnormalities and even the mortality of this awful disease are corrected by the administration of zinc. From these and other experimental studies, we have learned that zinc exerts a profound effect on T-cell function. Similar abnormalities, for example, can be produced in animals just by restricting the element zinc.

As we better understand the development and function of the immunological system, we will be able to make cellular engineering a much more proximate and simpler process than it is today. But even today we are seeing the potential, essentially, of creating life by understanding the immunological system well enough to exercise cellular engineering. This will develop rapidly in the years ahead.

Discussion

Q: What, if any, abnormalities or changes do you see in B-cells in cases where large amounts of autoantibodies are produced?

Dr. Good: The best way to look at the effects of autoimmunity is in inbred mice where we can actually work with cells in culture and with pure B-cells as well as all the stages of development of B-cells. First there is an excess of plasma cells and then a very marked increase in clonability of the B-cells. We can show that B-cells of these animals are abnormal. Rather surprisingly, Jyonouchi has found the pre-B cells and B-cells actually decrease in the marrow and lymphoidal tissue even before clinical disease begins. We believe that the same type of abnormality is present in some of the autoimmune diseases in our patients. The disease is not limited to B-cells because we find that as early as we can culture fetal liver cells there is an abnormality of granulocyte/monocyte development. Moreover, in confirmation of others' work, we find abnormalities of function of T-cells. These abnormalities are different in the different genetically determined autoimmune diseases. All the cellular abnormalities are corrected by total body radiation plus bone marrow transplantation, when you take the bone marrow from a donor that does not develop that type of abnormality. We think that the basic disease resides in the stem cells that can develop into granulocytes/monocytes, B-cells, or T-cells. There are abnormalities in all these circuits.

Q: Might you be able to predict what would happen if bone marrow transplantation were used in lupus or in Hashimoto's disease?

DR. GOOD: I do not know, but from what we have seen, I certainly think we can make bone marrow transplantation safer and avoid graft vs host reaction. It might then be conservative treatment to approach those diseases with bone marrow transplantation after treatment with massive doses of cyclophosphamide or total body radiation. The mortality in those diseases at the moment is not high enough to justify bone marrow transplantation and has the hazard of graft vs host reaction, but if we can avoid that reaction by bone marrow transplantation from donors who would not be sufficiently different from the patients genetically but would not be likely to carry the same genes, we might be able to correct those diseases in humans as we can treat and prevent them in mice.

DR. GILBERT: Do you have an age limitation for transplant recipients?

DR. GOOD: Yes. So far, bone marrow transplantation is a young person's game. Ninety percent of our successful marrow transplants are in persons under 20. We have had some success up to the age of 40, but mortality is much higher. The problem probably is that, in older patients, when the thymus begins to involute, the reconstruction of the immunological system is so slow (or does not occur at all) that infections cause problems. There is also more trouble with graft vs host reactions in older donors. We are now working on this problem with monkeys to see how the age range of potential recipients can be extended. In mice, if you do both a thymus and bone marrow transplant, you can reconstruct the immunological abnormalities that have developed with aging.

Ethical Aspects of Therapy for Genetic Diseases

Marc Lappé

The dramatic progress in devising therapies for previously untreatable diseases is to be welcomed as an advance that promises great alleviation of human suffering. But these same developments in genetic science also raise grave questions of how best to make the first experimental forays towards clinical application and to decide which therapies deserves our highest priority. These challenges bring us to a juncture where health imperatives, legal quandaries, and ethical dilemmas deserve our closest—and wisest—reflection.

It may be useful to recount how ethical questions have evolved over the last 10 years. The primary concern 10 years ago centered on the issues posed by compulsory genetic testing and screening. Among the disturbing prospects was the concern of some ethnic groups that mass genetic screening for the carrier state of serious disorders like sickle cell anemia could become the forerunners of a quasi-eugenic movement.

At that time I directed the Genetic Research Group at the Hastings Center, at Hastings-on-Hudson, NY; we had to decide whether it was more appropriate to talk about these problems or about the ethical issues generated by genetic engineering. We opted for the former, in large part because we could not fathom that genetic engineering was as near on the horizon as it so obviously is now. Nor did we appreciate the subtleties of ethical analysis that would be needed for justifying the types of therapies now being considered.

In the recent past the issues of prenatal diagnosis and abortion concentrated on the questions of disclosure and consent. For whom should prenatal diagnosis be offered? Should it be only for those women over the age of 35 at risk for chromosome aneuplody, particularly Down's syndrome? Now we have to ask how, if, and when should we move from offering an intervention that is essentially negative (selective abortion) to one where the same projected disease-state is considered for treatment. It is precisely at this juncture that the first major ethical questions of gene therapy are raised.

Ethical Issues in Therapy of Genetic Disease

Metabolic disorders (e.g., Niemann–Pick disease) or, indeed, some of the X-linked disorders (e.g., Lesch–Nyhan disease) have only recently become subject to intra-uterine diagnosis. They may now be subject to therapeutic intervention. We also have reasonable prospects for therapy of severe combined immune deficiency. These prospects pose major ethical questions in clinical judgment and patients' rights.

When do you disclose to an expectant mother that you have an experimental therapy on the near horizon? Initially, you may have techniques that have proven efficacious only in animal models, or in the first human cases. According to some researchers, where intra-uterine diagnosis has confirmed the presence of a fetus with a now potentially treatable disease, it will be difficult in all but a few cases to offer the uncertain option of an experimental therapy, when the certainty of diagnosis and abortion promise a clearer and simpler solution to the problem. Williamson (1) has observed that "the correction of a disease by gene therapy will be worthwhile only if there is no other, simpler and more effective technique available." Yet, ethicists might argue that the presence of even a potential therapy diminishes the acceptability of at least one "simpler technique," late abortion.

Clearly, this is a circumstance calling for the most heightened ethical sensitivity. It is entirely likely that parents who have had an affected child are less than ideally situated to give a free and voluntary consent to the therapeutic procedure instead of an abortion.

Many of the conundrums posed by gene therapy resolve to a basic dilemma: How can parents be helped to determine when measures that may or may not promise benefits outweigh their choice of a selective abortion? Is it ethically acceptable to opt for selective abortion to avoid the prospect of an infant's facing a life fraught with suffering when potential therapies have reduced that likelihood substantially? When do the uncertainties regarding the lifelong value of an intervention reach the point of sufficient assurance to warrant routine offering of the therapy?

Characteristically, ethicists do not have many more answers to this type of problem than do physicians or parents, but they sometimes help in framing the balancing considerations these kinds of questions need to be resolved. Just acknowledging that there will be dilemmas of this magnitude for a substantial number of genetic diseases that will be in line for experimental therapies is important in itself [*cf.* (*1*)].

Perhaps the greatest ethical dilemma is posed by the very grave and irreversible character of the clinical course of most genetic diseases. The belief is widespread that extreme suffering calls for extreme interventions and equally extreme therapeutic modalities. For many disciplines, particularly oncology, it has become a traditional precept to use those individuals with the most advanced, incurable, and irreversible disease as the first subjects for therapeutic intervention. Consider the therapies that have been proposed for individuals with leukemia or other forms of incurable cancer—for instance, radical neck dissection and radiation therapy for head and neck tumors. In these instances, the most extreme therapeutic interventions are reserved for individuals nearing the terminus of a disease process.

Ironically, clinicians now recognize that some of these experimental modalities are most effective or, sometimes, *only* effective when introduced *earliest* in the disease. Such cases undercut the rationale for using terminal patients as the subjects for novel interventions. The message to genetic therapists is clear: Do not wait until a child has the full ravages of a heritable disorder before instituting therapy.

This, however, raises the joint questions of proxy consent and the readiness of a particular technologic intervention for treating a disease. Formal guidelines for the orderly and ethically acceptable generation of genetic therapies based on recombinant DNA techniques do not yet exist except by reference to existing guidelines from the Department of Health and Human Services and the National Institutes of Health for experimentation (*2*). While these guidelines identify the importance of having appropriately defined techniques with reasonable prospects for therapy based on animal or primate models, the first attempts at human gene therapy have been done *without* having suitable models or proven animal test systems (3, 4).

Ethical and sound medical precepts dictate that genetic therapies be preceded by adequate pre-human testing. Once requirements of efficacy have been satisfied, the safety of these techniques must also be proven—a process hampered by the dearth of animal models for important human disease. The possibility of iatrogenic illness must be balanced against the consequence of the illness that ensues from failure to intervene. Thus, there must be some procedure and process for delineating the relative risks of intervening vs the consequences of not intervening, even when benefits cannot be completely detailed.

Issues of Public Support

Given the extraordinary progress in this field, it is not too early to begin to consider the question of how we should best move genetic therapies into the mainstream of clinical medicine [*cf.* (5)]. In the very near future genetic therapy for diseases like those discussed by Drs. Good and Desnick will attain widespread public importance. Previously therapy-resistant disease such as childhood-onset diabetes may call for treatment modalities that include genetic and nongenetic interventions (e.g., vaccination programs). Which approaches require wholesale public support through federal funding or new insurance programs? How can treatments be used on the scale necessary to achieve genuine public health objectives? Some, but not all, programs may pass the test of a positive benefit-to-cost ratio. Others may be justified on more humanitarian grounds. Which therapeutic advances deserve the highest funding priorities?

Questions of resource allocation are as critical now as are the issues raised by experimentation directed at the individual patient, and it is here that traditional ethical norms begin to fray at the edges. Weighing public and individual good is a delicate exercise at best. One test of the appropriateness of allocating public resources for an intervention has relied on measurements of the public consequences of disease entities, usually by some crude measurement of the cost/benefit ratio (e.g., the costs of intervention times the frequency of the occurrence of a particular disease and its cost were it to be left untreated). A significant portion of genetic diseases are by their very nature exquisitely rare disorders; thus, if one uses a measurement of human suffering multiplied by the relative frequency of any individual genetic disease, the "burden" of that disease would provide a poor basis to justify investment of public funds in developing modalities of treatment. However, all major mendelian recessive genetic disorders *together* comprise a significant burden of disease, particularly in childhood, where they account for a large portion of pediatric hospitalizations (up to 30–40%) and affect considerable numbers of individuals [estimated to be as many as 1% of the population (*1*)]. Hence, as I will argue below, it may be important to encourage research strategies that may lead to universalizable models, in preference to those earmarked for single, rare genetic disorders.

Distinguishing Basic Values from Those of Applied Research

A fundamental problem in identifying techniques with universalizability is that they rarely can be separated from less valuable approaches when they are at an experimental stage. Sometimes, early experimental approaches that appear promising as general treatment modalities are rushed into application, with deleterious effects on basic research (*6*). When clearly experimental techniques are applied prematurely to treatment modalities, as occurred in the work of Martin Cline (*3, 6*), a gap opens between scientific credibility and public support.

Public agencies have also reinforced a view that identifies single diseases as appropriate funding targets rather than whole classes of diseases. We have seen incommensurate decisions made in garnering statewide support for a few rare genetic diseases (e.g., a special program for Huntington's disease in California) or for some that are not so rare. The more common coagulation disorders (e.g., hemophilia), which are amenable to treatment, have repeatedly been proposed for support in the state and federal law-making bodies. As a counter to this trend, however, some legislators point to the fiscal debacle that ensued when renal transplantation and support for end-stage renal disease was given total federal support. Let us hope we do not perpetuate this "disease-of-the-year" dilemma for hereditary disorders. I suggest that part of the solution is to encourage funding priorities that encourage the development of those techniques that have the greatest prospect of generalizability. To do so means establishing effective treatment models for whole classes of molecular or biochemical disorders.

Specific Treatment Modalities

How close are we to developing therapies with this kind of general applicability? Indicators of early prospects for successful models suggest that we should grapple with that problem of assigning priorities right now. The following discussion indicates research avenues capable of bringing us to developing therapies that might lead to a more general solution for genetic diseases.

The five genetic interventions in Table 1 demonstrate the feasibility of inserting specified gene sequences into rapidly developing embryos such that there is a reasonable prospect that these gene sequences will become encoded in the somatic cells and, in one case, in the germinal epithelium and germinal tissues of the resulting organism. Although human embryo therapy has ethical problems of its own [*cf.* (*1*)], success in this area is a harbinger of the greater likelihood of effective treatments that regularly insert functional genes into living tissues.

The first study, demonstrating the technical feasibility of insert-

Table 1. **Reported Gene Transplantation Attempts**

Human insulin gene transplanted into fertilized mouse egg cells.	Collaboration between scientists in Switzerland and California.	The transplanted gene persisted through embryonic development.
Human interferon gene transplanted into fertilized mouse egg cells.	Yale University.	The gene persisted into the next generation of mice.
Virus genes for thymidine kinase transplanted into fertilized mouse egg cells.	The Institute for Cancer Research, Fox Chase, PA.	Thymidine kinase was produced by the mouse embryo cells.
Two people given blood-forming cells containing a gene for a component of hemoglobin.	Scientists at UCLA, in collaboration with doctors in Italy and Israel.	No conclusive result reported; a scientist reprimanded by the National Institutes of Health.
Two infants infected with a virus to treat an enzyme deficiency.	Scientists at Oak Ridge National Laboratory collaborating with doctors in West Germany.	Treatment failed to prevent mental retardation (did not provide enzyme to the infants).

Adapted from *The New York Times*, September 8, 1981.

ing a gene for human insulin into fertilized mouse eggs and obtaining postzygotic expression of this gene, was done by Kurt Burke at the University of Geneva in Switzerland and, coincidentally, by Axel Ullrich of Genentech Inc. [see the review by Ullrich et al. (*7*)]. A related experiment, by Frank Ruddle at Yale, was even more dramatic in that the interferon gene was transplanted into fertilized mouse eggs; subsequently, he and his co-workers demonstrated incorporation of this gene into the germinal epithelium and the transfer of the gene into a second generation [*cf.* Gordon et al. (*8*)].

In the third study a well-characterized viral gene, the gene for thymidine kinase, was transplanted into a fertilized mouse egg by Beatrice Mintz of the Institute for Cancer Research, Fox Chase. Dr. Mintz and her co-workers demonstrated the expression of viral genes in a murine test species, thereby opening the prospect of gene therapy by overcoming of the major obstacle of ensuring expression of heterologous genetic material. Her work also affords an avenue towards resolving the problem of how to get enough cells transfected to develop a sufficiently numerous population of transformed cells to make the necessary gene product. Apparently, you can be quite successful if you can start this process early enough [*cf.* Pellicer et al. (*9*)].

The next study involves the principle used by Dr. Mintz—namely, trying to get a clonal population of cells (in this case, bone marrow cells) to pick up a specified gene sequence and looking for evidence of expression. Martin Cline at UCLA attempted to use bone marrow treated with cloned DNA sequences to repopulate the leg bones of two young girls in Italy and Israel. His work was apparently both unsuccessful and ethically questionable [*cf.* (*3, 6*)].

The last example was the use of the Shope papilloma virus to infect two arginase-deficient infants so that they would thereby regain the ability to produce arginase. Neither child showed clinical improvement attributable to the virus treatment, perhaps because sub-infective doses were used [see Rogers (*4*), for a full discussion and defense of this protocol].

Ethical Issues

These examples, as heady and exciting as they are for the prospects of therapy, raise major ethical questions. According to some ethicists, such as Paul Ramsey of Princeton (*10*), the inviolability and presumed right to normal existence of a person have mistakenly been taken to imply an obligation to intervene. Thus, if one can specifically identify at an embryonic or even zygotic stage an affected individual for whom one has a possible gene therapy, one may believe he is morally obligated to try to "rescue" that individual. Others find it equally defensible to perform an abortion through the fifth month of gestation for any hereditary or chromosomal disorder.

Research on fetuses also overlooks the problem of absent consent, possible harms outweighing benefits, and the knotty, unresolved question of our obligation to treat at any cost. Moreover, treating persons in advance of successful animal experimentation denies those individuals respect by making them experimental subjects to unproven techniques for the sake of experimentation alone.

Issues of Social Justice and Strategic Considerations

We have seen that the optimism we may bring to advancing these therapeutic models is tempered by at least three broad sets of problems. The first is that there are no agreed-upon norms or guidelines for setting priorities in genetic research. Some may argue that this is exactly the right moment to have an open-door policy for encouraging the broadest possible avenue of therapeutic experimental ventures. Others would point out the importance of moving cautiously with regard to "rescuing" those individuals who have fatal, incurable diseases because of attendant excesses.

A second major problem, which we may encounter in the next five years, is how to allocate resources to treat genetic diseases. The third problem is how to decide, after an array of alternative therapeutic modalities has been developed, which one is the most appropriate for treating groups of related genetic diseases.

All of these issues are still in embryonic stages. Each turns on the question of how to define the readiness of a technique to be moved first into an experimental arena and then into an applied public health arena, where it becomes an acceptable modality for treatment.

But underlying all of these problems is a fourth and perhaps more critical dilemma: how do we assure that social justice will be reinforced and not undermined as these techniques proliferate? I have already shown (*11*) that where new modalities of prenatal medical technology have become available, they are used first and most extensively by the upper socioeconomic groups. A new case in point may be juvenile-onset diabetes. Although most researchers recognize the complex etiology of diabetes—e.g., its apparent dependence on certain HLA phenotypes and the possible role of viral infection and autoimmune phenomena in generating the disease (*12*)—until recently, few have proposed interventions to prevent its pathogenesis (*13, 14*). Instead, clinicians have relied on the apparent success of treating the pathological manifestation of the disease with insulin. Some would argue that insulin therapy had led to a "hyperfocus" on chemotherapeutic intervention in preference to other treatment modalities. Other interventions, such as the use of immunosuppressive agents to dampen the immune-mediated damage to the islets of Langerhans (*13*) or immunotherapy to prevent type I diabetes (*14*), are just now being attempted. All such new modalities must now compete for funding with the recombinant DNA technologies that have been developed for making pure human insulin.

It would be naive not to recognize that substantial investments in the last three years have gone into developing efficient ways to synthesize pure human insulin. At the same time, proportionately fewer dollars have been allocated to fewer scientists for basic research that could define the actual structure of the insulin gene and its relationship to other genes. In principle, this latter approach is the more valuable, because it can lead to prevention rather than palliation strategies.

From the viewpoint of public health, investigating the control and function of the insulin gene may more likely give long-term benefits than the application of insulin as a chemotherapeutic, after-the-fact treatment. Yet, our present investments are heavily skewed in favor of reaping immediate financial rewards, instead of being directed toward preventive strategies with possibly greater long-term health benefits. The likelihood that significant funding would go to this latter course of intervention is substantially diminished by the fact that most of the dollars for research in the area of insulin production and treatment of diabetes are concentrated in the private sector, and out of public-sector control.

This trend, should it continue, has two very negative consequences. First, the normal modalities of allowing scientific feasibility and heuristic appeal of experimental approaches to guide the direction of research would be displaced by the financial incentives to develop therapies that could be quickly monetized. This kind of displacement could mean that the initial stages of development of long-term solutions to complex polygenic diseases like diabetes and hypertension may not be evolving in the most efficient, least costly, or scientifically most desirable directions.

A related problem, the development of single-gene products that are attractive to private sector investors, is likely to be contingent on the existence of a very large population of affected individuals in economic need of this therapy. Development of such a posture by industry would ignore the possibility that the therapeutic modalities that work best and have the greatest potential for generalization to other disorders may well be model systems developed for treating very rare human genetic diseases. For instance, an approach for treating hypoxanthine–guanidine phosphoribosyltransferase deficiency in Lesch–Nyhan disease from cloned gene segments that code for this enzyme could very well provide a model for treating a large spectrum of otherwise rare inherited disorders [see (7) for a review of this problem]. But no corporation in its right economic mind would invest heavily in developing a specific therapy for that rare an entity. The notion that therapies directed at more prevalent diseases are more justified than those directed at rare ones should not be an ethical norm for basic research. It may be important to distinguish among which therapies are going to provide the most useful models for generalizable interventions and which ones are going to be left at way stations, albeit effective ones, for treating rare genetic diseases. But in the absence of reliable techniques for distinguishing which approaches have the possibility of extension to closely related diseases, it is foolish, and perhaps even unethical, to allow short-term gains to direct research priorities. As a society, we have discussed providing incentives to drug companies to develop otherwise uneconomical drugs for rare disorders—why not take the same approach for rare genetic diseases?

One promising approach has centered on interventions involving transplantation of clonally proliferating cells that can potentially restore the deficiencies or defective gene products that ensue from a broad constellation of disorders. Two inborn errors of metabolism, α_1-antitrypsin deficiency and combined immune deficiency states, are now being successfully treated by bone marrow or fetal liver transplantation (16). These procedures provide the basic research paradigms both for understanding the more widespread problem of deficiency states and for studying more closely heterozygous individuals who have more moderate clinical problems.

Private vs Public Sector Funding

These triumphs of therapeutic invention may become less rather than more common as the result of a wholesale shift into the private sector of technologies that would otherwise be supported by the public. Where economic incentives become mixed with scientific ones, basic research can get skewed into applied research by "priority" schedules and policy decisions that come to be made by boards of directors rather than scientific panels. As a result of the present funding climate for genetic research, the very techniques that offer so much promise for understanding basic science are being jeopardized. "Cost-effective" programs designed to generate profits will almost always be those that generate hard commodities, e.g., drugs that alleviate symptoms of disease states, rather than the soft commodity of knowledge.

This situation leads to a possible premature collapsing of basic science into applied science. Scientists would do well to maintain the distinction between those elements of their work that are basic research and those that are projected for early application. It may also be critically important for funding agencies to foster and promote basic research. Retaining a modicum of recombinant DNA research, e.g., for plumbing the structure of the human genome, may be more important in the long run than are technologically elegant techniques for inserting economically or medically desirable gene sequences.

Possible Solutions

As a first step, it makes good ethical and scientific sense to have competing approaches for treating genetic diseases—some of which focus on basic scientific strategems and others that are designed to promote development of specific new therapies. Second, it is important to acknowledge that competition between alternative modalities of treatment or diagnosis is to be encouraged rather than quelled through monopoly control of gene products, as may now be happening with human insulin. Third, the value of doing basic research should not be obscured by economic incentives to develop a technique for the sole purpose of reaping early rewards or short-term gains: such techniques may not provide the most long-lasting contributions to scientific knowledge *or* health. For example, it may be much more attractive to develop approaches and techniques that lead to the recolonization of a genetically deficient individual, through marrow, liver, or kidney transplants, than to design specifically engineered gene-product therapy. Unfortunately, the economic imperatives of the marketplace have led to the proliferation of micropackaging industries that purport to develop liposome or other membrane packages for delivering enzymes or other structural genes to individuals who lack them, long before there is any real evidence that such approaches are successful.

Although I am criticizing private-sector approaches, I do not purport to know which group—public or private—necessarily has the "right" approach to a given genetic problem. But I can conclude that financial incentives serve as a constant skewing device that may set priorities with regard to financial imperatives rather than medical and scientific readiness.

Supporting evidence for this view is expressed in a statement by the President of Exxon's Research and Engineering Company, Dr. E. E. David, Jr., in a speech before the New York City Bar Association on April 21, 1981, addressing the issue of private involvement in recombinant DNA research. Dr. David, a former president of the American Association for the Advancement of Science stated: "A company must bet more money on a particular program if that program is to have enough scope to make a difference. Consequently, as part of its fiduciary responsibility to the stockholders, company management must have a voice in deciding who performs the research, and what the research addresses in order to ensure that it has a bearing on company interests."

It is this last point I would hold up for review: Is it in our best interests to have interventions increasingly in the hands of those whose incentives for developing them is often tempered by issues of both medical efficacy and financial return, or in the hands of those in the public sector who receive funds from the public weal? Only the latter group is likely to consistently base its research on science's internal guide rules and to be relatively value-neutral. Yet, science is freely conducted when scientists begin by looking for the most useful scientific approaches to solving a problem, and only secondarily with public policy makers, either federal or state, deciding which modalities provide the greatest public benefit.

The disparity between private- and public-sector research also leads to a critical tension between the selection and choice of patients of individualized therapy in contrast to considering therapies that can be generated for *communities* of patients with like diseases. The absence of formal acknowledgment (circa 1981) of this problem underscores the fact that a discussion of distributive justice, scientific freedom, and public vs individual good has not yet taken place at a national level. As we begin to disband the budget of the specific National Institutes directed at looking at genetic diseases, arthritic diseases, or diseases of circulatory systems, in favor of allowing *laissez-faire* economics to move research priorities, we are left with a real quandary. How much scientific freedom and creativity do you lose when you abandon a federal base of support for disease entities? The full impact may also depend on the degree to which we sacrifice public accountability and public control for regulating how technologies are allocated to the medical sector.

Recommendations

That then leaves a major ethical problem in moving towards genetic therapies. It would be desirable to consider having a public agency, perhaps as a subdivision within the National Institutes of Health's Genetics Disease Branch charged with the funding and oversight of genetic therapies. It may be necessary to maintain rules and procedures (e.g., patentability or marketing of proprietary drugs) that allow the private sector to reap benefits. But if we do, the public has a right to request that the benefits that are going to be reaped, both medically and economically (for instance, in the synthesis of insulin), be returned proportionately to *them*, rather than to the stockholders of the corporations involved. Thus, while it was public monies that supported the research leading to the basic patents awarded to Stanford and the University of California at San Francisco, the companies who make the recombinant DNA precursors and products based on these patents return only a meager user fee to the schools, and still less to the public at large, to whom they are able to charge whatever the market will bear.

Issues of social justice are raised when genetic therapies become wholesale commodities to be sold in the marketplace, rather than being used as models for therapies for broad ranges of diseases. Although they have now gone into the private sector, the origins of some of these techniques were in the public sector. In allocating these exquisitely effective and elegant modalities, it will become important to recognize that the issue of justice and fairness demands greater equity and profit-sharing in their distribution.

Supported by NEH/NSF Grant No. 1SP-8114338. The views expressed in this paper are those of the author and do not necessarily reflect the policies or opinions of the sponsoring agency. The secretarial assistance of Ms. Alice Murata is gratefully acknowledged.

References

1. Williamson, B., Gene therapy. *Nature* **298,** 416–417 (1982).
2. 45 CFR 46.
3. Anonymous, NIH censure for Dr. Martin Cline: Tighter rules for future research plans. *Nature* **291,** 369 (1981).
4. Rogers, S., Reflections on issues posed by recombinant DNA molecule technology. *Ann. N. Y. Acad. Sci.* **265,** 66–70 (1976).
5. Mercola, K. E., and Cline, M. J., Sounding boards: The potentials of inserting new genetic information. *N. Engl. J. Med.* **27,** 1297–1300 (1980).
6. Anonymous, Cline stripped of research grants. *Nature* **294,** 391 (1981).
7. Ullrich, A., et al., The structure and function of the human insulin gene. *Science* **209,** 612–615 (1980).
8. Gordon, J. W., Scangos, G. A., Plotkin, D. J., Barbosa, J. A., and Ruddle, F. H., Genetic transformation of mouse embryos by microinjection of purified DNA. *Proc. Natl. Acad. Sci. USA* **77,** 7380–7384 (1980).
9. Pellicer, A., et al., Introduction of a viral/gene and the human beta-globin gene into developmentally multipotential mouse teratocarcinoma cells. *Proc. Natl. Acad. Sci. USA* **77,** 2098–2102 (1980).
10. Ramsey, P., *The Patient as Person,* Yale University Press, New Haven, CT, 1970.
11. Lappé, M., Justice and prenatal life. In *Justice and Health Care,* E. Shelp, Ed., D. Reident, Dordrecht, Holland, 1981, pp 83–94.

12. Woon, J. W., Austin, M., Onodera, T., and Nothins, A. L., Virus-induced diabetes mellitus. *N. Engl. J. Med.* **300,** 1173–1179 (1979).
13. Vialettes, B., Beaume, D., Simon, M. C., Lassmann, V., and Vague, P., Assessment of the role of immune reaction in EMC virus-induced diabetes by the effect of early and delayed cyclosporin A treatments in mice. *Diabetologia* **19,** 322–232 (1980).
14. Kolb, H., Greulich, B., Kiesel, V., and Gries, F. A., Immunotherapy of type I diabetes. *Lancet* **ii,** 97–98 (1982).
15. Dillon, M. J., et al., Problems in diagnosis and treatment of adenine and hypoxanthine–guanine phosphoribosyltransferase deficiency in childhood. *J. Clin. Chem. Clin. Biochem.* (in press).
16. Tourraine, J. L., Treatment of severe combined immunodeficiency with bone marrow or foetal liver transplants. *Nouv. Presse Med.* **13,** 2215–2219 (1979).

Discussion

Q: To tie this in with Dr. Shaw's talk, is this going to lead to another round of malpractice suits of, say, physicians who do or do not advise people as to their alternatives or do not institute an alternative?

DR. LAPPÉ: I take a very chary view of the ethical responsibility of physicians to disclose and inform. It is very unfortunate that there have been these nine cases. Individual discretionary judgment and standards of practice have not been developed for what would constitute an acceptable disclosure when a therapy just reaches a point of application. Failure to disclose information that would lead to selective abortion is an ethically complex legal notion. The failure to provide information about the availability of therapies when they are at an experimental stage is a totally untested area of law. I think it would be very unfortunate in this litigious society to encourage patients to file suit for failure to provide experimental modalities of therapy. This could very well come to pass, however, if no clear line is drawn between experimental therapies and those that are clinically acceptable and proven.

That line could be drawn very clearly when one was dealing with drugs under the Food & Drug Administration guidelines.

In the standard case, a drug moves from (*a*) receiving a permit as an investigational new drug to (*b*) receiving approval as a drug with proven safety and efficacy. Only at that latter point, when it is accepted by the medical community, would malpractice for *not* offering it in treatment be accepted as legally proper. There is no guideline currently of how you would do that, say, in terms of transplantation. Do all children with myelogenous leukemia or all adults with an acute myelocytic leukemia, both of which might benefit from intervention with transplantation, deserve to get that treatment? Consider that this is a very rare and expensive commodity and perhaps of proven value only for younger children. Most physicians would rather spend their resources in trying to rescue a child who has 35 or 50 years of life remaining, if they can be rescued, than a 60-year-old individual, except as that person might be an appropriate test for the therapy. It is not an easily answered question. By analogy to cases like this, it would be very unfortunate to have or to encourage suits of this sort early in the development of genetic therapies.

DR. DIETZ: Could not rules be set up to prevent such suits?

DR. LAPPÉ: It might be possible to develop legislation that more precisely defines what type of therapy is in fact experimental and thereby requires careful informed consent procedures to protect both individuals and their attending physicians. There can also be contracts drawn when companies develop new products. For instance, when the influenza vaccine was developed, a federal exemption from liability was a critical clause for those companies. You can well expect that lawyers in corporations that have developed genetic therapies may have developed similar strategies to avoid liability. For clinicians in daily practice, when these techniques are in the gray area of promising but unproven modalities, failure to provide identification of where an individual can go to receive that therapy might very well be a litigable issue, but I think a very unfortunate one.

DR. GOOD: Could you touch on the ethical issues involved in the increasing involvement of industry with academic institutions? Very large grants are being given to academic institutions by companies that have a real interest in the developments of science. Are we getting into problems with that?

DR. LAPPÉ: I have been following those issues from the viewpoint of a health official in the State of California. I drafted legislation some years ago both to protect the development of these techniques within academic institutions and to ensure that guidelines would apply equally across public and private sectors. It is a very unsavory amalgam to have corporate entities, whose incentives are primarily financial, melded with academic institutions, where the principles of freedom of inquiry have been the touchstone that has led to the flourishing of this panoply of medical interventions. At the same time, many of the scientists who have been caught up in these corporations have accepted their offers with what the scientists believe to be very few strings attached, with the exception of requirements for co-patenting or "first look" policies. But, if you look at the actual language of these agreements, which claim not to carry any restrictions on academic freedom, there really are some strings: the choice of problems to be addressed, the researchers whose work will selectively be underwritten and endorsed by the funding organization, and the resulting competition within and among academic institutions and between departments for funding all reduce academic freedom. The ultimate requirement that the intervention yield a measurable economic benefit to the corporation as a whole is, in my judgment, the most ethically troubling unwritten requirement. It skews the priorities that might be set by more appropriate criteria of basic science. In this regard, I think Harvard's initial decision not to participate is very laudable. The decisions that we have seen at other institutions are less so.

Dr. Good: But at the same time Harvard makes that adjustment, it accepts $50 million from Hoechst; it gets very tough.

Dr. Lappé: Indeed so, particularly as the ability of the public sector to support institutions dwindles. It is a very, very difficult problem, and it will be a thorny one for the future.

Q: Do you think it is ethically preferable for the politician to take the money away from the corporation and give it to the university than for the corporation to give it directly to the university?

Dr. Lappé: If those were really equivalent options, I think you would have me in an end game where I could not give you a good answer. But I do not think those are the only options available. Theoretically you could have both funding systems working, one from the corporate sector, the other in the public sector. But what is happening now is that potential support from the private sector has been proportionately so overwhelming that it has displaced what dwindling support is available from the public sector and has led to an infusion of corporate funds to the universities. The issue of whether it is preferable to have some funds come in vs no funds at all is a difficult problem.

The current reshaping of the structure of financial institutions and their tax structure as a whole is creating more and more incentive for this kind of investment from the private sector to public institutions. As universities lose their base of support in the federal government, we ought to recognize that we are creating very strong forces that are pushing the privatization of knowledge into corporate rather than university settings, a very unsettling and disturbing process.

Q: Are there any guidelines in cases where, for instance, 10 patients need a bone transplant or kidney transplant and you find a single donor who may be the proper donor for each of these patients: who decides who is going to get the transplant? Are there any guidelines? What is the policy?

DR. LAPPÉ: I can answer this very generally by saying that the most unfortunate consequence of having a rare commodity needed by a substantial number of people is that it can lead to attempts to apply criteria of merit for who is the most deserving on grounds other than medical need. In your case, we would assume an equally good tissue match for all 10 transplants and that the disease in each person was in the same state of possible remediation. In such circumstances, ethicists say that you really have two general choices. You can begin to apply criteria of human worth, as was done by the Seattle group that had to decide allocation of renal transplants—for instance, you might factor in the age of the individual (how many potential years of life remained) times the social contribution of the individual to get a ranking—or you could use the medical criteria of the efficacy of the treatment times the number of years of usable life or worthwhile life left for that individual. Those are all in one category of determining the social utility of medical decisions. The counterpoise to these calculations is to use a lottery. In a situation of comparable medical indications and probable clinical success, some ethicists believe you are morally required to use an approach that does not discriminate on the basis of social usefulness.

However, the "lifeboat ethics," of the lottery-type approach, only begins when you are really sure you are in a lifeboat. I maintain there is probably no situation where you would find 10 equally deserving people, in a medical-biological sense, with the same disease at the same level of pathogenesis such that you cannot make a medical decision as to which is the most appropriate person to give the therapy to. When you cannot make a medical judgment, some ethicists would say you ought to apply a measure of benefit that would accrue in terms of life—the number of days left in an individual's life. Others say it is more appropriate to do it purely by lot. Lastly, you can ask the affected individuals—and this is a bit of moral cruelty—to devise a system of their own. I happen to opt for the middle course, saying that on the course of equal biological and medical indications, doing it by lot is most ethically acceptable. It is not a simple question. Ethicists will provide you with the framework for resolving problems of this sort, but will rarely tell you which is the best. I will suggest that it is more often acceptable, in my judgment, to use a random process of selection and make that clear to everybody who wants to participate in the process in the first place, rather than make ability to pay or social worth in the community a test for acceptability.

Dr. Nickel: I am interested in the gene pool. If we are doing therapy interventions of genetically or transmittable diseases, what are we doing to ourselves down to road via our gene pool?

Dr. Lappé: This becomes a significant question only if you begin to salvage substantial numbers of individuals who are now unable to reach reproductive age. The answer has to be divided into three categories of inheritance: those that are mendelian recessive or X-linked; those that are dominantly inherited; and those that are polygenic in origin. For autosomal recessive conditions the lion's share of the genes each generation, 75–80%, are reintroduced into the pool by the heterozygote, where that individual survives. Thus any dysgenic effect of treating the homozygote with sickle cell anemia will be years and years away before it is seen. In fact it will be swamped by the modestly dysgenic effect of selectively aborting the homozygote but allowing the carrier for an autosomal recessive to reproduce. Reproductive compensation of this sort only modestly increases the incidence of disease.

However, for dominantly inherited disease, this is a very germane question. The successful intervention and treatment of retinoblastoma, which as you have heard is not strictly dominantly inherited but involves deletions of chromosome 13 in the q area, for the bilateral type of retinoblastoma, which would have been fatal before reproductive age, has already led to an increase in the frequency of individuals who have this disorder. Half of the offspring of each of those affected with the bilateral form of retinoblastoma will again be at risk for that bilateral form.

We now know that we have an at-risk population for retinoblastoma who can be detected by early screening and pre-emptively treated early enough to salvage most of them. For this type of disease, you are going to have to bite the bullet, because the dysgenic effect will be very rapid—a doubling each generation if you include every individual who would otherwise have died. Compare that with the frequency that is reintroduced by spontaneous mutation and you will find that medical salvage through gene therapy is a very serious problem. To a lesser extent, this effect would also be true for some X-linked disorders.

For polygenic disorders, the issue is still much too complex to project the degree of dysgenic effect. For instance, the etiology of diseases like diabetes appears to me to be sufficiently complex, because of the role of susceptibility states that might be determined by HLA-linked genes, that it would be very hard to predict what the effect would be of allowing individuals who have juvenile-onset diabetes to reach reproductive age. A more general problem in these individuals is the apparent teratologic effect of the hyperglycemic environment for diabetics generally during pregnancy. There should be and is some attempt to disclose this type of information as part of genetic counseling.

The long-term effects of therapy for diseases with onset before reproductive age is nonetheless very germane and should not be passed aside the way I and other ethicists may have done in the past before the advent of feasible approaches to therapy.

Gene Therapy—Is It Inevitable or Necessary?

Theodore Friedmann

At this conference we have heard about some remarkable advances in the diagnosis and treatment of human genetic disease. These developments are all the more stunning when we remind ourselves that not many years ago, no one knew how genetic information was stored, whether encoded in DNA or protein or RNA, how genetic information flowed through these molecules, and in fact how many chromosomes were present in humans. Now, our understanding of genetics in general, and the diagnosis and therapy of human genetic disease in particular, are on the verge of revolutionary changes, and I want to extrapolate from our current state of knowledge of genetics to the potential future uses of genetic manipulation in diagnosis and treatment of a growing number of human diseases known to have a major genetic component. First, however, some words of caution about most predictions.

In science we are occasionally seduced by elegant methods and techniques, and may trap ourselves into self-fulfilling prophesies and into arguments of the technological imperative: "If something can be done, it should be done." As a result, we are occasionally tempted to fit new technical approaches into inappropriate settings. If we are to avoid that pitfall in the field of the potential treatment of human disease at a genetic level, we must show that there is a need for such a novel approach. Secondly, science is often forced, under political or societal pressures, to promise too much. Dr. Shaw reminded us that physicians must never promise too much for the effectiveness of their therapy, and they must not guarantee good results. The same is true of biomedical science in general, and some of us are distressed at the current tendency to overinflate and exaggerate information disseminated to the general public about the promises of genetics. Our recent experience with interferon is an example of such overpromising, and in almost all cases it is destined to disappoint.

On the other hand, there is no question that there is staggering new science here, and it clearly will continue to explode at an ever-increasing rate. The ability to understand and manipulate genetic material is growing at a dizzying pace, and what seems fanciful and wishful thinking today will become commonplace tomorrow. Just 10 short years ago, one of this country's most eminent nucleic acid chemists predicted that no appreciable length of nucleic acid would be sequenced before well into the twenty-first century, because of apparently insurmountable difficulties of determining the sequence of only four units over a total length of thousands or hundreds of thousands of units. And yet in the five years since the introduction of rapid sequencing methods by Sanger et al. (*1*) and Maxam and Gilbert (*2*), full nucleotide sequences have been determined for several simple prokaryotic and eukaryotic viruses, for mitochondrial DNA, and for many isolated prokaryotic and eukaryotic genes; and the sequences for more complex genomes of adenovirus, Epstein–Barr virus, and others are certainly coming.

To predict where the field of human genetics is going, we must know its current state and identify the forces acting upon it. To examine the potential for gene therapy, we should know, of course, what the therapeutic needs are, and what can be done, and we should eventually understand the ethical components to the decisions we make.

As a result of the discussions here, I think we all have a fairly good idea of the nature of many genetic diseases, and how they can be diagnosed and treated according to the Garrod-inspired model of inborn errors of metabolism (*3*). We have tended to think of the basic genetic defect as a mutation in the coding region of a gene encoding a specific polypeptide, and that such a protein is involved in important metabolic pathways. The absence of a functional gene product, an enzyme, causes metabolic derangements associated with the absence of vital metabolites, the accumulation of other metabolites, or both. We have heard of the design of rational therapy based on supplying the missing product (Factor VIII for hemophilia A, perhaps the use of insulin for insulin-deficiency diabetes mellitus, etc.), removing accumulated products, and decreasing production of metabolites by limitation of input into pathways by means of dietary restriction. We have heard of providing enzyme cofactors, as for methylmalonic acidemia and multiple carboxylase deficiency and others, and Dr. Cederbaum has told us of the new concept of "diversion therapy" for argininosuccinate lyase deficiency. We have also heard of disease management through large-scale screening programs, the possibility of targeted enzyme replacement therapy, and the new exciting possibilities of organ transplantation through the use of cyclosporin A and similar drugs for more effective immune suppression. I suspect that all these approaches will continue to fill some therapeutic need. We have also heard about the expanding power of chromosome studies for the diagnosis of increasingly numerous disorders, especially those related to the development of cancer, and the use of restriction fragment-length polymorphism for many disorders in which the defective gene product is completely unknown and in many examples of retardation syndromes, including the fragile-X syndrome.

The Need for New Kinds of Therapy

But for each of these successes there is a much larger list of diseases for which there is no adequate diagnosis or therapy, for which dietary restriction doesn't work, for which product replacement or treatment with agents designed to remove toxic metabolic products is not effective or feasible. Despite the conceptual difficulties of using diabetes mellitus as a disease model, for the reasons pointed out by Dr. Rimoin, treatment of diabetes mellitus with insulin is far from perfect and the incidence of complications of this disease is still unacceptably high. Similarly, despite the availability of enriched cryoglobulin preparations for the treatment of hemophilia, many patients still suffer painful and crippling bleeding episodes. Patients with cystinosis still die of their disease despite renal transplantation and reasonable chemical control. McKusick's compendium (4) is full of genetic disorders that are virtually unapproachable, both diagnostically and therapeutically. The reasons for such failures are certainly not always the result of inadequate understanding the pathogenesis of the disease. There is probably no molecule whose structure and whose role in disease is better understood than hemoglobin, and yet the therapy for most disorders of hemoglobin production, such as sickle cell anemia and the thalassemias, is product replacement by blood transfusion—a treatment of only limited usefulness that carries its own morbidity, including the occurrence of hepatitis and iron accumulation.

Despite some striking successes, we are simply not sufficiently knowledgeable in the diagnosis and therapy of many or most human genetic diseases. This constitutes in my view one of the forces acting on human medical genetics today: the real need to develop better methods of diagnosis and therapy for most human genetic diseases. That being so, the advent of powerful new molecular genetic tools for understanding, diagnosing, and treating genetic disease should be welcomed.

Using these tools, we have recently learned a great deal about the organization of mammalian genomes and how genetic material is controlled and expressed. We have been forced to discard our notion of the human genome as a fixed and static structure, recognizing now that it is dynamic and "breathing"—undergoing sequence rearrangements as normal features of immunoglobulin gene expression and probably in many other events related to development and differentiation. We have just begun to understand the differences between expressed and nonexpressed chromatin, to understand the conformational differences, the changes in DNA–protein interactions, the effects of base modification (such as methylation) on the molecular events that turn genes on and off. The point is, we will soon very likely know a great deal about how gene expression is controlled. Detailed knowledge of the mechanisms of regulation of gene expression is a requirement for the human use of gene therapy, and such knowledge is coming very rapidly indeed.

Our new knowledge of gene expression and of the organization of genetic information forces us to expand our definition of genetic disease to include many more disorders as being caused by sequence alterations and rearrangements in noncoding regions of genes. Without much doubt, many aberrations of differentiation and aging will be shown to result from sequence rearrangements. With respect to cancer, very good evidence supports the idea that sequences coding for transforming functions are found in normal cells but are turned off in the non-neoplastic state (5);

as a result of the movement of promoter-like sequences or of other rearrangements, such cancer genes are activated. One should therefore think of cancer in many of its forms as a disease whose understanding and treatment may be achieved at the genetic level.

To summarize, we clearly need new kinds of diagnostic and therapeutic techniques for some human diseases. Our failures with many diseases may be because therapy and diagnosis are aimed at a point distant from the defect. In at least some genetic diseases, therapy aimed directly at the genetic defect itself will be useful and effective.

Diagnostic and Therapeutic Applications of New Techniques

Probably the most immediate application of "genetic engineering" methods will continue to be toward a more profound understanding of the structural or sequence defects that cause many diseases. Mutant genes will be isolated and characterized, and the simple point mutations of some genes, the deletions, the rearrangements, and even the nature of what we now call multigene defects will be understood. Our experience with the globin genes, however, should again convince us that this knowledge may not lead directly or quickly to improved therapy.

Diseases in which we have identified neither the mutant gene product nor the nature of the genetic defect—and this includes the vast majority of human diseases—will now be subject to characterization through gene mapping and linkage analysis.

The isolation of human single-copy genes and the preparation of gene libraries will enable us to identify a large number of restriction fragment-length polymorphisms (so-called RFLP analysis) and to correlate these polymorphisms with many genetic disorders for which no other markers exist. Pedigrees can then be analyzed for the inheritance pattern for such polymorphisms, and linkage to an inherited trait can be used for diagnosis, as has already been done for thalassemia and type 2 diabetes (6, 7). One can foresee the detection of individuals at risk for disorders linked, e.g., to HLA or other markers, such as multiple sclerosis, diabetes, some forms of arthritis, for the enormous problem of cystic fibrosis, and for many of the other diseases in McKusick's compendium (4) that are not yet subject to screening or accurate diagnosis.

From a therapeutic point of view, obviously, the large-scale production of hormones and other products is already well advanced, as in the production of insulin, growth hormone, and various other important gene products. Other human hormones, vaccines, and products with improved activity and decreased side effects will be produced and will become readily available.

The most controversial applications of genetic manipulative methods, of course, involve the potential use of exogenous genes in humans for gene replacement or modification therapy. For some years, many of us have expected that the first attempts to carry out this kind of therapy would occur in disorders of hemoglobin production, as in sickle cell anemia or thalassemia, and we have all recently been aware of the experiments of Cline and his group at UCLA in several patients with thalassemia (unpublished). These first, perhaps faltering steps in the development of genetic therapeutic techniques have drawn criticism on several grounds, including the contention that we do not yet know enough scientifically to proceed with these approaches. We need to learn and understand more about the fate of newly introduced genetic information, how those new genes are regulated, and how to target incoming sequences to the organ, tissue, and cellular sites of the defect if we are to have full control over genetic manipulations in humans.

Although it is certainly true that medicine and science should always be able to understand and justify their actions on the basis of knowledge, at times physicians are required to act even in the face of imperfect knowledge, without the luxury of time or distance from real clinical problems. This sort of justification is, of course, subject to abuse and has been used to support clearly impermissible and unethical work, but the principle is important and valid and needs to be kept in mind during a discussion of the uses of new techniques in clinical settings. I wonder, in fact, whether there isn't a real moral obligation in some cases to use new methods if currently available techniques are known to be in principle and in practice ineffective and inadequate. On the other hand, what seems to be an important new therapeutic direction today may become somewhat less compelling as technical advances appear in other fields. For instance, the problems of graft rejection or of graft vs host response are likely to be reduced or even eliminated in the near future by the impressive new advances in transplantation immunology. Because of these improvements in transplantation techniques, treatment of diseases by replacement of affected organs, such as bone marrow, liver, and others, may become much simpler and more effective than the still more difficult techniques of gene manipulation. The clinical and therapeutic need to act will always have to be balanced by the need to know and to anticipate developments in other fields—and this balancing procedure will not get easier in the near future.

The potential advent of genetic manipulation as a part of therapeutic techniques for human disease is not a simple extension of current techniques, and carries with it possible ethical costs. We may have the ability to bring about in an evolutionary instant genetic changes in many species, including humans, that previously had been designed, tested, and modified over billions of years; such power is likely to come before we are wise enough to anticipate and understand fully the genetic consequences. Genetic knowledge, like all knowledge, is also likely to be abused by unscrupulous and self-serving demagogues, and we are already seeing the propensity of some of our political and religious leaders to muddy the waters for their own self-serving and at times nefarious purposes. Their temptations will probably increase with our increasing knowledge, but an enhanced general societal awareness of the issues, of the pros and cons, of the benefits and the dangers, will help to assure that these and other technical advances will be applied as wisely and knowledgeably as possible. Symposia such as this will help.

References

1. Sanger, F., Nicklen, S., and Coulson, A., DNA sequencing with chain-terminating inhibitors. *Proc. Natl. Acad. Sci. USA* **74,** 5463–5467 (1977).
2. Maxam, A., and Gilbert, W., A new method for sequencing DNA. *Proc. Natl. Acad. Sci. USA* **74,** 560–564 (1977).
3. Childs, B., Sir Archibald Garrod's conception of chemical individuality: A modern appreciation. *N. Engl. J. Med.* **282,** 71–77 (1970).
4. McKusick, V. A., *Mendelian Inheritance in Man,* 6th ed., Johns Hopkins Univ. Press, Baltimore, MD, 1982.
5. Perucho, M., Goldfarb, M., Shimizu, K., Lama, C., Fogh, J., and Wigler, M., Human tumor-derived cell lines contain common and different transforming genes. *Cell* **27,** 467–476 (1981).
6. Orkin, S., Alter, B. P., Altay, C., Mahoney, M. J., Lazarus, H., Hobbins, J. C., and Nathan, D. G., Application of endonuclease mapping to

the analysis and prenatal diagnosis of thalassemias caused by globin gene deletion. *N. Engl. J. Med.* **299,** 166–172 (1978).
7. Rotwein, P., Chyn, R., Chirgiwin, J., Cordell, B., Goodman, H. M., and Permutt, M. A., Polymorphism in the 5'-flanking region of the human insulin gene and its possible relation to type 2 diabetes. *Science* **213,** 1117–1120 (1981).

Index

abortion, 12, 15–16, 27–32, 34–36, 40, 43, 60, 62, 64, 65, 282–284, 296
abortion laws, 17, 34–35
acanthosis nigricans syndromes, 95
acatalasemia, 148
acetylcholine esterase, 22
N-acetylgalactosamine, 61
N-acetylhexosamine, 70
acrodermatitis enteropathica, 195, 278
acromegalia, 53
actinic keratasis, 121
acute intermittent porphyria, 200–201
acute lymphocytic leukemia, 106–107, 109, 110, 112
acute myeloid leukemia, 271, 297
acute nonlymphocytic leukemia (ANLL), 106–107, 109–112, 119
adenosine deaminase, 205, 208, 269–270
adenovirus, 303
adenylate cyclase, 95
adrenocortical insufficiency, 202
adrenogenital syndromes, 13, 92, 96
agammaglobulinemia, 73, 136–137, 141
aging, 125–126, 277, 305
agranulocytosis, 273
albinism, 6
aldosteronism, 194
alimentation, enteral, 170
alkaptonuria, 6
allotransplantation, 184, 185, 201–208
  see also transplantation of specific organs
Alport's syndrome, 206
American Board of Medical Genetics, 66
amino acid studies, 149–154, 166
δ-aminolevulinic acid, 200–201, 205
amniocentesis, 12–13, 21, 22, 28, 30, 60, 62, 64
androgen, 199–200

anemia, aplastic, 269, 271, 273
anencephaly, 93
aneuploidy, 93, 283
angioneurotic edema, hereditary, 199–200, 278
animal models of genetic disease, 71, 72, 172, 212, 223, 256, 258, 284–285
aniridia–Wilms' tumor syndrome, 106–108
α_1-antitrypsin deficiency, 169, 171–172, 175–177, 199–200, 205, 292
aplastic anemia, 269, 271, 273
apoenzyme–coenzyme binding, 196
arginase, 288
argininosuccinate lyase, 159, 304
argininosuccinic acid (ASA), 159, 190
arthritis, 306
artificial insemination, 32–33
ascorbate, 197, 198
Ashkenazi Jews, 21, 26–27
ataxia telangiectasia (AT), 55, 73, 81–86, 95, 121, 136, 138, 141
autoimmune disorders, 86, 93, 126, 266, 277, 279–280, 290
autosomal dominant inheritance, 7, 75
autosomal recessive diseases, 60–61, 73, 300
autosomal recessive inheritance, 6–7
autosomal trisomy, 10
azathioprine, 173, 174, 180, 181

Barr body, 10
Bartter's syndrome, 194
basal cell nevus carcinoma syndrome, 73, 99
B cells, B lymphocytes, 86, 134–139, 264–268, 270–271, 275–276, 279–280
biliary atresia, 205
bilirubin, 176–177, 199

biotin, 197, 198
blood–brain barrier, 181, 212, 216–217, 257
Bloom's syndrome, 73
bone marrow transplantation, 113, 173, 183, 202–204, 258–259, 268–277, 280–281, 288, 292, 293, 299, 308
branched-chain ketoaciduria, 188, 197
Burkitt's lymphoma, 106–108, 110–111
bursa of Fabricius, 163
busulfan, 272

cancer, 72–87, 105–119, 121, 273, 277, 284, 304, 305
  breast, 74, 76, 80, 112, 118
  colon, 80, 112, 118
  skin, 121
cancer susceptibility, 72, 74–79, 81, 84–85, 130
  gene for, 76–81, 84, 105–119, 306
carboxylase deficiency, 197, 198, 304
carcinogens, 75, 105, 111, 118–119, 122
carcinoma, 24, 106–108, 112, 118, 121
carcinoma–pheochromocytoma syndrome, 99
carcinoma, small cell (lung), 106, 107, 119
cardiovascular disorders, 169, 171, 198
carrier detection, *see* heterozygote detection
cartilage–hair hypoplasia, 273
catalase, 108
ceruloplasmin, 175–176, 195, 205
C1 esterase inhibitor, 199–200, 278
Chediak–Higashi syndrome, 203
chimeras, 204, 225–227, 229, 259, 269–270, 275
cholesterol, 169, 171, 189, 192, 193
chromatography, 150–154, 224
chromosome
  abnormalities, 9, 12, 21, 43–51, 105–119, 121, 124, 141
  analysis, 8–9, 50–51
  banding techniques, high-resolution, 9, 12, 106, 109–111
  fragile sites, *see* fragile sites
  Philadelphia, 12

chromosome—*cont.*
  translocation, 32, 49, 81, 107–110, 112–113, 180
  X, 7–8, 10–11, 44–48, 50, 84, 93, 141, 225
chronic granulomatous disease, 203
chronic myelogenous leukemia, 12, 106, 109, 110, 112
"class switching," 132, 137–138, 140
clear cell carcinoma, 24
clofibrate, 193
cobalamin, 197, 256
Colcemid, 109
collagen lysyl hydroxylase, 198
colonic polyposis (polyposis coli), 14, 73, 99
complementary DNA (cDNA), 13, 15, 220, 224–226
complement components, 278
congenital adrenal hyperplasia, 100, 194
congenital goitrous cretinism, 92
congenital neutrophil dysfunction, 272–273
consanguinity, 6, 149
copper, 13–14, 175, 189, 194–195, 205
coproporphyria, 200–201
cretinism, congenital goitrous, 92
Crigler–Najjar syndrome, 176–177, 199
cyclophosphamide, 272, 280
cyclosporin A, 172–175, 177, 179–181, 205, 278; 304
cystathioninuria, 196, 197
cystic fibrosis, 68, 306
cystinosis, 207, 304
cystoadenocarcinoma, 106, 107

danazol, 199–200, 278
demecolcine, *see* Colcemid
diabetes insipidus, 92, 98
diabetes mellitus, 94, 206, 285, 290–291, 301, 303, 306
dialysis, peritoneal, 157–158
dietary management of genetic disease, 3, 13, 156–161, 183–189, 191, 257
Di George's syndrome, 202, 204, 267, 270
dihydropteridine reductase, 162, 187

DNA, 4, 44, 48, 50–51, 108, 118, 142, 147, 226, 288, 303, 305
  complementary (cDNA), 13, 15, 220, 224–226
  polymorphisms, 84
  rearrangement, 109, 132, 134–136
  recombinant, vii, 13, 22, 50, 67, 131, 183–184, 220, 223–224, 226, 285, 290, 292–294
  repair mechanisms, 82–83, 120–130
dominant/recessive, 7, 97
Down's syndrome, 9, 26–27, 30, 43, 46, 54, 121, 283
Duchenne's muscular dystrophy, 32
dwarfism, 91, 194

Eck fistula, 168
Ehlers–Danlos syndrome, 197, 198
electrophoresis, 11, 13, 15, 150, 200, 224
emphysema, 200
encephalopathy, infantile glycine, 194
endocrine-deficiency disorders, 89–96
endocrine gland disorders, 73, 88–100
  modes of inheritance, 97–99
enteral alimentation, 170, 193
enzyme entrapment, see erythrocyte; liposome
enzyme replacement therapy, 209–224, 304
  delivery strategies, 212–223
epidermodysplasia verruciformis, 121
Epstein–Barr virus, 141, 180, 303
erythrocyte-entrapped enzymes, 215–218, 222–223
erythrocyte transfusion therapy, 208–209
esterase D, 11, 15, 108
ethics of genetic therapy, 282–301, 307–308
eugenics, 59
exons, 4–5, 131–132

Fabry's disease, 191–192, 202, 205, 207, 210–211, 217–220
Factor VIII, 206, 304
Fanconi's anemia, 73, 121, 202–203, 271, 273
fertilization, in vitro, 32–33

fetal liver transplantation, see liver transplantation
fetal testing, see prenatal diagnosis
fetal therapy, in utero, 198–199
α-fetoprotein, 21, 22, 82
fibroblast transplantation, 207–208
folate, 197–199, 201
follicular lymphoma, 106–107, 112
fragile sites, chromosomal, 44–48, 51
fragile X syndrome, 44–48, 51, 54, 304
Friend virus, 72
fructose intolerance, 188

galactosemia, 3, 13, 157, 160, 162, 187, 205
α-galactosidase, 207, 210, 217–220, 225
gangliosidosis, 71
gas chromatography/mass spectrometry (GC-MS), 154–155, 163
Gaucher's disease, 69, 191–192, 202, 206, 210–211, 217–218, 222–223
gene mapping, 11–12, 138–139, 142–143, 306
gene pool, viii, 124, 300–301
gene products, 183, 184, 196–199, 201–202, 224–227, 290–291, 293, 303–304, 307
gene therapy, 184, 224–230, 302–308
genetic counseling, viii, 17–19, 23–25, 28–32, 34, 36, 40–42, 59–60, 62–65, 96, 99, 163, 184, 301
genetic screening, 17–18, 22, 28–29, 36, 60, 62–68, 258, 282, 304
gene transplants, 13, 138–139, 227–230, 287–288
Gilbert's syndrome, 199
glandular hyperplasia, neoplasia, 96–97
globin gene, 13, 15, 143, 224, 228, 287, 306
glucocerebrosidase, 211, 218
glucocerebroside, 206, 210
glucose-6-phosphatase, 169
glucose-6-phosphate dehydrogenase, 14, 224
glucosidase, 210–211, 213–214, 217–218, 220–223
β-glucuronidase, 203, 212
glucuronyl transferase, 176
glycine encephalopathy, 194

glycogenosis, 192–193, 210–211, 217–218, 220–221
glycogen storage disease, 169–170, 176, 177, 192–193
glycosphingolipids, 192
GM₂ ganglioside/gangliosidosis, 61, 70–71, 210–211
gonadotropins, 99
gout, 172, 190, 193, 202, 206
graft vs host reaction, *see* transplant rejection
Grave's disease, 97
Gross virus, 72
growth hormone (somatotropin), 91, 95, 98, 100, 194, 225, 227, 307
gyrate atrophy, 188–189, 197, 198

Hashimoto's disease, 280
hematin, 200–201
heme synthesis, 200
hemochromatosis, 93
hemoglobin gene, *see* globin gene
hemoglobinopathies, 7, 15, 22, 93, 147, 204, 307
    see also sickle cell; thalassemia
hemophilia, 32, 206, 286, 304
hepatic, *see* liver
herpes simplex virion, 227–228
heterozygote detection, 22, 33, 62–64, 66–68, 70, 184, 258, 292
"heterozygote index," 82–84
hexosaminidase A (Hex A), 61, 70–71, 210–214
hexosaminidase B (Hex B), 70–71
high-density lipoprotein, 192
histiocytosis X, 93
histocompatibility, 203, 204
    see also major histocompatibility complex
HLA-linked genes, 301
HLA markers, HLA typing, 76–81, 85, 306
HLA-matched transplants/transfusions, 259, 268–269, 273–274, 276
homocystinuria, 150, 166, 182, 197
homology, gene, 126, 136, 142
hormone receptors, 94–95
    see also target cells
hormones, lipid-soluble and water-soluble, 88–89, 94–96

hormones, polypeptide and nonpeptide, 88, 90–93, 95, 96, 98, 225
Huntington's disease, 286
Hurler's disease, 203–204, 256, 258
hybridoma, 264
hyperammonemia, 157–158, 160, 188
hypercholesterolemia, familial, 170–171, 189, 192–194
hyperglycinemia, 194
hyperlipidemia, 169–171
hyperlipoproteinemia, 193
hyperparathyroidism, 96, 196
hyperphenylalaninemia variants, 155, 162, 166, 187, 197, 198
hyperplasia, glandular, 96–97
hypertension, 92, 121, 291
hypogammaglobulinemia, 136–138
hypoglycemia, 148, 157, 170, 193
hypogonadism, 99–100
hypophosphatemic rickets, 96, 195
hypopituitary dwarfism, 91
hypoplasia, 92, 93
hypospadias syndrome, 95–96
hypothyroidism, 92, 162, 194
hypoxanthine–guanidine phosphoribosyltransferase, 193, 291

α-L-iduronidase, 203
immunodeficiency, 81, 84, 125–126, 136–139, 205, 278–279
    see also severe combined immunodeficiency
immunoglobulin genes, 81, 131–143, 305
immunoglobulin heavy chains (IGH), 81, 85, 109, 132–134
immunoglobulins, 131–143, 216
immunological system, development of, 134–137, 263–266
immunosuppression, 75, 86, 172–174, 177, 179–181, 205, 272, 278, 290
inborn errors of metabolism, 5, 13, 97–98, 147–166, 169–172, 175, 183–230, 267, 271, 277, 283, 303–304
indomethacin, 194
infantile glycine encephalopathy, 194
inheritance patterns, 6–8
insemination, artificial, 32–33
insulin, 91, 92, 95, 169, 170, 206, 225, 227, 287–288, 290, 293, 303, 307
interferon, 226, 227, 287–288, 303

introns, 4–5, 132
in utero therapy, 198–199, 204
in vitro fertilization, 32–33
IQ, 10, 151, 256
iron, 93, 189, 305
isovaleric acidemia, 188, 190–191, 257

Kallmann syndrome, 99
ketoacidosis, 191
ketonuria, 150
kidney disease, end-stage, 278, 286
kidney transplantation, 14, 75, 86, 172–174, 182, 201–202, 206–207, 278, 284, 293, 299, 304
Kleinfelter syndrome, 10, 99
Kostmann syndrome, 203
Krabbe's disease, 69, 71

lactose intolerance, 188
legal problems associated with genetic disease, viii, 17–42, 67
leprechaunism, 95
Lesch–Nyhan syndrome, vii, 32, 54, 193, 283, 291
leukemia, 105, 118, 276–277
  acute lymphocytic, 106–107, 109, 110, 112
  acute myeloid, 271, 297
  acute nonlymphocytic (ANLL), 106–107, 109–112, 119
  chronic myelogenous, 12, 106, 109, 110, 112, 297
  lympholytic, 121
  viral-induced, 72–73
life span, genetic determination of, viii, 125–126
life span, maximum (MLS), 124–126
light-chain genes, 132–137
liposome-entrapped enzymes, 213–215, 217–218, 221–222, 293
liver transplantation, 172–177, 180–182, 201–202, 204–205, 274, 292, 293, 308
LOD, *see* log odds determination
log odds determination (LOD), 78–80
"longevity genes," 125
low-density lipoproteins (LDL), 171, 189, 192, 193, 213, 217–218, 220–221

lung carcinoma, small cell, 106, 107, 119
lupus, *see* systemic lupus erythematosus
lymphocytes, *see* B-cells; T-cells
lympholytic leukemia, 121
lymphoma, 105–112, 174, 180, 181, 265
lysosomal storage disorders, 61, 191–192, 204, 208–224, 259, 277

major histocompatibility complex (MHC)/site/locus, 72–73, 76–80, 126, 266, 268, 273, 275–277
malpractice, 17, 19, 21–22, 24, 26–27, 29, 296–297
mannosidosis, 71, 197, 198, 204, 258
maple syrup urine disease, 157
marrow transplants, *see* bone marrow transplantation
Mediterranean fever, familial, 206–207
medullary cystic disease, 206
melanin, 6
melanoma, 112
meningioma, 106, 107
Menkes' disease, 194–195
mental retardation, vii, 6, 10, 11, 16, 43–54, 155, 161, 188, 287, 304
messenger RNA, *see* mRNA
metallothionein, 195
methotrexate, 109–110, 228
methylmalonic acidemia, 160, 161, 166, 188, 196, 197, 304
β_2-microglobulin, 225–226
mixed parotid gland tumor, 106, 107
Moloney virus-induced leukemia, 72
monoclonal antibodies, 264–265
mRNA, 4–5, 132, 135, 138, 200, 224–226

organ transplants, *see specific organ transplanted*
orotic aciduria, 194
osteopetrosis, 203, 273

pancreas transplantation, 202, 206
parathyrin, 92, 95

"penetrance," gene, 75, 78, 84
penicillamine, 13–14, 189
peritoneal dialysis, 157–158
phakomatoses, 99
phenobarbital, 199
phenylalanine, 5–6, 152, 161–163, 184, 186–187
phenylalanine ammonia lyase, 187
phenylalanine hydroxylase, 5, 161–162, 184–185, 187
phenylketonuria (PKU), 3, 5, 22, 148, 150, 152, 155, 156, 160–162, 166, 172, 184–187
pheochromocytoma, 99
Philadelphia chromosome, 12
phytanic acid, 191
pituitary hormones, 88, 90–93
plasmapheresis, 177, 184, 191–192
polycystic kidney disease, 27, 206
polygenic inheritance, 8, 88, 291, 301
polypeptide hormones, 88, 90–91, 95, 96, 98, 275
polyposis coli (colonic polyposis), 14, 73, 99
porphobilinogen, 200–201
porphyria, acute, 200–201
portacaval shunt, portal diversion, 167–172, 192–193
Prader–Willi syndrome, 48–49
prednisone, 173, 174, 180, 181, 278
prenatal diagnosis, 12, 21, 25, 28–30, 35–36, 62, 64–68, 155, 163, 184, 258, 282–283
procarbazine, 272
progeria, 121
pro-insulin gene, 91
prolactin, 95
prostacyclin, 194
prostaglandin, 194
pseudovaginal–perineal–scrotal hypospadias syndrome, 95–96
public vs private sector genetic research, 292–295, 298–299
pyridoxal phosphate, 198
pyruvate dehydrogenase, 157

recombinant DNA techniques/probes, vii, 13, 22, 50, 67, 131, 183–184, 220, 223–224, 226, 284, 290, 292–294

Refsum's disease, 191
Reifenstein syndrome, 99
rejection, *see* transplant rejection
renal, *see* kidney
renin, 194
resistance genes, 277
restriction endonuclease polymorphism, 22
restriction endonuclease polymorphism analysis, 13, 91, 142–143, 304, 306
retardation, *see* mental retardation
retinoblastoma, 11, 15, 16, 73, 106–108, 118, 301
rickets, 96
RNA, 4–5, 134, 140

Sandhoff's disease, 71, 210, 257
screening, *see* genetic screening
sea blue histiocyte syndrome, 177
severe combined immunodeficiency (SCID), 73, 136–137, 141, 202–204, 208, 268–271, 273–274, 276, 279, 283, 292
sex selection, prenatal, 30–31
Shope papilloma virus, 288
sickle cell anemia, sickle cell trait, 3, 7, 13, 14, 67, 70, 282, 300, 305, 307
somatotropin (growth hormone), 91, 95, 98, 100, 194, 225, 227, 307
spherocytosis, 14
sphingolipid-storage diseases, 61, 71
sphingomyelinase, 181, 205
splenectomy, 14
splenic transplantation, 201, 206
strychnine, 194
substrate depletion therapy, 184–187, 189–193, 201
superoxide dismutase, 126
SV40 virus, 123, 226–227
systemic lupus erythematosus, 121, 126, 280

target cell insensitivity to hormones, 94–96
Tay–Sachs disease, 21, 26–27, 61–68, 70, 210–212, 257

T-cells, T lymphocytes, 81–82, 86, 136, 137, 179, 205, 208, 264–268, 270–272, 275–276, 278–280
testosterone, 96
tetrahydrobiopterin, 162, 187, 197, 198
α-thalassemia, 21, 68
β-thalassemia, 67–68, 189–190, 204, 305–307
thymidine kinase, 228, 287–288
thymoma, 136–137
α-thymosin gene, 225
thymus, 86–87, 126, 263–264, 266–268, 270–271, 274–278, 280–281
    transplantation, 202, 204–205, 266–268, 270, 277, 281
thyroliberin, 92
thyrotropin, 92, 97
thyroxin, 92, 96, 98, 194
transfer RNA, 4, 225
translocation, Robertsonian, 81
transplantation, *see* gene transplants *and specific organ of interest*
transplant rejection (graft vs host reaction), 172–175, 179–180, 269, 271, 274–277, 280, 307
trisomy, 10, 15–16, 43, 93, 112
tuberculosis, 70, 74, 274
tumors, 12, 105–119, 121, 134–135, 285
Turner's syndrome, 10, 16, 33
tyrosine, 5–6, 162, 176, 187, 205
tyrosinemia, 176, 177, 188, 205

UDPglucuronosyltransferase, 199
urea cycle, disorders of, 147, 155, 157–160, 188, 190
uric acid, 172, 190, 193, 209

vasopressin, 98
viral genes, 226, 229, 288
virus, 72, 119, 123, 226–227, 230, 288, 303
virus-induced leukemia, 72–73
vitamin B$_6$, 166, 188–189, 198
vitamin B$_{12}$, 160, 161, 166, 188, 198, 256
vitamin D, 94, 96, 197

Werner's syndrome, 73
Wilms' tumor, 106–108, 118
Wilson's disease, 13, 175–177, 181, 189, 205
Wiskott–Aldrich syndrome, 73, 202–203, 272–273
Wolman's disease, 93

xanthine dehydrogenase, 229
xanthoma, 169, 171
X chromosome, 7–8, 10–11, 44–48, 50, 84, 93, 141, 225
xeroderma pigmentosum, 73, 99, 121
X-linked inheritance, 7–8

zinc, 195, 197, 198, 279